# A Woman's
# BEST MEDICINE

# *A Woman's*

# BEST MEDICINE

## Health, Happiness, and Long Life Through Maharishi Ayur-Veda

Nancy Lonsdorf, M.D., Veronica Butler, M.D.,
and Melanie Brown, Ph.D.

Jeremy P. Tarcher/Putnam
a member of
Penguin Group (USA) Inc.

The views represented in this book are those of the authors and do not necessarily represent those of Maharishi Ayur-Veda Universities. For the most complete presentation and understanding of Maharishi Ayur-Veda, it is recommended that you participate in the courses and programs of the Maharishi Ayur-Veda Universities.

Jeremy P. Tarcher/Penguin
a member of
Penguin Group (USA) Inc.
375 Hudson Street
New York, NY 10014
www.penguin.com

First Trade Paperback Edition 1995

*Library of Congress Cataloging-in-Publication Data*

Lonsdorf, Nancy.
    A woman's best medicine : health, happiness, and long life through Maharishi
Ayur-Veda / Nancy Lonsdorf, Veronica Butler, and Melanie Brown.
        p.   cm.
    Reprint. Originally published: 1993.
    Includes bibliographical references and index.
    ISBN 0-87477-785-2
    ISBN 978-0-874-77785-7
    1. Women—Health and hygiene.   2. Medicine, Ayurvedic.
I. Butler, Veronica.   II. Brown, Melanie.   III. Title.
RA778.B8794   1995                94-8619   CIP
613'.04244—dc20

*For Maharishi Mahesh Yogi*

*In gratitude for the profoundly nourishing
knowledge he gives and lives*

*for his boundless compassion
and for his supreme dedication to creating perfect health
for the world family*

# CONTENTS

# CONTENTS

# ACKNOWLEDGMENTS

We are in awe of the medical wisdom of Dr. Brihaspati Dev Triguna, Dr. V. M. Dwivedi, and Balaraj Maharshi, along with that of Dr. J. R. Raju and Dr. H. S. Kasture, and express our deep appreciation for their vast knowledge. We are extremely grateful to our wise, clear-headed, and exuberant editor, Connie Zweig, for her sensitive editing, and to Jeremy Tarcher and Rena Wolner for their gracious support. We also thank Allen Mikaelian, Coral Tysliava, and Katherine Pradt for their kind help. We express our deep gratitude to our agent, Muriel Nellis, whose heart is as brilliant as her mind, for her abiding care and wisdom, and we thank her delightful associates, Jane Roberts and Karen Gerwin. We also offer our profound thanks to Donna Seibert, Renata Hartmann, M.D., Chris Clark, M.D., and Barry Charles, M.D., for their heroic help in the preparation of this book.

We are very grateful to the following people for their far-reaching work in establishing Maharishi Ayur-Veda in the world (in alphabetical order): Skip Alexander, Ph.D.; Richard Averbach, M.D.; Uli Bauhoffer, M.D.; John Boncheff, D.SI; Chris Clark, M.D.; Michael Dillbeck, Ph.D.; John Douillard, D.C.; Jay Glaser, M.D.; John Hagelin, Ph.D.; Renata Hartmann, M.D.; George Jensen, M.D.; Bevan Morris, D.SI.; Tony Nader, M.D.; David Orme-Johnson, Ph.D.; Cathy Poole, representing the Maharishi Ayur-Ved Health Center technicians; Atsuko Rees, M.D.; Brian Rees, M.D.; Stuart Rothenberg, M.D.; Robert Schneider, M.D.; Hari Sharma, M.D.; Amy Silver, M.D.; Bev Sprague R.N., representing the Maharishi Ayur-Ved Health Center's nursing and administration staff; Keith Wallace, Ph.D.; Ken Walton, Ph.D.; the Badgett family and the Zimmerman family, representing those dedicated individuals creating the Raj and the Maharishi Center for Perfect Health and World Peace.

And finally, we extend our heartfelt thanks to those who have so lovingly contributed their help and support (in alphabetical order): Karin Aarons; Vicki Alexander, J.D.; Bryan Aubrey, Ph.D.; Bija Bennett; Clara Berno; the Braunstein family; Carla Linton Brown, Ph.D.; Annabelle S. Brown; Wells S. Butler; Lucy Clark; B. Mawiyah Clayborne, Ph.D.; Susie L. Dillbeck, Ph.D.; Richard Eidson; Paula and Ralph Gilbert; Julie Guttmann; Bettye Jacobs; Maureen Kelleher, Ed.D.; Carolyn G. King, Ph.D.; Gail Koplow; Suzanne and Tony Lawlor; Emily Levin; Sam Lewis; Heidi M. Lloyd; David Lonsdorf; Jan and Michael McCutcheon; Beverly Merson;

# ACKNOWLEDGMENTS

Margaret Mullins, R.N.; Rhoda Orme-Johnson, Ph.D.; Victoria Peterson; the Poneman family; Christina Rawley, Ph.D.; Judy and Victor Raymond; Joncie Rowland; Margaret Scarborough, Ph.D.; Claudine Schneider; Christina and Peter Sterling; Aquilla Wells; and our clinical staffs and professional colleagues.

# INTRODUCTION

Good health is such a natural part of our lives that we often pay attention to it only when we *don't* have it. If we are diagnosed with an illness or someone close to us is, we may set out to learn all we can about that illness. Many of us become experts in one illness or another, and that's not necessarily a bad idea. Certainly, it gives us a way to gain some mastery over the illness. But why not instead become an expert in health?

We would like to propose that you can learn to master health with the same vital, absorbing interest and expertise. You can learn to reawaken your healing abilities to prevent sickness altogether, no matter how healthy or ill you are. Since it's the most natural thing in the world to be healthy, it doesn't matter how long you have waited or how inadequate your preparation may seem. The more healing you can activate in the present, the less past habits and ailments will dominate. A healthy present can eliminate an ailing past.

In this book we introduce you to Ayur-Veda, specifically Maharishi Ayur-Veda, a complete system of health, in light of its application to women today. Ayur-Veda (ah-yuhr-vay-duh) means "knowledge (*Veda*) of the totality of life *(Ayus)*." Having its roots in ancient India, it is not only a system of medical knowledge but also a comprehensive, scientifically documented body of knowledge of all life. It offers knowledge about your senses, mind, emotions, body, and relationships—with others, with the environment, and with yourself, and is based on the development of consciousness that underlies and integrates all aspects of life. It brings you the wisdom, the core memory, that this "body of knowledge" is none other than your own.

In recent years, medical doctors, researchers, and patients alike have recognized that the ability of your body to heal itself, based on the integration of the physiology, mind, and emotions, is the real essence of the healing process. Yet the knowledge of how to tap into the source of this healing mechanism is not developed or available in Western medicine. Ayur-Veda remedies this situation. It contains the time-tested techniques and vital information needed to reawaken your innermost nature, your innermost responses. So although Ayur-Veda originated as an ancient health system, its prescriptions for health are remarkably contemporary.

Ayur-Veda is not simply another piecemeal approach to healing, but a complete system of customized health, addressing every part of life. It supports a health model, not a disease model, of medicine. It enables you to recognize that your physical well-being resides not only within your body, mind, and emotions, but is fully connected to the biological cycles of nature, to the seasons, to the universe itself, to the deepest laws of nature. Once you can tune in to these basic patterns of nature operating within you, you can stir the biological memory in all the cells to behave in their own collective best interest, enabling you to achieve a natural state of excellent health, deep happiness, and long life virtually without effort.

*Essentially, the fundamental healing principle of Ayur-Veda is to restore balance in mind, body, and emotions simultaneously by reawakening your own resources of biological intelligence.* It offers a full program of prevention based on your individual constitution, which you can enjoyably incorporate into your daily routine to bring about significant changes in your physiology, your psychological health, and your behavior. Even the most serious imbalances resulting in autoimmune disorders, cancer, and heart disease can benefit from an Ayur-Vedic program designed to rebalance your healing system. Once you start to live this integration, you experience a sense of deepening personal freedom and may begin to enjoy the most desirable by-product of radiant good health: twenty-four-hour-a-day bliss.

# INTRODUCTION

## The Origins of Ayur-Veda

Ayur-Veda originated within the Vedic tradition of India, the oldest tradition of knowledge in human history. Although written texts exist, the tradition of the Veda (literally, "knowledge") primarily has been passed on verbally. The Veda is not the formalized objective knowledge we emphasize in the West. The Western scientific method of discovery of the laws of nature relies primarily on observation and experimentation conducted by scientists in laboratories. The Veda was "discovered" by scientists of consciousness, enlightened seers, men and women, who directly cognized the structures of the universe within their own awareness. As Einstein cognized the theory of relativity in his mind years before its existence was proved in the laboratory, these great Vedic masters, sinking deep into the silence of their minds in meditation, perceived how the laws of nature function. That knowledge is contained in the Veda. It offers precise descriptions of the laws of nature and how they function at every level of creation. And it offers techniques to apply this knowledge to every area of your life in order to give you a means to gain happiness, health, peace, and harmony for yourself and for society.

Vedic science covers a vast range of knowledge, from spiritual philosophy to logic, mathematics, music, speech, astronomy, architecture, and health. It was the Vedic seers who first recognized the unified field, now described by quantum physics, who first understood the science of the integration of human consciousness and the material world. They discovered that this field, even in its unmanifest state, is not a void but a fullness containing everything, every possibility of life, the potential for the entire universe. They called it *samhita* (sung-hee-tah), a unified wholeness that appears as the knower, the known, and the process of knowing. They discovered that all interactions in life are simply expressions of the self-interacting, self-knowing samhita or unified field unfolding within itself.

The Vedic tradition defines itself as timeless because, although there are written Vedic texts such as the Upanishads, the Veda is an *internalized* knowledge, nature's script preserved in life itself—

**3**

perhaps best understood as the "DNA of knowledge." Vedic knowledge is neither a philosophy nor a religion nor even a set of aphorisms about life. It is ongoing, living, experiential knowledge, although forgotten and revived from time to time, of the unfolding of natural law in all its phases. Embedded in human consciousness, these timeless laws of nature can be cognized by anyone whose consciousness is fully awake.

From the Vedic tradition comes Ayur-Veda, a powerful and detailed body of knowledge about health, which focuses specifically on restoring balance within your psychophysiology through enlivening the interaction of consciousness with all aspects of your body, mind, and emotions. Ayur-Veda is referred to as the "mother of all healing" because it predated and directly influenced Chinese, ancient Greek, Western, and holistic medicine in general. Along with profound principles of prevention and healing, the eight medical subspecialties of Ayur-Veda are: internal medicine; surgery; eye, ear, nose, mouth, and throat problems; children's illnesses; toxicology; rejuvenation therapy; reproduction; and spiritual healing. Much of what we know of Ayur-Veda is available in writings of the physician Charaka (chuh-ruh-kuh), a text known as the Charaka Samhita.

Although techniques of Ayur-Veda are widely practiced in India today, these practices generally do not incorporate the full understanding of Ayur-Veda from the original tradition. The passage of time and the influence of the Western medical model have led to the dilution or loss of much of the ancient Ayur-Vedic system of medicine and its prescriptions for healing.

In the early 1980s, the preeminent Indian scholar and teacher in the Vedic tradition, Maharishi Mahesh Yogi, founder of the Transcendental Meditation program, gathered together many of the most knowledgeable and distinguished Ayur-Vedic physicians, Western physicians, scientists, and researchers. Their mission was to delve deeply into the theory and practice of the ancient Ayur-Vedic system in order to restore Ayur-Veda to its original purity. By exploring the knowledge of how consciousness interfaces with matter, a specialty of Maharishi's Vedic Science, the Ayur-Vedic healing prescriptions and ancient techniques were revived in full in their original precision and integrity. This revival of Ayur-Veda is known as Maharishi Ayur-Veda, and when we speak of Ayur-Veda in this book we are referring to its modern restoration as Maharishi Ayur-Veda. And when we speak of Maharishi Ayur-Vedic approaches to healing, the most significant technique we refer to is Transcendental Meditation (TM), which is essential because the principal focus of Maharishi Ayur-Veda is on the rebalancing of your physiology through direct experience of the unified field of consciousness.

## What Maharishi Ayur-Veda Offers

*Ayur-Veda is a very precious and practical aspect of the Veda. Its purpose is enlightenment. It restores balance in order that a very balanced state of intellect is generated. In that state, activity and silence are coordinated to make the full value of life a living reality.*

Maharishi Mahesh Yogi[1]

The secret to reawakening the organizing principles of health within you is to locate and access that most powerful uniting healing connection: the junction point between consciousness and your body, mind, and feelings. Maharishi Ayur-Veda provides twenty approaches to tap into this powerful inner resource. In this book we will explore a number of these scientifically based approaches and the principles underlying them, including all daily and seasonal home-care routines. The programs offered here are simple. You can easily incorporate any of them into your daily life to produce significant benefits, not only in physiological functioning, but also in psychological health and emotional stability. We'll address specific concerns, ranging from heart disease, cancer, obesity, chronic fatigue, PMS, and menopause to substance addiction, relationships, pregnancy and childbirth, and infant care. We will not discuss every specific disease, nor will we try. Because Ayur-Veda is a nondisease-based health system, it does not suggest that everyone who has the same symptoms receive the same treatment. You will be able to understand the Ayur-Vedic approach and apply it to any aspect of your own health. Please note, however, that this book is not a substitute for professional medical treatment.

As women, we are often aware of early imbalances, a sense that things are "not quite right," before they are named as specific diseases by the lab report. Yet we are just as often frustrated by our inability to communicate our vague symptoms to specialists because "pre-disease" symptoms are not classifiable, testable, or always treatable by the modern medical approach. Ayur-Veda offers a deeper, subtler kind of medicine, confirming your own self-diagnostic awareness and providing you with ways to maintain basic good health and treat both expressed and unexpressed conditions of physical, mental, and emotional illness and pre-illness on the basis of your individual constitution.

The Ayur-Vedic system identifies seven types of constitution. Each constitutional type predicts the kind of imbalances to which you may be most susceptible. The individual daily and seasonal routines for each type focus on food, rest, exercise, behavior, and specific therapeutic modalities to restore balance and eliminate impediments to good health. To illustrate how each of these programs can work, you'll also read brief personal stories of women with various health problems who were helped by specific Ayur-Vedic treatments. Their stories may seem oversimplified or appear to be "quick-fix" tales, but in each case the woman had undergone other medical treatments without much success. In each case she tried Maharishi Ayur-Veda and found that, to her surprise, her symptoms improved and she started to enjoy a deeper sense of well-being. We present these stories not as miracle tales but as very ordinary examples of how the Ayur-Vedic approach works in a variety of situations, and why.

At root, all illnesses simply reflect a loss of connection with a unifying inner source. To facilitate this reconnection, Maharishi Ayur-Veda offers a three-part approach to medical care based on the link between consciousness and matter. First-class Ayur-Veda works to reconnect the body and mind with the underlying field of consciousness. Second-class Ayur-Veda enlivens biological memory and enables your body's intelligence to reset its own inner healing mechanisms. Third-class Ayur-Veda uses outside products and techniques to help rebalance the body and mind.

Let's look now at how Ayur-Veda supports what scientists today call mind-body medicine.

## INTRODUCTION

### What Is Mind-Body Medicine?

One of the essential discoveries of Ayur-Veda, as well as of other ancient traditional medical systems such as the Chinese and Native American, is the realization that the mind and body are intimately connected and that consciousness is inseparably merged with both. The behavior of molecules and immune cells thus cannot be predicted on a solely physical basis, but is influenced strongly by our mental and emotional states of consciousness. Now modern medicine is beginning to recognize this interconnection as well, although several Western thinkers, such as Aristotle and Darwin, were aware of it centuries ago.

In 1964, psychiatrist George Solomon and his colleague Rudolph Moos at Stanford University published a landmark study demonstrating a link between emotional conflict and the onset and course of rheumatoid arthritis, a study that provoked great skepticism in the scientific community. A decade later, Dr. Robert Ader, working with Nicholas Cohen at the University of Rochester School of Medicine, conducted a series of experiments in which rats were trained to depress their immune systems when given sweetened water. The researchers found that just a mental association could suppress the functioning of the immune system. Ader called this field of research "psychoneuroimmunology," or PNI, which has quickly grown into one of the most exciting fields in modern medicine. PNI, writes author-physician Michael Crichton, "will become a vitally important clinical field—perhaps the most important medical field in the 21st century—supplanting our current emphasis on cardiology and oncology."[2]

PNI describes the intimate relationship between the activity of your brain and the activity of your immune system, suggesting that, in a very basic sense, your health is the result of the relationship between your mind and body. PNI proposes that we can no longer consider mind as one thing and body as another, or mental health as separate from physical health. Your mind is not just sitting up there in your brain but is joined with and informs every single bodily cell. Every cell, we could say, contains a "piece of mind." Conversely, each of your thoughts, feelings, desires, ideas—any as-

7

pect of your intelligence—results in the production of a chemical messenger from your brain called a neuropeptide, which translates your thoughts into a physical state. So your thinking really does structure how you feel. This is why even the thought of medicine can have an effect and why placebos so often work well.

The discoveries of psychoneuroimmunology also challenge the classical view of the body as three separate systems: the endocrine system, the central nervous system, and the immune system. PNI research has demonstrated how these three systems are interconnected closely via messenger molecules.[3] We've learned, for example, that people with a high degree of mental and emotional stress get colds more easily, and that people experiencing hardening of the arteries can benefit from a stress reduction program—whether or not they are eating a healthy diet, exercising regularly, and taking medications as needed. Dr. Ed Blalock at the University of Alabama has shown that the immune system really functions like a sensory organ, just like our eyes or noses, sensing stimuli such as bacteria and viruses via our white blood cells and influencing our behavior by unleashing a surge of powerful biochemicals. One of the most eminent PNI researchers, Dr. Candace Pert, has demonstrated "that the human body is an impressive pharmacological factory," that we have a psychosomatic network wherein the cells of our minds and bodies chatter constantly back and forth in a language of biochemicals, resulting in the full range of our human emotions. According to Dr. Pert, since neither your mind nor your body really can be understood independent of the other, we need one term to describe how minds and bodies join together to create an information system that has a biochemical basis. She calls this system a "bodymind," explaining that "your body is the outward manifestation of your mind."[4]

As a consequence of PNI, there is now a new kind of medicine, mind-body medicine. As a further consequence, the materialistic, technological approach to medicine, which views the body as a mechanical machine completely separate from the mind or consciousness of the person, is now understood to have reached, in many ways, the limits of its applicability. There is no doubt that the technological medical approach is of great benefit in trauma and acute life-threatening conditions, but it doesn't secure real prevention and the depth of immunity necessary for maintaining our good health on a lifelong basis. The sad truth is that although modern medicine has spent countless billions of dollars on synthesizing and developing a host of chemical treatments to manipulate the body from a state of disease to one of health (a practice known as allopathy), the real essence of healing has been missed.

Mind-body medicine is beginning to identify that missing element. We're finally seeing that the only reason most chemical treatments work is because *the body itself produces similar chemicals.* Mind-body medicine has discovered that the body is a pharmacy stocked and run by the body's own intelligence. And the compounds in this interior pharmacy are created as much by your emotions, viewpoints, attitudes, behaviors, and social relationships as by your physiological responses. With every thought and feeling, you are either nourishing or weakening your physiology.

The new medicine can thus help you envision healing not simply as the necessary repair of a body that breaks down and needs to be fixed, but as a beautiful thinking, feeling "bodymind" that is the source of its own healing.

This is the specialty of Maharishi Ayur-Veda.

It is our great fortune to be able to share the knowledge of Maharishi Ayur-Veda with you, along with our thoughts and experiences of teaching and practicing Ayur-Veda through this book. We welcome hearing your thoughts and experiences. May yours be the healthiest, most joyful life and may you serve our world well by moving to awaken a profound degree of love, healing, and wholeness in all humanity.

# Chapter 1

### ❀

# WHOLENESS

## Reuniting Our Physical, Mental, and Emotional Lives

*From the center of Reality, the whole circumference of life is seen to be completely harmonious, for when the center is found, it becomes clear that the innumerable radii all converge from the circumference towards a single point.*[1]

Maharishi Mahesh Yogi

Sometimes we in the West forget that we are intimately connected to nature; we tend to think of nature as the flowers, the birds, the rivers, the mountains, and the stars. Somehow we've convinced ourselves that "human nature" is something separate and distinct. We take vacations "to be in nature," but we often forget that nature is in us. We forget that in reality, our psychology and physiology are material expressions of natural law, and that we are direct participants in the design of the universe. While regulating our heart rate, adjusting our body temperature to remain nearly constant despite the climate, and sculpting the depth of our perceptions, the laws of nature also breathe compassion into our hearts, and structure a sense of social and even global responsibility into our thinking, making us aware that thoughts of our environment are the same as thoughts of our own health and our own personal quality of life.

If you want to be healthy, what you really need to remember is how to go "back to nature," not to the great outdoors only but to the great *indoors:* back to nature inside yourself.

Healing, after all, is not something that *you* do; it's a phenomenon orchestrated by the laws of nature in your mind, heart, and body, in the same way that nature conducts repair after a forest fire or regenerates the earth after a hard winter. You need only to allow that repair and regeneration to occur, to let healing take place without interference. You need only to set up the proper conditions and routines to promote this inner harmony and allow your physiology to remember what good health really feels like. If there is one single secret to becoming completely healthy, it's recognizing that you have access to those laws of nature hidden beneath the surface of life and you can learn to use them well.

## Self-Referral Healing:
## A Remembrance of Things Whole

There is a Vedic proverb, "What you see, you become." Think about the last time you looked out over the ocean, your attention captured by the waves. Did you ever have a moment where you found yourself, instead of looking at wave after wave, becoming aware of the magnitude of the whole body of water? That feeling of expansion that you experience when you stop noticing only the waves and "remember" to notice the ocean is akin to a way of feeling, knowing, and being in the world that is called "self-referral." You refer back to your deepest self, to the most expansive aspect of selfhood where everything is already connected, and experience life from that place where you are most whole. It's that deeply comfortable place we arrive at when we move beyond all the shifting elements, past the boundaries of experience to a feeling of no boundaries, beyond the inner self-talking that distracts each of us from ourselves and also from those we love. It is the essence of the feeling of being "at home," connecting with nature inside. In Maharishi Ayur-Veda, it is understood as the unified field of pure consciousness.

By referring back to this inner wholeness from where all the intelligence and orderliness of your bodymind's functioning first develops deep in your awareness, you discover the universal source of knowledge for creating and maintaining invincible health. Once there, you regain the experience of the inseparability of nature inside you and nature outside you. And when you regain this integrity, this memory of who you really are, of inner wholeness, life begins to feel complete rather than piecemeal, as though everything has fallen into place at last.

Healthiness is maintained far more by this deep integration of mind, body, and emotions than by intentionally cultivating positive attitudes or by trying to change outer circumstances. Neither your good will nor your optimistic thoughts, your emotions nor your mind alone can heal your body. Healing affirmations, visualizations, and the like that do not tap into the orderly intelligence of nature within can be only partially effective. Nature wants you to be whole as much as you do, guiding you through your DNA, yearning to keep you on the track of good health at every moment of life. All you need is a way to make contact with the full range of nature's self-repair and self-healing program, which lies within every cell of your body, within your own consciousness.

This is the knowledge Maharishi Ayur-Veda brings.

The basic approach is to restore the body's natural intelligence and therefore its full ability to heal itself. You learn to tap into nature's orderliness within you, where you are at once patient, medicine, and doctor. It teaches you how nature flows within you and out from you, in the same way it flows throughout the universe. It describes how you can reconnect with this interweaving flow to enliven your good health. And although the self-healing mechanisms of Ayur-Veda are taught through a number of specific techniques and guidelines, none is more important than this essential truth: *This knowledge is already there inside you, or you wouldn't be able to remember it, awaken it, and put it to good use.*

Ayur-Veda thus offers a process of remembrance, not of things past but of things unshakable and eternal, of your own healthiness. And this is the sweetest medicine, which teaches your body to remember what glorious health feels like, your mind to recall what unbounded wisdom feels like, and your heart to remember the joy of the constancy of tender love.

## The Harmony of Healthiness

"Healthiness" reflects a unified life, an order and balance of things. When you see a woman who is very healthy, you might notice that she gives the impression of total radiance, expressing a quality of internal energy. You might also notice that her intelligence is bright and lively, her thinking expansive and clear, and her emotions stable and easily accessible. Her friends may describe her as "the picture of health." It's almost as if her healthiness were visible in every cell of her being. And if you could see into the cellular level of her body, you would find that each cell functions individually and collectively in a highly organized manner. She seems to be at one with herself, integrated in all aspects of her life. When you ask her how she feels, she may well tell you she feels deeply happy. She isn't describing an absence of disease or reporting the results of a negative lab test. She's identifying the joyful feeling of well-being, the feeling of bliss, the experience of her body, her mind, and her emotions working effortlessly and fully together, the experience of being a truly healthy woman.

Internal harmony is perhaps the most salient feature of all living systems, expressing the intelligent growth and regulation of all aspects of nature, from the blossoming of a rose to the rising of the tides to the movements of the planets. From cells to galaxies, all matter of life is arranged to uphold and express nature's intelligence in a vast universe of balance and cohesion. In this way the organized intelligence of the universe is a collection of many forms or bits of expressed intelligence, all life but all organized in different ways. Without this intelligence, gold wouldn't always be gold wherever you find it and flowers wouldn't always bloom in the spring.

In humans, the material essence of nature's intelligence is called DNA (deoxyribonucleic acid), the densely organized genetic code built into our cells that structures both our individuality and the memory of our collective humanness, which is capable of tremendous flexibility.

One way to look at your health is to understand that the healthier you are, the more fully you're expressing the intelligence of

**13**

your genetic potential. When you're expressing your DNA as it most wants to be expressed, your cells grow and move around just where and when they're supposed to, perfecting the flow of orderliness in your entire physiology, and the more balanced you feel inside and out.

Illness, on the other hand, has a certain disorderliness about it. You may say, "I'm not feeling myself" because "myself" feels better balanced, more stable, and more integrated. Or if you are quite sick, you may have a feeling of chaos and the accompanying thought, "I'm falling apart." (But no one truly falls apart, because nature is still kindly keeping us together even when we're too sick to notice or care.)

The harmony factor in health shows up in every part of your psychological and physical life. When you are functioning optimally, your heart rate is steady, your blood flows evenly through your veins and arteries, and the internal metabolic thermostat in your hypothalamus keeps your temperature at exactly or very close to 98.6° Fahrenheit, whether you are at the Equator or at the Arctic Circle. At the same time, your pancreas is regulating your blood sugar at a nearly constant level while your lungs, kidneys, and brain orchestrate the exact amounts of oxygen and carbon dioxide needed to keep your physiology in balance. So it is with every aspect of your body's functioning, because that incredibly well-organized package of nature in you, your DNA, is maintaining its precision operations through a constant self-referral feedback process and readjusting every moment accordingly in order to maintain perfect balance within and between every cell of your body.

This functional integrity applies not only to the inner workings of your body but also to your perceptions of the world. Human physiology adores orderliness and automatically constructs order out of disorder whenever it has the chance. When you observe a moiré pattern in silk taffeta, for example, you don't merely see a bunch of lines; you experience a pattern, a wholeness. Your eyes search the field and your brain spontaneously connects the points of intersection that make the patterns. It's not that you can't see the individual lines, it's simply that, being a healthy human, you "prefer" the pattern. It's more natural for your order-seeking physiology to take in.

When we choose bedroom wallpaper, most of us tend to want

a uniform pattern that is not too demanding, something we can live with peacefully on a daily basis, because then we ingest less chaos and disorder into our nervous systems. Certain colors—soft greens and blues, for example—have been found to create more quiet harmony within. Researchers say this is why we prefer them when we are ill.

We favor harmony *because* it is more life-supporting and more health-giving. It is so satisfying to us, in fact, that the continual integration of new experience and thinking into larger and more all-encompassing patterns has been identified throughout history as the basic quest of all human life—the desire for the single pattern, the complete picture, the Theory of Everything, the desire to take in the basic design of the universe, the desire for wholeness itself.

Even from the moment of birth we seek this grand unification. In his *Journals,* Emerson observed, "Every child is filled with a desire for the whole; a desire raging, infinite." So it is no surprise that the origin of the word "healthiness" comes from "wholeness" and that "to heal" really means "to make whole."

## How Nature's Wholeness Nourishes Our Health

The desire for wholeness is far more than a psychological yearning; it is the desire for life to seek more of itself, to find, take in, and maintain even more life. Such desires are an important part of our evolution, of the biological mechanics that create reality through our very existence. In this way, it is perfectly natural to want more and more and to expect these longings to be fulfilled. Wholeness itself is most nourishing, involved in every aspect of our physiology. But it is often forgotten when we start to lose ourselves in specific health problems. And if we lose access to the intrinsic organization and intelligence of nature, we lose that lifeline to our own possibilities for total health. No love relationship, no quest for success or power or money is more compelling than the desire to feel the full depth of our own healthiness, because it rejuvenates all other aspects of our lives.

The healing value of nature's wholeness has been acknowledged by every culture. The Eastern cultures have perhaps appreciated this healing interaction most fully and have been able to integrate it into daily life.

According to recent research, we heal more quickly and efficiently when we connect to nature in even the most basic ways. In a study of postsurgery recuperation, for example, researchers found that patients whose rooms faced a small grove of trees needed less recovery time than those in rooms facing a brick wall. They also required less pain medication and reported that they were less emotionally upset. And simply watching fish swim in an aquarium lowers blood pressure so effectively that it even works in a dentist's office with people who are about to have a tooth pulled. If such minor interactions with nature bring such positive benefits, imagine what full direct contact with the laws of nature inside you could do to revitalize your health.

Perhaps no one is more aware of the need for this revitalizing contact with natural law than women today.

## A Mutual Recognition

There is a poignant moment in Wendy Wasserstein's Pulitzer Prize-winning play, *The Heidi Chronicles,* when the heroine, a noted art historian, is giving a speech to her high school alumnae association on "Women, Where Are We Going?" She confesses that in spite of her success, she is unfulfilled, and she adds, "I don't blame any of us. We're all concerned, intelligent, good women. It's just that I feel stranded." Heidi Holland seems to be speaking for many of us. Although important changes have taken place in the personal and professional lives of women in the past several decades, the progress is often double-edged: The breakdown of old barriers has uncovered new ones. While women's professional opportunities and obligations have greatly expanded, there has not been an equivalent societal support to help with familial and household responsibilities.

In trying to stitch work and family lives together, we can't avoid the realization that each day still has only twenty-four hours in it. Long after midnight, many of us are trying to catch up with our commitments instead of our sleep, and we are simply running out of time and energy. The more we seek to expand our lives, the more we seem to encounter physical, mental, emotional, and social conditions that restrict or negate the value and pleasure of that expansion.

As we search for ways to hold such complex lives together, a collective realization is quietly emerging: We are becoming aware that it is time not simply to move ahead but to move *deep,* to regroup from within. This collective "Aha!" among women today is the recognition that what we need most, to accomplish what we want most, is to recall that voice of deepest awareness, our connection to nature's harmonizing influence within, to reawaken our personal repository of inner wisdom and healing. We may each have our own name for it, but whatever we call it, what is essential is that we recollect it.

If we lose access to the deeper field of reality, we may end up feeling stranded, unfulfilled, and incomplete. For this reason, this inner connection to nature should be our most prized possession. But most of us no longer can hear that inner voice. We have deafened ourselves through incessant activity, through constantly focusing our awareness on people and matters outside ourselves. It is only when we repossess that inner voice—really listen to it and flow with it—that we can enjoy a feeling of completeness and full participation in our own lives. If we lose contact with it or decide to ignore it, life may well become a series of fragments and disappointments. And this chips away at our ability to be healthy and can lead to a whole range of effects of a fragmentary life, which we frequently call illnesses.

## The Health Consequences of "the Big Juggle"

We may recognize that most aspects of women's lives have improved, but women's health is not among them. Our health problems are increasing dramatically. As we've begun to enjoy the advantages of traditionally male occupations, we've become subject to a marked increase in "male" illnesses, such as lung cancer, heart disease, and drug addiction. Indeed, heart disease is now the leading cause of death for women as well as men.

Working women today have higher rates of illness than men and require more disability days. Smoking, drinking, and illegal drug use are increasing among women, as are a variety of eating disorders, from unnecessary dieting to bulimia and anorexia. Although women still live six years longer than men on average, the gender gap in mortality is closing as well: Women's life spans, while still longer, are not increasing at the same rates as men's.

In particular, stress-related symptoms in women are on the rise, owing perhaps to the increase in role-strain and overload, as women attempt to be all things to all people. Over half of the women in the United States with children under six are in the work force. Over half of new mothers are working outside the home or looking for work within a year of the birth of a child. It is not entirely surprising that 50 percent of the women surveyed by the National Center for Health Statistics reported that some kind of stress had negatively affected their health in the past year. Workplace stresses alone are not causing the increase in stress-related illness; women are equally susceptible whether working to care for a family at home or working at an office.

The effects of stress are even more severe among professional women: Women physicians and women psychologists, for example, have three times the suicide rates of their male counterparts, and in the general population, twice as many women as men currently suffer from depression. Women take far more tranquilizers and antidepressants and also more prescribed mind- and mood-altering drugs than men; 70 percent of all psychoactive medications are prescribed to women.[2]

Because it is women today who are most susceptible to stress, resulting from a complex balancing act between family, career, emotional and financial needs, it is women who are most seriously in need of a more all-encompassing form of health care. Despite all our good intentions, activities such as aerobics, low-fat diets, or any of the other approaches we responsibly incorporate into our lives, while useful, do not touch our deepest health needs.

These deeper needs are caused in large part by the loss of the connection to nature inside, by the loss of the feeling of being so completely stable that it doesn't matter what changes come along. When our activities are divorced from this innermost sense of who we are, life can become unbalanced and eventually unhealthy. Our hearts ache, our minds feel frazzled, and, as more and more research shows, our bodies develop one disease or another to remind us how out of balance we have become.

We not only become prone to physical, mental, and emotional illness, we also tend to make mistakes, as we stop trusting ourselves. When you lose this inner integrity, it's as if a dimmer switch had thrown a darkening shadow across your awareness, and you don't see the consequences of your choices clearly. When your mind tells you one thing and your heart another, you may find that you can no longer rely on the marriage of your judgment and feelings. If your mind is clouded and your body tired, you may be highly emotional about or passionately committed to something or someone terribly wrong for you. Or you may be sharp intellectually while making a presentation at work but feel so depressed and emotionally unavailable that you are incapable of enjoying your success. Success thus may breed anxiety and illness, the very opposite of what it ought to create.

When you have a high degree of inner integration, you don't have to make uncomfortable choices: Your mind, heart, and body act in harmony and cooperate to fulfill your desires. Everything you think, feel, and do ultimately has to connect; otherwise, you feel scattered and unstable. This little understood but key component of healthiness cannot be put into a small white pill.

### On Being a Wise and Healthy Woman: Reunion with One's Self

We may believe that nurturing anyone anytime it is needed is one of the great and powerful traditions of being a woman. But who, we may ask ourselves or our friends, nourishes *us?* Are we fated to label ourselves forever "codependent" because we've lost touch with the ability to self-nurture?

It isn't really true that women "love too much"; it's simply that we've become separated from our own inner source of love, segregated from the laws of nature that support self-nurturance. As a result of this inner splitting off, we may experience one of the most painful and unhealthy consequences of a fragmented life: the loss of a loving heart at the basis of all our relationships.

Only when we are reconnected inside, when we feel ourselves

to be, as the poet Goethe expressed it, "a grand, beautiful, worthy and worthwhile whole," can we satisfy our hearts' desires, enjoy our daily experiences at work and at home, revel in our leisure time, and share the kind of full intimacy with our spouses, children, parents, partners, and friends that we and they so richly deserve.

Reconnecting with ourselves need not be a gear-grinding event for any of us; what we require is not so much a change of outer scenery but a revisioning of the inner landscape. Rejoining with our deeper selves, we discover this healing, unifying support awaiting us, a reliable and steadfast resource for self-nurturance which was never truly lost to us, but which may have been hidden, unexpressed, or simply forgotten.

This knowledge of a powerful, loving, health-promoting inner source of life is not new. It is what the sages have been telling us about throughout history. It is the *Wakan* of the Sioux Indians; it is Plato's "everlasting loveliness which neither comes nor goes, which neither flowers nor fades"; it is Jung's "boundless expanse with no inside and no outside . . . no mine and no thine." It is at the sacred heart of the Goddess traditions. And in the Vedic tradition, it is the home of all the laws of nature, the home of that tender force of creation, in its feminine form, that all-loving mother who is always there for us, even when we are unaware.

We believe that women have had remarkable access to this inner resource of self-referral awareness. Reconnecting with it enables us to reunite our minds, bodies, and emotions and establish the basis for a lifetime of psychophysiological well-being.

### Knowing in Your Heart:
### Women's Intuitive Development

When we consider the differences between males and females, we may think about the obvious physical, hormonal, and reproductive differences. But subtler differences exist as well. Why, for example, are women in particular thought of as intuitive?

Both ancient Ayur-Vedic physicians and modern researchers agree that intuition is very real and that, although it can be developed by both men and women, women have an apparent built-in physiological capability for developing subtle perception, abstract thinking, and refined feeling, the essential components of intuition. Such a developed physiology can enable any woman to support and maintain an inner awareness of wholeness along with any activity. It provides a great health advantage. By keeping inner awareness lively, your activity becomes nearly frictionless, offsetting the process of wear and tear on your bodymind.

You are using your intuition when you need to *feel* if an idea makes sense, when you require something beyond "the facts," when you say, "I know it in my heart." Intuition enables you to know something *directly,* without relying on external data. It results from the deeper, more cooperative flow of mind and heart together, supported by a balanced and integrated physical body. Intuition offers a way to cognize the laws of nature directly, to perceive reality with an "inward eye."

Women's psychophysiology has been found specifically to support intuitive functioning, but we can't credit either nature or nurture alone. It may be given by nature, but women also have had the requisite "intuition practice." The desire for knowledge is a basic human quest, and we are all seekers. When a person is deprived of a formal education and kept isolated from the affairs of the world, as were so many women throughout the centuries, she develops a way to educate herself by tapping into knowledge on the *inside;* she learns to "know" life from within.

Relying on subtle states of awareness to be informed, it may be that women evolved a way of knowing that we call women's intuition. This developmental process could have come about in very much the same way that all inward development comes about, reminiscent of the journey that cloistered priests, nuns, and monks may have experienced as they consciously embarked upon an inward spiritual life. Lacking the "objective" world, the knower learns about life through the inner experiences and revelations of self-awareness.

Even for the most educated women, the intuitive processes were the primary direct avenues for knowledge. Going within, women poets such as Elizabeth Barrett Browning and Christina Rossetti were able to bring what writer Virginia Woolf called "trophies" to "the surface": to discover the meanings of life by "magnifying everything that was within." St. Teresa of Avila, founder of the

Carmelite order, described her own experience of this process of intuitive knowing: "It was as if a person who had never learned anything, nor yet was able to read, suddenly found himself [sic] in possession of all the data of science."[3]

With the need to develop a *feeling* way of knowing, enhanced through the strengthening of the heart through devotional service—whether to family or within the "acceptable" professions of teaching, social service, nursing, or religious vocation—women became the traditional guardians of inner knowledge. The historical legacy of women's development is in large part this integrating of inner and outer life, trusting intuition, the heart and mind merged, the finer levels of awareness opened up. And this legacy— whether cause or effect—provides us with a distinct women's psychophysiology.

## The Benefits of Women's Psychophysiological Development

The parameters for intuitive functioning are now being identified in research on developmental differences in men's and women's physiology. The results of brain physiology studies, such as those conducted by Christine de LaCoste-Utamsing and Ralph Holloway in 1983 and by UCLA researchers Laura Allen and Roger Gorski in 1991, indicate that the corpus callosum, the part of the brain that connects the left and right hemispheres, is as much as 25 to 40 percent larger in women than in men. This provides what the researchers describe as greater neural flexibility or "plasticity," enabling one hemisphere of the brain to take over the functions of the other with more ease. Women apparently use both hemispheres in a number of ordinary activities. For example, they most often use both sides of the brain when they spell words while men primarily use the left side.

The plasticity of the female brain is said to begin *in utero* and continue throughout life, bringing some important benefits in health. For example, as people grow older, it is the left side of the brain that deteriorates most. But a recent study at the University of Pennsylvania concluded that women's brains stay sharper several times longer than men's. Women also recover from strokes more quickly and more efficiently, particularly with regard to speech. This speedier recovery process may be the result of the development of the larger corpus callosum, creating inherent flexibility in the mediating processes of brain functioning. Or it may be, as other research on brain differences has indicated, that females tend to process language within the frontal lobe of the brain while male language skills are focused more in the parietal lobe, in the mid-portion of the brain, so that strokes in that area would be more damaging to the recovery of speech in men than in women.[4]

There are other possible explanations why the female brain experiences less severe consequences after injury. When Dr. Norman Geschwind and his colleagues at Harvard University studied the influence of male hormones on brain function, they noted that testosterone seems to affect the development of right-brain functioning, increasing the likelihood of a more specialized brain and minimizing integrative functioning. They noted that the influence of testosterone may prevent neural recovery after injury. This may explain the results of the following experiment: A research team at Columbia University trained a group of male and female rats to cross an elevated runway and then removed the sensorimotor cortex to extinguish the memory of this training. When the rats were retested weeks later, only the males were unable to cross the runway; the females showed little if any impairment.

We also know from brain research that intuitive thinking occurs best when the two hemispheres of the brain are functioning in an integrated, synchronous way. Overall intuitive awareness in women may thus be a very real function of our normal psychophysiology. When understood in this light, "women's intuition" is no longer very mysterious; women are simply using their ordinary perceptual and abstract thinking abilities.

Other research on physiological differences between men and women further clarifies specific developmental abilities in women, particularly in perception. Studies undertaken by neuropsychologists Diane McGuinness and Karl Pribram at Stanford University indicate that women are more attentive to sounds in conversation and to their emotional meaning, and more empathetic and more accurate than men in perceiving subliminal messages.[5] In addition, women's hearing is far more sensitive on average than men's: At 85 decibels and above, sound seems twice as loud to a woman as it seems to a man. Apparently, women listen equally with both ears, while men generally rely more on the right ear. Women are also more sensitive to and more aware of touch, taste, and smell.

We are also learning that gender differences in physiological functioning lead to different ways of interfacing with the world: Simply speaking, women and men screen the same information in different ways. Whereas men are generally more interested in objects, women are generally more interested in people and remember names and faces more easily. While women are better at taking in verbal information, men are better at visual information gathering—at least in daylight (women have better night vision on average).

There is also evidence that women respond with finer attention to conversation, are better listeners than men, have greater empathy, and are not as easily distracted by the intervention of visual sights. Newborn girls utter more sounds than newborn boys and maintain a larger variety of sounds throughout the first years of life. They speak their first words and sentences earlier and have larger vocabularies by age two. Researchers speculate that perhaps because everyday speech in females is enhanced by emotional and visual input from other cerebral regions, verbal skills develop sooner and more easily. Possibly as a result, during the school years girls have one-sixth the reading problems that boys have and are found to develop more complex thinking skills at a younger age than boys.

In adulthood, women process information faster on average than men and can make more rapid choices on the basis of that information. Cognitive studies further indicate that men seem to have better developed right-hemisphere functioning and excel in spatial reasoning, enabling them mentally to rotate three-dimensional objects, while women have the ability to think more abstractly and more globally. If we begin to wonder whether this has anything to do with our physiology, at least one study confirms that it does: Women improved their spatial rotation scores by 50 to 100 percent during menstruation, when their estrogen levels were lowest, while men improved their scores in the spring when their testosterone levels were highest!

A number of theories suggest reasons for these various physiological gender differences. But what is important for us is that women and men do have identifiably different physiological capabilities, whether the brain is determining behavior or whether behavior is creating the brain's structures. And it seems clear that our health care must reflect and make use of those differences. We must consider the idea that a physiology that is more integrative than specialized may require medicine that is more integrative than specialized.

## Better, Not Bitter, Medicine

Clarifying and appreciating these gender distinctions brings up the possibility that women, having a unique physiological set-up, may heal differently and therefore may require other healing technologies. If we are endowed with the gift of a flexible physiology that can support heightened perceptual and intuitive awareness, we must learn to use it properly for our own health care. With a fully developed integrated physiology, we could live the life of complex diversity required today while remaining settled and stable inside, enjoying any change that comes along without losing our psychological or physiological equilibrium. What a powerful opportunity for creating an invincible state of the best of all possible health.

The only thing that can prevent us from tapping into that magical balancing resource within is forgetting that it exists. And the forgetting is not solely an intellectual loss; it is also a heart-wrenching loss. It can cause us great fear and paralyzing doubt, a feeling of being all alone and without resources, and this inevitably shatters some or all aspects of the integrity of our physical, mental, and emotional health. As our physiology tries to adjust to a baseless, unconnected life, we can become susceptible to all the possible forms of illness we can name and even some we can't.

It is apparent that all of us, and especially women, require a health-care system that incorporates self-knowledge and self-referral medicine as a means to unite mind, body, and heart, a system that can serve us on a deeper level of health. We believe the most important understanding that the medical community can achieve in accommodating a woman's way of healing is the recognition that a woman's physiological and psychological development—because it is more flexible than determined, more

25

integrated than specialized, more open to thinking and feeling in wholes than in parts—may necessitate a deeper, more unified level of care.

We suggest that Maharishi Ayur-Veda offers and delivers this kind of unifying in-depth care to women and men alike because it delves more deeply into healing beyond cells and tissues. It provides the means to tap into nature's healing resource inside. Coming home to nature within ourselves provides the most effective house call of all. Coming home to the inner self, we create our own best medicine.

Before we explore how the processes of Ayur-Veda bring about a reunion of mind, body, and heart and reawaken our inner healing resources and responses, let's look at what is available for women within the practices of conventional medicine today.

## Chapter 2

*Chapter 2*

DEPTH

### The Need for Deeper Care
### of Women's Health

*Avert the danger which has not yet come.*

Yoga Sutras

*Taking recourse to my own self-referral nature,*
*I create again and again.*

Bhagavad-Gita

Medicine should be the very process that makes us feel whole. But like so many other fragmented aspects of our lives today, we are medically attended to "in pieces." We run (if we can) from our back doctor to our psychotherapist to our eye doctor to our gynecologist. Many of us see at least ten doctors a year. From head (doctors) to toe (doctors), we are being treated part by part, but with no sense of integration of our health concerns or the feeling that one doctor knows us well or even knows what another is doing. And although we are told that all these levels of specialization mean better medical care, or at least better treatment of specific ailments, this has not been the case. It is no news to anyone who has had conventional medical care in the past decade that the system itself has become unhealthy, and at times separated from its health-giving purpose. We propose that this has happened primarily because the basic premise implies an essential distrust of nature's ability to heal, thereby robbing us of the very essence of recovery. As is widely understood, the entire modern medical system is set up to address the problem, not the cause; the ailment, not the person who develops the ailment.

## Shortcomings of Disease-Model Medicine

Western or allopathic medicine is based on the diagnosis and treatment of disease, not on its subtler, underlying causes. While we can successfully (and thankfully) replace a damaged knee joint with a titanium mechanism, we still cannot arrest the development of osteoarthritis and we still cannot advise someone how to avoid it entirely. Perhaps of most concern, we still pay little attention to how a knee operation affects an entire human being, psychologically as well as physically. We have not dealt with the fact that a *person* has a knee operation, not a knee. We do not ask, how does a person deal with a decade of pain? What happens after the surgery? There is no theoretical basis whereby we can set such an operation in a context of overall healing.

In addition, when we employ a disease model of medicine instead of a health model, only known illnesses are considered treatable. In order to be treated, diseases must be named. "New" diseases are identified to explain a host of constitutional symptoms that defy ordinary diagnoses, but we may simply be renaming groups of symptoms. In the early 1900s, there was a "disease" known as "circulatory neuraesthenia"; in the 1970s, another called "hypoglycemia"; and in the 1990s, groups of similar symptoms have been called variously Chronic Fatigue Syndrome, Epstein-Barr disease, food allergies, mercury poisoning from dental fillings, and environmental hypersensitivity.

These symptoms raise some serious questions: Are there actually myriad new diseases? Or are there collections of less well-defined symptoms representing *degrees* of illness—more or less severe forms of other illnesses? Are there underlying disturbances in ongoing bodily functions that may not yet be identifiable as known diseases but that are nonetheless disabling? Why must a disease be named in order for us to receive care? These are questions rarely addressed by Western medicine, where the interest in the diagnosis is primary.

We can summarize the limits of the modern medical system within two areas of medical attention:

*Diagnosis:* Conventional medicine lacks the means to diagnose symptoms that do not fall into specific disease categories associated with a specific constellation of physical signs and laboratory values.

*Treatment:* Conventional medicine does not have a subtle enough framework for understanding functional problems lacking medical names. In the absence of an objectively verifiable disease that shows up on a lab test, an X ray, or during a physical exam, doctors have little to offer patients who may be experiencing distressful symptoms.

Missing the forest for the trees, this illness-based perspective narrows the vision of good health by defining it as a "lack of disease." And this has an unfortunate effect. If we can't identify a known illness, we don't attempt to recognize subtle changes in our state of well-being, such as the onset of indigestion, fatigue, a headache, or a heartache. Relatively little attention is given to understanding and promoting those basic but less dramatic factors responsible for keeping us healthy. Moreover, by treating mind, body, and emotions as separate, we are discouraged from seeking the healing value of wholeness, of experiencing a more orderly level of wellness through the integration of our psychophysiological functioning. We learn to separate the functioning of our body from the functioning of our mind, from our emotions, and ultimately from a daily, self-healing process.

The disease model of health has entirely dominated the Western medical field and left little room for other perspectives on healing within medical practice. It appears that the responsibility for this unhealthy confusion lies far less with the diagnoses and treatment offered by the individual doctor than with the orientation of the medical system itself. As a result, an increasing number of doctors today are entering the unifying field of psychoneuroimmunology (PNI) and/or experimenting with other alternative approaches.

## Questioning Invasive Medicine

Medicine is a localized, culturally influenced profession; its practice is supported by the values and biases of the people it treats. As a result, it changes dramatically from era to era, as well as across cultures. And progressive though the march of medicine may seem, it doesn't necessarily consistently improve health. We sometimes forget this. We forget that the majority of health transactions within a given medical framework are based on the interests of a given society and not necessarily on absolute principles of healing. It is the culture which determines wellness and disease, the agreed-upon treatment methods, and the healing messages in the patient-doctor relationship.

Every nation thus holds a different vision of what medical care means. As a predominantly high-tech nation, the United States supports high-tech medicine. Whether effective or not, technology determines practice. For example, researchers have found that physicians with diagnostic imagers in their offices order four times more exams than their counterparts, but don't necessarily get four times more useful information. Patients are said to have more confidence in a doctor with a well-equipped office. As a result, no matter what they may personally advocate, doctors have been fully encouraged to adopt a "part-by-part" method of defining and treating illness because modern medical research, practice, and training have been overwhelmingly skewed toward the diagnosis and treatment of disease using the latest high-tech interventions, especially drugs and surgery.

In her eye-opening book *Medicine and Culture,* Lynn Payer, a medical correspondent for *The New York Times,* compared the American outlook on medicine with the French, British, and West German perspectives. The differences are striking. For example, chronic and degenerative illnesses in the elderly, such as Alzheimer's disease and arthritis, have comparatively little specialist support in the United States; although there are approximately 11,000 cardiologists practicing in the United States, there are fewer than 900 geriatric specialists.[1] In England, however, there are nearly identical numbers of cardiologists and geriatric specialists. One can conclude that the medical focus in England is equally concerned with the quality of life in elderly citizens as with treating heart disease in the general population.[2]

Payer suggests that the American system promotes a far more invasive, aggressive kind of medical treatment—which may well serve certain kinds of medical problems, but which may not always be appropriate or even helpful for others. Because this model is used almost exclusively, it may also account for the increase in treatment programs where the cure turns out to be worse than the disease in terms of the overall health of the patient. This situation shows up in an overreliance on surgery.

The United States is very much a "surgical" nation. Its surgery rates are two to three times higher than those in Europe. For example, despite similar rates of breast cancer in the past several decades, three times the number of mastectomies were performed in New England than in England or Sweden. Even U.S. diagnostic tests are more invasive, cutting open and drawing blood more frequently than any other nation. The French, for example, almost never do a dilation and curettage (D & C), but in the United States it is the third most common medical procedure.

Furthermore, the United States is a drug-oriented nation. Besides prescribing drugs more often, American physicians frequently prescribe higher doses than are prescribed in other parts of the world, and, as a result, there are higher rates of side effects. Americans are particularly keen on getting rid of mental illnesses with drugs; the recommended dosages are often ten times higher in the United States than elsewhere.

The radical, intrusive, and often unnatural care—whether surgical or chemical, whether curative or not—that the modern medical model upholds undeniably brings more risks with it. Both patients and doctors have to address this situation with an open mind and decide if this is the kind of medicine we want to rely upon exclusively. It is true that many diseases such as cancer, heart disease, and autoimmune diseases demand intensive treatment such as potent drugs and surgery. But is this because we have developed a medical system that mostly treats later-stage illnesses? We must also ask: *Could these diseases have been found and treated at earlier stages or prevented entirely under a broader health-care system that includes other kinds of medical knowledge and intervention?*

## The Quick-Fix Disillusionment

There is no doubt that the fragmented, overspecialized medical system in the United States has taken its toll on our health care and therefore on our health. But it has caused a further problem: a lack of trust in physicians themselves, many of whom feel at least as disconnected from the deeper healing values of the profession as their patients. The glory and joy of being a doctor may be fading.

There is no clearer sign of the times than reports of the large number of doctors who are seriously disenchanted with current practice in the United States today. A recent series of articles in *The New York Times* focused on some of the factors. A Gallup Poll for the American Medical Association indicated that, despite the money they might earn, "almost 40 percent of the doctors interviewed . . . would probably or definitely *not* enter medical school if they had a career choice to make again."[3] Moreover, applications to medical school have dropped 25 percent over the past five years. The malpractice suits, the paperwork, the regulation by outside agencies, the lack of opportunity for caring doctor-patient relationships are cited as the reasons for the disillusionment.[4]

It is hardly the fault of doctors alone; many Americans have come to think of good medicine as "taking action." An aggressive course of treatment is perceived as more useful than a less active course, even though medical research does not often justify major interventions. But most patients consider a good doctor to be someone who "does something." We are more suspicious of a physician who wants to wait and see than of one who proposes a "cure."

The current situation is clear: Americans demand a quick medical fix and are supporting a quick-fix system, at an unprecedented cost. The United States spends more than any other country (12 percent of the gross national product) on health care, with the costs escalating at $50 billion a year.[5] By the year 2000, Americans will spend $1.5 trillion on health care or 15 percent of the gross national product. Yet in two critical measures of health, infant mortality and life expectancy, U.S. citizens are worse off than citizens in most industrialized nations, with life expectancy ranking twenty-second in the world for men, and sixteenth in the world for women; U.S. minority populations are falling even farther behind.

Moreover, the United States hasn't made much headway in halting its two most lethal illnesses, cancer and heart disease: Overall cancer rates are still rising annually and heart disease is still the biggest killer, resulting in one out of three deaths. Expensive heart surgery procedures have not proved to be very effective. It seems clear that something is terribly wrong with a system that is costly, unproductive, and unappealing to doctors and patients alike. We must face the fact that disease-model medicine has had limited success in improving the overall health of our nation. And women especially are paying the price.

## Why Modern Medicine Is Not Serving Women Well

The "part-by-part" system of medicine has led to a number of often inappropriate treatments for women. "As doctors, we think we're helping women when we may actually be harming them," says Dr. Mary Guinan, a recent assistant director at the Centers for Disease Control.[6] Cesarean section is the most common surgical procedure in the United States, and hysterectomy is in second place. Both are women's operations and both are extremely questionable when undertaken in such numbers. According to a *Consumer Reports* research review, these are the two most frequently performed *unnecessary* procedures; half of the cesarean sections and 27 percent of the hysterectomies were deemed not needed.

A stunning 600,000 hysterectomies are performed each year in the United States, several times the rate of hysterectomies performed in European countries, such as France and Germany. So common is this operation that an American woman has just about a fifty-fifty chance of reaching sixty-five with her uterus intact. There are some serious consequences to her health: She is exposed to infection during surgery; if her ovaries are also removed, her risk of heart disease is increased; she may suffer from depression, fatigue, and other overall debilitation from having an important part of her physiology removed and her hormones thrown into chaos.

Then there are the increasing numbers of cesarean births—now 25 percent of all U.S. births[7]—many of which are at best unnecessary, for hospital or physician convenience, and at worst cause real damage. They are often recommended following sessions of electronic fetal monitoring, which have not been shown to benefit either the baby or the mother but which do pave the way for a threefold increase in cesarean procedures. According to a report in the *New England Journal of Medicine,* "Fetal monitors are more likely to make you a candidate for a cesarean operation than to help reduce the chances of birth-related problems."[8] In addition, as at least twenty studies have demonstrated, a woman who has delivered via cesarean section is perfectly capable of delivering her next child vaginally. But despite such consistent evidence, many obstetricians continue to favor a surgical delivery for subsequent births.

Obviously, hysterectomy is a safe and necessary procedure for treating uterine cancer[9] and other life-threatening illnesses, and many women have gratefully undergone much-needed cesarean procedures. Nevertheless, the fact remains that more women than men have their reproductive organs surgically invaded or removed as a treatment for *non-life-threatening* illnesses. Endometriosis, fibroid tumors, prolapsed uterus, even severe menstrual pain are often "solved" by hysterectomy, even though there are safer, less invasive (and less expensive) treatments available.

Another of the most common procedures in Western medicine performed on women is episiotomy, or surgically enlarging the birth canal, which is routinely done during 70 to 80 percent of North American births. Results of a recent major study at McGill University in Montreal suggest that such cutting procedures are of no major benefit either to the prevention injury to birth canal tissues or to the birth outcome or to the enhancement of sexual functioning, although they decrease labor time by about nine minutes.[10]

Overall, women seem to be perceived as a different kind of patient than men, and while we are advocates for researching and recognizing medical differences between women and men, we are concerned about how women are treated within current practices.

Currently, women's health issues are at the heart of some of modern medicine's most controversial treatments. As we will discuss in chapter 11, while hormone replacement therapy (HRT) does seem to prevent severe symptoms of menopause and may reduce the risk of death due to osteoporosis and heart disease in women, there are studies that argue against its use. Besides its long-known potential risk for increasing the incidence of endome-trial cancer, as well as the incidence of gall bladder problems, liver tumors, and blood clots, hormone replacement therapy may also increase the risk of breast cancer by as much as 36 percent. Such were the findings of Dr. Graham Colditz's research team at Harvard Medical School, which has been conducting one of the largest ex-isting ongoing studies on women's health, with 121,700 women participants in the Boston area.[11] There are no clear answers yet regarding HRT, but at the very least, individual considerations be-yond family history, such as dosage and the woman's own feel-ings and responses to treatment, have not yet been sufficiently addressed in this controversy. Furthermore, less threatening hormone-balancing techniques and new approaches to heart dis-ease and osteoporosis need to be fully explored.

The medical profession's approaches to women's mental health issues are also problematic. It is known, for example, that women are twice as likely to suffer from depression as men. (Approxi-mately one in four women and one in eight men will experience a major depression at least once in a lifetime.) A recent twelve-year study at Johns Hopkins indicated that women are ten times more likely to be affected by non-major depression related to emotional stress. Yet women's "raging hormones" or menstrual cycles can't al-ways be cited as cause; social factors are now understood often to be at the basis of such debilitating feelings. If hormones are over-emphasized, social issues are often ignored. However, cultural fac-tors, including poverty, unhappy marriages, infertility, and sexual and physical abuse, are more major factors than biology in account-ing for the difference in depression rates between men and women, according to a 1990 American Psychological Association research report. For example, at least 20 percent of all U.S. adult women have had a significant experience of sexual or physical abuse.

But sadly, the medical world has not handled women's mental and emotional responses to such events well. The most typical treatment has been to hand out prescription drugs. Valium and other tranquilizers were the drugs most frequently prescribed for women throughout the 1950s, '60s, and '70s, not curing anything but resulting in a kind of prescribed drug addiction for a large and unsuspecting group of patients. Many of these women are now facing the crisis of addiction and the detoxification process, and must now deal with the original problems against which they have been anesthetized for decades. Even today, women are still prescribed more drugs than men.[12]

## Identifying Female Illness

Underlying the above statistics is one essential fact: Our medical system tends to overdo invasive gynecological intervention (while sometimes neglecting symptoms in other parts of women's bodies, such as the heart). Even women's normal reproductive functioning is frequently viewed in the dim light of the disease model and treated as illness, generally with drugs. Many normal female conditions, particularly those associated with maturation processes, are thus considered ailments. Menopause, for example, has been called an "estrogen deficiency disorder" in all women, regardless of whether or not any disease is present. Male maturation symptoms, on the other hand, are not considered illnesses; baldness, for example, is simply baldness, although it is occasionally positively linked to virility.[13]

Apart from such inappropriate concerns, there *are* real medical problems associated with being a woman today. Women are experiencing more "female" illnesses than in the past: The incidence of PMS (premenstrual syndrome), dysmenorrhea (extreme menstrual pain), fibroids, ovarian cysts, ectopic pregnancies, infertility, and breast cancers is increasing at rates that cannot be accounted for by better diagnosis alone. These increasing rates are truly frightening, more so because we don't know why this is happening. There is as yet no medical explanation why one out of every 8.5 women today is subject to breast cancer; or why its incidence has doubled since 1960 and increased over 25 percent in the past ten years alone. What is equally frightening is that, as recently as 1989, out of the approximately $700 billion spent on health care in the United States, only $16 million was given to researchers by the National Institutes of Health to find out why.

Environmental causes, life-style conditions, and other factors seem to be taking their toll on women's health, but reliable answers to the "why" questions are hard to come by. Why has the number of American males increased faster than the number of females (even though there are still 7 million more women than men in the United States)? Why has the death rate declined slightly more for men than for women, a phenomenon that has not happened in a century, according to the U.S. Census Bureau?[14]

The most fundamental reason for the crisis situation in women's health today appears to be the narrowness of our medical model. Within this model, one issue stands out even more starkly than others: We are all subject to the misunderstanding that good health depends not so much on how we live our daily lives but on how well we respond to the structures and priorities of the current health-care system. Having regular checkups, mammograms, PAP smears, and so on. is somehow meant to assure us that we won't get sick if we are "good" about being tested regularly.

Many of us are diligent about breast self-examination. In fact, 90 percent of all breast tumors are discovered by women themselves.[15] But what we may not be told is that by the time a cancerous breast lump of less than one inch in diameter is detected, a tumor will have been growing for five years. Even mammograms are not as useful as we have been led to believe, for many cancerous tumors already have spread by the time they are detected on mammogram. Fortunately, mammogram detection can help reverse the disease in other cases and therefore continues to be of value. But it is *not* a completely reliable solution.

It's clear that early detection of cancer or of any other serious illness, although certainly better than late detection, is not really the answer we want. Such preventive testing measures, while helpful, are overrated and can lead to unnecessary guilt on the part of a woman patient for not having made an early enough discovery and undeserved blame of a physician for the same missed detection. What we need is a far earlier detection system, *before* the illness becomes severe enough to be identified as cancer. Because whether or not we take the tests, we are in fact getting sicker. And modern medical research can't really tell us why.

## Research in Women's Health

Despite the mushrooming need for health care for women, and although women spend proportionately more money on their health than men, comparatively little research has addressed women's health problems in particular. "Women have felt abandoned," reports Dr. Mathilde Krim, cofounder of the American Foundation for AIDS Research (AmFAR), in discussing the amount of AIDS research focused on women. Her statement applies equally well to all aspects of medical research in America. Reviews of research on women's health in *The New York Times* and *The Washington Post* indicate that the U.S. government has expended a far smaller amount researching major illnesses in women than in men.[16] Only 13 percent of the National Institutes of Health (NIH) budget was spent over the past decade to study health issues concerning over 50 percent of the population.

Women indeed have been abandoned on almost every research front, often entirely left out of clinical trials of new drugs because of concerns of interference from menstrual cycle fluctuations or possible pregnancy complications. As a result, much of the medical research on which doctors base their treatment has been conducted with men only. For example, a recent NIH study on aging, *Normal Human Aging,* has *no* data on women for the first twenty years of the study.

Fortunately, the tides are now turning, thanks to more professional and public attention on this lack of research on women's health issues. For example, in 1992, the National Institutes of Health, under the leadership of Dr. Bernadine Healy, undertook a ten-year, $500 million "Women's Health Initiative" to study several vital women's health issues, including the link between dietary fat and breast cancer, and hormone replacement therapy and its effects on heart disease, cancer, and osteoporosis. Women's exclusion from new drug trials is also starting to be addressed through a few new entities, such as the creation of a federal Office of Women's Health at NIH. In this area, some important concerns are being raised, not the least of which is safe treatment: Metabolic differences between the sexes have rarely been taken into account in drug research. According to a 1993 study reported in the *Journal of NIH Research,* "Drugs designed to relieve pain in men may not necessarily be effective in women."[17] Should women receive the same dosages of a new drug as men, if no women subjects have been tested? Does the new drug have the same effects on a woman? The necessity for such questions indicates a more pervasive lack, a lack of knowledge about women's health concerns within the medical establishment.

### Are Women's Health Concerns Taken Seriously?

In the complex psychosocial structure that has emerged to treat men's and women's medical problems with differing degrees of urgency, the current system seems to fail women more consistently. Apart from reproductive concerns, neither women's conditions nor their complaints are likely to be taken as seriously as those of their male counterparts. According to Gena Corea, in her powerful book, *The Invisible Epidemic,* the underreported and misdiagnosed cases of AIDS in women is indicative of a deeper problem: Women are generally if quietly marginalized within current medical practices. In this regard, there is a great deal of medical mythology that perpetuates the way things are supposed to but may not, in fact, be.

• *Point 1:* Women's subjective experiences of health awareness and self-diagnosis have not been given much credence. Women's symptoms even for common complaints such as headaches, back pain, dizziness, chest pain, and fatigue, although exactly the same as men's complaints, are addressed with less concern by male doctors.[18] Researchers have also identified troublesome communication problems between women and their male physicians.

• *Point 2:* Five hundred thousand women a year die from heart attacks and strokes in the United States, ten times the number that die from breast cancer, and these diseases are now the leading cause of death among women as well as men. After the age of sixty, women are more likely than men to die of heart disease or stroke. But studies suggest that doctors are not as quick to diagnose heart disease in women. Women tend to get heart attacks later in life, and this has diminished physicians' concerns that women suffer from heart disease.

Dr. William Castelli, director of the Framingham (Massachusetts) Heart Study, says, "Because of the myth that women don't get heart attacks, doctors may not take women's signs and symptoms seriously."[19] As a result, women are more ill if and when they do have heart surgery, and their recovery is less complete and less likely. Indeed, so "male" is heart disease that even the instruments used in the delicate procedures of heart surgery are currently designed for men's larger arteries.[20] We don't know whether women have been helped or hurt by this overall lack of intervention, for there is almost no research on aggressive treatment for women's cardiovascular diseases.

• *Point 3:* AIDS is among the top five causes of death for women ages fifteen to forty-four, and the group of women with AIDS includes a disproportionate number of poor and minority women. And although women are the fastest-growing population of AIDS patients in the world, representing approximately 50 percent of new cases, and often die sooner than men from distinctly different infections, meaningful research on women and AIDS took many years to get under way. The research is pointing out that women die sooner from AIDS because of inadequate treatment. According to a *Journal of NIH Research* report, "Some manifestations of HIV-1 infection are different in women from those in men. But such differences remain poorly understood, and AIDS patient advocates charge that the health-care system fails to address women's needs."[21] It is only recently that the conditions in which women in particular manifest the virus are being identified as AIDS-related.

### Specializing in Women's Health

To alleviate some of these concerns, there is growing support for a medical specialty in women's health beyond obstetrics and gynecology. Ideally, such a specialty would be "unspecialized" and include an integrative or holistic approach to all health issues. It would enable a woman to see one doctor regularly, not one doctor for the reproductive system only and others for everything else. It would address a woman's physical, mental, and emotional well-being and would require a physician trained at least in gynecology, psychiatry, nutrition, orthopedics, urology, and preventive medicine.

In contrast to emphasizing this specialty, some physicians feel that making medicine generally more responsive to women throughout the entire medical system ought to be the essential goal, rather than the creation of a new field. We believe that a women's health specialty, while helpful in providing a woman with one physician for most of her health concerns, would still support a piecemeal and fragmented treatment approach, albeit under one roof. Her menstrual problems would still require a separate treatment from her back pain; her depressed mood would still call for yet another treatment, as would her irritable bowel syndrome. Even within this specialty, we would still need a deeper approach to go beyond body parts or even "person" parts to understand and clarify why a woman has fallen ill in the first place.

We need a medical system that can help the doctor and patient to understand the genesis of any symptom in terms of all the possible mind-body-environment interactions. If this primary cause is not addressed, no full restoration of health or avoidance of further symptoms can occur. If we continue to do medicine in pieces, we will succeed in making one set of symptoms go away only to await the next and never truly deal with underlying health. What really needs to be addressed in health care for both women and men is how to activate nature's powerful healing system at the deeper levels of our functioning, where our body, mind, and emotions are united and balanced and reinforce one another, going deeper than our organs, tissues, biochemicals, or even our DNA. We believe that the purpose of a women's health specialty ought to be to provide medical knowledge, however its delivery is organized, that teaches women real prevention, self-care, and complete healing from a more profound level.

It is clear today that women not only want a deeper approach to medicine but indeed may have no other choice if we are going to get well and stay well. That approach would also make the best use of our own detection and healing abilities.

## A Woman's Ability to Detect Illness

Research has shown that women are the primary health-care purchasers and are more likely to respond to information to improve their personal health care. Women today are more likely to do the following:

- Report and become aware of illness earlier than men. A health study conducted in Detroit demonstrated that women tend to report more days of symptoms than men, perhaps indicating an earlier awareness of the onset of illness.[22]
- Seek more help for health care than men.[23]
- Request more communication in the medical process.
- Report many symptoms that men do not report. Both women and men have the ability to diagnose themselves, but research indicates that women are more likely to do so.

A woman may not be able to identify a condition by name, but she can generally identify its composite symptoms and give a physician a clear picture. As we've seen, however, most doctors today are trained to concentrate on finding a diagnosis. As a result, they too often treat the lab results, not the patient. If no surface signs appear and no doctor can verify an illness, we assume good health and are shocked if later something else happens, and a friend reports: "Can you believe it? Joan just died all of a sudden. And she was in perfect health!" Apparently not.

Early on, illness can actually begin to be noticed as the faintest subjective feeling that something is not quite right. Subjective health assessment therefore ought to be a very important part of diagnosis and treatment. Your subjective feelings actually can be more accurate than any "objective" medical assessment. This was demonstrated in a seven-year study of 3,500 older people who were asked to evaluate their own health. Not surprisingly, those subjects who rated their health as poor were three times as likely to die as those who perceived themselves to be in good health. What *was* surprising, however, was that subjects whose physicians assessed them to be in poor health but who rated *themselves* as healthy lived longer than their more pessimistic counterparts.[24]

As we saw earlier, most women have been culturally supported to develop a very real intuitive capacity, built into psychophysiological functioning, that results in heightened sensitivities to physical and emotional conditions. It's natural, then, that women would be aware of subtle levels of disease that, because they are not diagnosed as such, are not treated effectively before they worsen. Often women who seek out a doctor's help early on are told, "It's all in your head" and/or given pills that mask the vague symptoms, which may later manifest in more observable but also more serious ways. This is a common experience when doctors are oriented to look for specific diseases and have no tools to deal with less than normal health that is not yet full-blown illness. As Linda Hughy Holt, M.D., head of the obstetrics and gynecology department at a Chicago hospital, observed, "I think women get very frustrated looking for a doctor who is not going to brush them off because they can't explain the problem."

Essentially, if doctors can't identify your symptoms in terms of a disease, they can't treat them. If a diagnosis cannot be made, then no real illness is acknowledged. "You won't get much sympathy for a nameless problem like 'not feeling good' or 'under the weather,' especially if it happens too often," author Barbara Ehrenreich observed.[25] If a physician is unable to find any visible signs of health impairment, he or she may assume that a patient's physical discomfort is caused by an emotional or mental hypersensitivity and refer her to a psychiatrist or quickly assure her that nothing's wrong.

But something *is* wrong. Patients who arrive in a severe state of distress, although not yet ill on an observable physical level, may be dealing with an early stage of physical disease and/or with thought processes and anxieties that could easily create (further) physical deterioration. This is what the most recent research on mind-body interactions suggests.

Of course, expectations of what being healthy feels like differ for all of us and are constantly redefined throughout our lives. In some cases, our anxiety may be the result of how we have interpreted symptoms, of how we expect to feel at a given age or time of life. Some of us brush off fatigue as meaningless; others of us define it as a cause for concern. By including our own interpretation of a baseline of healthiness in our intuitive self-diagnosis, we can offer doctors and ourselves continuity in the assessment of our current health status.

> *Susan R., a forty-six-year-old corporate executive who was accustomed to feeling in control of her life, found herself deeply frustrated when trying to solve a medical dilemma without adequate support from the medical specialist she had been seeing. After many months she sought the help of another physician who, she thought, might be more open to her own self-knowledge, her concerns about a potential thyroid problem.*
>
> *She said, "I know my endocrinologist says that the lab test indicates that my condition is not severe enough to treat, but I'm convinced I'm not feeling myself. He just doesn't seem to believe me when I describe how I'm feeling. I know I'm not as clear-thinking. I've been dragging myself out of bed even after nine hours' sleep; I've gained ten pounds in the last three months without changing anything in what I eat or how I exercise. Worst of all, my memory is not good and, as a corporate official, I just can't afford that."*
>
> *On repeat testing, it was found that indeed the early indications of hypothyroidism had progressed, and by now, Susan was clinically and verifiably hypothyroid. But she had known months before that something wasn't right.*

Our current medical model is not set up to deal with subjective diagnoses that empower the patient and not the lab. If no specific disease is identified, there are generally no treatments offered beyond some general words of advice to avoid stress or take a quickly prescribed tranquilizer. (Fortunately this latter practice is less prevalent now than a few years ago.) Whether dealing with subtle "functional" symptoms or full-blown disease, the modern medical approach is limited to treating disease rather than restoring balance to the bodymind from a deeper level. We treat tension headaches with pain relievers, heartburn with antacids, many chronic diseases with steroids, and dysmenorrhea with birth control pills. This is not restoring health; it's managing disease. And in many cases, we actually reduce the opportunity for healing to take place.

## The Patient-Doctor Healing Relationship

If subjective feelings of illness were to be taken seriously, respect for patient input would begin in the doctor's office and be considered not just anecdotal but vital. This could lead to a less static, healthier doctor-patient relationship. Generally speaking, the patient and the doctor form a partnership to attend to a health problem. If this relationship is not loving but is merely a formal arrangement, very little in the way of healing has a chance to occur.

To "doctor" originally meant "to teach" or "to mend," but now it has come to mean "to falsify" or "to adulterate." We can imagine that, somewhere along the line, "doctoring" moved from a healing model to a repair model (something from the outside required for mending) to a model of failure and distrust. As the outer healer moved away from the inner healer, the entire health delivery process became distorted—so much so, that patients now feel they must have legal rights to protect themselves from their doctors and doctors likewise from their patients.

Yet we know that a large percentage of healing occurs as the result of the nurturing responses generated in a patient-physician transaction: The relationship with a caring physician can produce effects as powerful as any prescription, but the mutuality has to be there. "When the patient and the physician agree on the nature of the problem," observed Adolph Meyer, the first professor of psychiatry at Johns Hopkins University, "the patient gets better."[26]

In Ayur-Veda there is a unity between the doctor, the patient, and the process of healing within the patient, for all three are understood to play an important and dynamic role in health care. This tends to produce a feeling of mutual love and respect between doctor and patient, not antagonism, fear, or any of the unhelpful and unnecessary blocks to healing. Having recognized that the bodymind itself has all the knowledge it needs to re-create itself within itself, and that the deepest laws of nature lively in every cell are the true coordinators of the healing process, the Maharishi Ayur-Veda doctor quietly guides the patient to the underlying reality of the healing field within. Once the mechanics of this process of self-knowledge are set in motion through the proper conscious-ness-awakening techniques of Maharishi Ayur-Veda, the healing process becomes fully effective and fully effortless.

## Wanted: A More Nurturing and Powerful Approach to Our Health

A very positive trend is emerging in women's health today: the awareness of a collective desire for better care, the desire for a system supporting the understanding of subjective symptoms that cannot be diagnosed or treated under the prevailing organization of treatment. Such a care system would utilize a patient's intuitive abilities, respect her awareness of her own illnesses, treat her as an equal in both the diagnostic and healing processes, and enable her to be medically supported and financially insured to participate in fully preventive programs to restore the basis for good health.

A physician practicing within such a system would give real consideration to the patient's self-assessment. For example, the physician would respect fear as a symptom. One woman said in a recent interview, "When you feel as desperately ill as I did, and doctors tell you that you're in excellent health, then you start to get frightened that no one can help you, that you'll be this way for-ever."

A disease does not just happen. Patients as well as doctors must be able to understand the "whys." Behind the inflammation of multiple sclerosis, arthritis, or thyroiditis, beyond the vasodilation of migraines or the prostaglandins of menstrual cramping is a more fundamental, causal level of functioning. Before a breast cell actually becomes cancerous, before a gallstone forms, or before a clinical depression becomes obvious, some everyday functions of the mind and body have become unbalanced and are no longer fully self-repairing. This level of biological functioning must be understood and accessed to effect true healing.

Women and men alike require medicine that heals at that place deep inside where a thought or an emotion becomes a neurotransmitter, where consciousness is most awake and precise: the junction point where the mind, heart, and body meet and interconnect and where the body begins to heal itself.

Our mind, body, and emotions, along with our society and our environment, are all interconnected, as the growing research in the field of PNI and our own experiences indicate. Our ideal medical system would reflect this, so that all aspects of health would be addressed within a unitary framework, totally reorganizing the current procedures for medical care which send the mind to one doctor, the arm to another, and the heart to a third. Only a system of unified medicine that goes beyond the molecules is going to help us get well and stay well.

Maharishi Ayur-Veda approaches health and healing on a deeply integrative level, guiding us to seek and find the answer to the most essential question: How to quietly re-enliven nature's already existing program within ourselves.

## Reawakening Your Body's Intelligence Through Maharishi Ayur-Veda

Ayur-Veda provides you with diagnosis and treatment dealing with both expressed and unexpressed conditions of illness and pre-illness on the subtlest levels of your psychophysiological functioning. As a woman, you are no doubt aware that your body, mind, and emotions are intimately connected to nature through certain biological cycles. Because these biological rhythms govern and balance all life, when your bodymind is reminded of these biological roots, an immediate physiological awakening occurs. Using specific Ayur-Vedic routines, you are able to tap effortlessly into the most basic level of healing so that your body, as well as your mind and heart, automatically supplies what is needed to maintain good health. As a result, you can quickly return to your "real self" and to the subsequent experience of spontaneous good health on every level of your life.

Maharishi Ayur-Veda takes medical care well beyond freedom from physical disease to a far deeper understanding than the "if it hurts, take it out" perspective. It offers you a way to reeducate yourself about what it means to be healthy; it enables you to shift your internal paradigm from a disease- to a health-based view. It reminds you that you can experience a health-producing state of consciousness that admits less entropy, wear and tear, fatigue, and stress; a state in which you don't need to replenish your energy be-cause you have no experience of losing it.

Maharishi Ayur-Veda offers earlier interventions in the health-care process, as well as treatment programs to eliminate any imbal-ance you may be experiencing when symptoms have become more obvious. Because it has methods of dealing with subtler symptoms than conventional medicine can, it does not often require high technology machinery to confirm your initial awareness of illness. Furthermore, Ayur-Vedic treatments and prescriptions do not prod-uce the kind of harmful side effects associated with many modern medical treatments. Yet if and when powerful chemicals or aggres-sive surgery are required, Ayur-Veda can be relied on to provide ways to minimize side effects and toxicity and to restore the body's self-healing capabilities quickly and efficiently.

Maharishi Ayur-Veda teaches you techniques and principles of self-repair, balance, and orderliness as means to experiencing not merely lack of disease but a joyous, blissful state of life. It also pro-vides a means to experience the integration of your mental, emo-tional, spiritual, and social lives, as well as your physical life, and that there is no distinction. In this way, the Ayur-Vedic medical model ultimately resolves the most pressing and most unfortunate lack in modern medicine: the loss of our connectedness to the reconstitutional powers of nature.

"If you don't know where you're going," said the Caterpillar to Al-ice, in Wonderland, "then it doesn't matter how you get there." Be-fore we determine "what to do" in Ayur-Vedic terms, it's essential to know where we are going. What do we mean by deeper levels of health? Why do we want to connect to nature within? How does consciousness marry our thoughts to our nerve cells? Let's take a brief look at the underlying territory—what we call the "physics of physical health"—before we explore how to get there.

## The Physics of Physical Health:
## From Classical to Quantum Medicine

*Mind and matter are essentially the same. The field experienced subjectively is the mind, objectively it is the world of material objects.*

Yoga Vasistha

You may wonder why you need to think about physics in order to think about healing. The answer is that thinking about physics is the most accurate way to think about your physical self. To imagine getting well, you really need to understand what it means to be completely healthy so you can put your attention on creating that condition. To comprehend the depth at which healing actually occurs in your body and mind, you need to get deeply physical, and that means discovering the innermost level of the physical universe, the essential field of healing inside you. Let's look at healing from this perspective.

As your thoughts are structuring health in the deeper regions of your physiology—in the DNA, hormones and neurotransmitters, and immunomodulators—the bodymind is structuring it from even deeper patterns of intelligence. United at the deepest levels of your being, the bodymind creates the basic patterns of psychophysiology that are the current blueprint of who you are. This "who-you-are-ness" is contained in every single cell of your physiology, in the same way that a tiny piece of a hologram contains the entire hologram.

PNI research has demonstrated that our thoughts and emotions change our body more swiftly and effectively than any external medicine, suggesting that *healing is a single organized process of thoughts, feelings, and cells working together,* all aspects of health occurring within the body and mind simultaneously. Before a spontaneous remission happens, usually a deep shift in mental and emotional outlook has taken place that restructures the underlying patterns of biochemical intelligence, producing change at the cellular and molecular levels.

While many physicians and researchers today have begun to acknowledge the interdependence of mind and body, modern medical practice in general has not fully embraced this connection. It continues to address the objective, measurable, "body" aspect of medicine, generally neglecting the interconnectedness of the physical with its subjective aspects. Thus, any illness without specific observable pathology remains untreatable by drugs or surgery. Even psychiatry, the medical field most responsive to the physical bases of mental illnesses and the mental bases of physical illnesses, lacks an appreciation of how these two are united at a deeper level of biological intelligence within the bodymind.

It seems clear that much of the current practice of so-called modern medicine continues to rely on eighteenth- and nineteenth-century medical "cause and effect" theories, the Newtonian model of classical physics, and the dualism of the French philosopher René Descartes. As a result, many illnesses go untreated because the classical system of medicine is unable to explore the underlying causes of illnesses that manifest on a deeper level than the cells and the tissues. Consequently, we continue to lack a complete medical practice that can diagnose and treat this underlying level of physiology, even though the new medicine, like the new physics, is there waiting for us to take advantage of its powerfully unifying technologies for healing.

With varying degrees of success, the field of holistic medicine has attempted to eradicate this lack through a number of programs, including a variety of herbal treatments, touch therapies, diets, and exercises to address mind and body conditions together. But however effective it has been, most holistic medicine has also approached healing in a piecemeal manner. Few holistic health modalities have offered a deeper theoretical framework for understanding how the healing processes work in a total system beyond the specifics of the cells and tissues. Moreover, although most holistic practices acknowledge and utilize various aspects of the mind-body connection, the majority have not moved beyond a universal symptom approach similar to the disease model's and do not recognize *individual constitutional differences* in their patients any more than modern medicine does.

In some ways, much of holistic medicine as practiced in our society is even less individualized than modern medicine; for example, although they don't cause the potentially harmful side effects of some modern medicine, not all herbs are good for all people. Without a complete holistic system, instead of running from one conventional doctor to another, we may end up running from one alternative practitioner to another, in order to address all our symptoms, again attending to the leaves and perhaps the branches, but not really to the roots of the tree.

## The Quantum Medicine of Ayur-Veda

The Ayur-Vedic system of medicine is surprisingly modern in that it approaches health from the vantage point of quantum physics and unified field theory. It essentially serves as a bridge between quantum physics and medicine. It further provides an internally consistent and theoretically complete framework from which to diagnose and treat. Like quantum physics, which does not negate but encompasses classical physics, it does not negate modern medicine but is able to complement, include, and expand it.

The ancient theory and practice of Ayur-Veda precisely describes the deeper functioning of our bodymind in terms astoundingly similar to those used by today's quantum physicists to describe the deeper levels of the physical world. We can think of the ancient Ayur-Vedic sages as the first "quantum doctors," practitioners of deep meditation and self-awareness who literally came to know the unity of the subatomic world, who silently cognized how nature functions and heals on the deepest levels of life. Their descriptions of human physiology as manifestations of transformative wave functions go far beyond the classical biochemical descriptions of cells and tissues, probing into the energy fields containing all the particles that interconnect our bodily, mental, and emotional functions. According to Maharishi Ayur-Veda, every cell in our body has a changing aspect but is also inseparably connected to the underlying quantum field. It thus has two modes of intelligence: a silent, eternal, unchanging value and an infinitely dynamic, creative value. Both these values are simultaneously upheld by nature's own administration. When the unified field of consciousness is accessed at this deepest level of life, the Veda (knowledge) is awakened in our physiology and we can enliven any of the laws of nature required to promote the most life-supporting influences and bring about a state of total healthiness.

On the basis of this deep understanding of life, Maharishi Ayur-Veda offers a healing program for the bodymind, a "quantum field approach" bringing the fundamental missing element to modern medical practice.

## The Quantum Continuum:
## The Health Underlying Any Sickness

When you understand the deep connection between the unified field of consciousness and your body, health and sickness take on a different character and move out of the realm of good vs. bad or lucky vs. unlucky. In the quantum world of perfect orderliness, these events are not the opposites they appear to be in the classical physical world; rather they are life events created out of a single immortal field, a single fabric of wholeness. Physician Larry Dossey has said, "All the carvings of life into bit-pieces of health and illness create an illusion that destroys the seamless existence of life."

From the vantage point of the unified field, where our own little bit of DNA is comfortably cradled in the bosom of "big DNA," the universal intelligence simultaneously taking care of everything in creation, we recognize that the universe is not really outside us. The unified field is within us, locatable in our own being. Indeed, we are nothing other than the unified field. And this gives us a grand way to understand the widely reported observation that the decisions, actions, and attitudes we maintain when we are sick are as important as the kind of diseases we have and the treatments we undergo in determining the outcome. The way in which medicine is received into our body, with what mental and emotional attitudes, becomes at least as significant as the medicine itself.

Research indicates that we have far more control over the effects of medicine than we may realize. If you take a pill and feel, "This pill is incredibly powerful and will really help me," it can create a very different physical result than if you ingest a pill with the attitude, "This probably won't do me much good." This is the placebo effect, the effect of your attitude of mind toward a "pill" that has no "objective" medicine in it. If a physician, trying to be "realistic," tells a patient that he or she has only three months to live, this too creates a physical effect, presumably a negative one. These events happen because *nothing is more powerful than the medicine that consciousness itself makes.*

From a modern medical point of view, a classically informed patient has a disease that is real, concrete—"the sad truth." The disease is more real than her thinking about it. From the quantum–Ayur-Vedic view, the ways in which we think about our health and illness are part of a larger picture that goes beyond the bodymind.

In quantum terms, you can maintain an overall condition of good health even as you deal with a specific illness. There are many dramatic examples of people who seem to be on the edge of death, whose bodies are wasting away, and yet who are completely serene, at peace, flowing in love. We often feel deep peace in their presence; expecting to cheer them up, we may find we feel cheered up. They do not appear mentally or emotionally overshadowed by physical illness but seem to be maintaining a deeper state of overall good health, the kind that produces joy.

We may have spent time with a friend who is ill, perhaps someone who has been treated with radiation for cancer; she is frail, she has lost her hair, but perhaps not her humor or her purposefulness. Her sense of *herself* remains intact despite what she is going through because she can step back and observe the bigger picture. She is accessing her quantum physiology, which underlies the disease, an inner field of no sickness / no health. She is experiencing that she is not her cancer; she's experiencing the innermost core of her being. This contact is waking up all the resources of her bodymind.

Sometimes such individuals have in a sense been able to "redesign" themselves from the level of the unified field, from consciousness, to reenliven their emotions, mental experiences, and even the most physical aspects of their bodies. This quantum restructuring is a possible underlying explanation for spontaneous remission. It is different from "positive" thinking or in any way keeping up a mood. It draws all the processes of our body, mind, and heart into a synchronous physiological purpose to support us in our desire to be of one piece, even when we are very ill and, in a sense, fragmented. The experience that many people report of being very healthy and very sick at the same time could be the result of being in contact with the unified field. This experience offers evidence that a quantum, "eternal" physiology can be maintained along with the classical phenomenon of bodily decay. This phenomenon is also called quantum healing. Let's look more closely at the kind of freedom it brings.

## Quantum Healing from the "Superposition"

Picture yourself looking up at the clouds and noticing a particular formation that looks like a small herd of elephants. Look again and you might notice an ornate painting of eighteenth-century cherubs. Depending on how you see it, your perception of the clouds can change instantly from one picture to the other. Sometimes right before the perceptual shift occurs, you can see both views. You see the "potential" of each formation right before you mentally choose one image.

In a similar way quantum physics represents the world as multiple possibilities. Until a choice is made, the world is a curious overlapping of all its alternatives, a phenomenon known to physicists as a "superposition." From the superposition, even seemingly opposing things can occur together simultaneously because they are potential and not concrete. If you can operate from the superposition in your own awareness, you can choose which reality you want. This freedom is yours in the quantum world because here, as physicist John Wheeler describes it, you are really in a "participatory" universe where nothing is independent of anything else. Whereas in the classical physical world, particles and waves are separate and distinct from one another, in the quantum world, the same things, say, light photons, can be observed to be either particles *or* waves, depending on how you wish to interact with them. It is your choice whether they are to become wavelike or particlelike.

These quantum processes also operate in higher levels of human physiological functioning and give you the ability to choose to experience two or more seemingly opposite things at the same time, such as being sick and being well simultaneously. In so doing, you incorporate more wholeness into your bodymind and function on a deeper, more unified level of awareness. When you start experiencing life from a deeper level of wholeness, you are in a superposition to "superheal."

Psychologist Albert Rothenberg calls the ability to hold two opposing concepts in mind simultaneously "Janusian thinking," from the god Janus, who simultaneously looks into the future and the past. Reentering the medical world with this quantum perspective, life is as much waves, thoughts, and emotions (mind) as it is particles, cells, and tissues (body). It is both, but neither can be left out. Modern medicine in practice leaves out consciousness and most of our subjective world. Focusing only on the particle choice, it leaves out the wave choice. It tends to treat the "particular" physiology but not the underlying wave patterns of intelligence. Ayur-Veda, however, addresses mind, body, and feeling together and sees all three as an expression of the same underlying reality.

Just as quantum physics incorporates classical physics and resolves many of its problems, Ayur-Veda incorporates the bodily approach to health, the hallmark of modern medicine, and resolves many of its concerns. While modern medicine treats and removes specific diseases on the structural, molecular, and biochemical levels, Ayur-Veda opens the deeper channels for the continuous flow of bodymind health primarily through unified field–level prevention techniques. Yet Ayur-Veda by no means negates drugs or surgery. Indeed, Ayur-Vedic physicians were the first doctors to bring surgery to the world. They recognized that gross structural and biochemical levels of repair are sometimes needed, for which surgery and drugs are perfectly suited. Broken legs and damaged retinas require repair at the structural level. But there are deeper levels of needed repair that neither drugs nor surgery can touch.

If we want to change the way our bodies physically behave and strengthen our overall health through a process of "health determination," we don't have to do anything dramatic; we just have to give nature a chance to move freely within us.

## Beyond Particular Medicine: Accessing the Healing Field

It is very possible that the discovery of the unified field will render other technologies of medicine less necessary. To promote healing, we can now look to the field (consciousness) as inevitably as we look to the particle (body), to the entire system deep within and beyond the body, as well as to the specific symptoms.

The first step is to change our thinking about medicine. We know we influence the functioning of our bodies through our thought processes, our intelligence, our emotions, our behavior, and our desires. But obviously these are not the only influences on our health. *Everything* has its influence and therefore everything has the potential to be medicine: the air we breathe, the friends we spend time with, the TV shows we watch, not to mention what we eat or drink. A certain movie may make our hearts race wildly in fear or make us feel depressed, depending on our individual bodymind. Even knowing this will happen, we feel obliged and even interested in taking it in. (Saying "I'm going to take in a movie" has real meaning for our physiology.) To the degree that we don't discriminate to avoid negative, stressful influences and rather expose ourselves to them, we get sick, and we don't really know why.

Medicine, whether good or bad for us, comes in all sorts of packages. Those kinds of "medicine" found to help the body stay healthy include the beauty of nature, the reciprocal attention of loving friends and family, extended social support, and hope. The healthier we are, the more we can take in the experiences of "good" medicine—medicine in accordance with and supported by natural law.

The research is bearing this out. For example, when a group of university students were shown a movie about Mother Teresa, their immune functioning, as measured by salivary immunoglobin A concentrations, increased and remained elevated an hour later. Even those students who did not particularly like Mother Teresa were still immunologically affected in a positive way by watching the film. The principal researcher, Harvard psychologist David McClelland, concluded that the influence of Mother Teresa's loving behavior was apparently "taken in" by the "disapproving" students on a deeper level of psychophysiology than their objections.[27]

When you add the quantum element of subjectivity, you add the most important ingredient of health, the "heart" of medicine, the pure climate in which healing can best take place. The techniques of Ayur-Veda are basically ways to enable you to "take in the good" as fully as possible and promote nature's orderly intelligence within as directly as possible. You could be ingesting a starry night sky, a piece of music, or a healing herb. But how you digest it, whether partially or fully, in fear or in love, cynically or openly, makes the difference to your healthiness.

Once you experience the innermost level of health, you can absorb fully the beneficial and coherent qualities in nature and turn from the destructive ones. You can learn how to really evaluate your own health, to be aware of how you're really feeling, not just in terms of aches and pains, but in terms of your thinking-feeling-being self. These are the intrapersonal lab tests of health, as well as the techniques for healing. Essentially, you can look for the bliss in any moment of experience as a sign of health. And you learn to recognize that you are practicing a significant form of self-healing when you feel a wave of happiness or feel an upsurge of tenderness or compassion for a friend.

By reconnecting to the fundamental tendency of nature to restore balance and health, *you reawaken the intelligence of nature within you to eliminate disease.* Once this connection is reestablished, all aspects of your life wake up, and good health takes on a far more comprehensive meaning. You realize that health extends far beyond physical well-being; it also includes happiness, self-esteem, an expansive state of self-development, the growth to personal greatness, and a profound desire for the health and happiness of others.

## The Self-Healing Process: Being Here

There is really only one kind of healing: self-healing. And nature has given each of us a wonderful setup for rapid and efficient self-healing. An "out with the old, in with the new" principle prevails, through which your cells and tissues are re-created daily. Designer-inventor Buckminster Fuller likened this process of regeneration to a cruise ship where new passengers come aboard and other passengers get off while the ship continues to sail. Just as you are not only particle but wave, your body is not only content but process. Your cells are not just *structure*—not just pieces of the cohesiveness of organs and bones. They are also agents of *renewal*, enabling your bodymind to regenerate consistently and purposefully. Nearly every atom in your body is replaced annually and therefore every piece of your brain, every ounce of your heart muscle and every tissue of your liver is renewed from within itself. All this change is governed by the orderly maneuvers of specific laws of nature conducting the flow of life within you.

What doesn't change in your body is the same thing that doesn't change in any aspect of the physical world: the patterns of intelligence underlying and governing these changes. So the ability to make a new, healthier body, the essential requirement for long life in the direction of immortality, is not so farfetched as it may first appear. By recalling the deepest memory of who you really are, you realize you are not only human, you are *being,* a living process of nature. You are not simply an object created *from* nature, you *are* nature at each moment.

Maharishi Ayur-Veda provides a model for diagnosis, treatment, and prevention that mirrors the whole of biological life. It teaches subtle medical techniques for levels of the bodymind that classical medicine does not reach. It offers a variety of approaches to health, including individualized bodymind eating regimes, exercises, and environmental or seasonal regimes, to help your individual physiology get in touch with its own nature and thereby stay in balance. You can thus enter your bodymind through any door; the inner sanctum of your own self-healing resources awaits you.

With the help of a few simple principles, you can learn to let nature flow through your psychophysiology and allow the organizing power of the unified field to impart a sense of "being" into every action, a sense of healthiness into every thought, gesture, and emotion, a sense of wholeness into every activity of your life.

The following chapter offers you specific information about your Ayur-Vedic constitutional "bodymind" type, how to identify it and use it wisely and well. You will learn how the unified field flows into your particular bodymind and how you can maintain awareness of its presence. You will also find out how you can use this information to give you a stable platform of real prevention through early awareness of imbalances, so you can attend to your own physiology and begin to make it invincible.

# Chapter 3

KNOWLEDGE

## Identifying Your Ayur-Vedic Constitutional Type: Women of Dynamism, Determination, and Substance

*Health results from the natural, balanced state of the doshas. Therefore, the wise try to keep them in their balanced state.*

Charaka Samhita

Why does one person get sick and another remain healthy? If we could find out what makes a person more robust and better able to resist invaders, we could prohibit disease from the inside and concern ourselves less with exposure from the outside. But modern medicine has focused attention mainly on the invader—the bacteria, virus, or toxin assumed to cause the disease. The "resistance of the host" approach suggests another possibility: There is something in the immune systems of healthy people that helps them to fight disease more effectively than those who are less resistant.

When the Common Cold Research Center in Salisbury, England, recently closed, after nearly fifty years of trying and failing to find a vaccine or antiviral compound to conquer the common cold, the researchers' main discovery remained as much a mystery as curing the cold. They had found that approximately one-third of the volunteers exposed to a virus that made the other two-thirds sneeze, cough, and feel miserable never showed any signs of a cold. But they never found out why.

No one seems to be able to predict who will become ill merely from an analysis of bad circumstances or habits. A century ago the eminent physician Sir William Osler observed, "It is much more important to know what sort of patient has the disease than what sort of disease the patient has."[1]

A focus on the person rather than on the illness has always been the main approach of Ayur-Vedic medicine, precisely discerning the individual characteristics of each patient, putting the "who" before the "why."

## Personal Health as Universal Balance

Ayur-Veda suggests that balance governs every function in the body and that all disease results from the disruption of this overall homeostasis, or overall balance. Where Western medicine focuses on destroying the invader, Ayur-Veda focuses on structuring invincible defenses through inner balance, as organized and governed by DNA. If life is filled with orderly intelligence, then DNA is like a microchip of pure biological intelligence inscribed in a chemical cipher called the "genetic code"—the dynamic blueprint from which your body is built. When your body is maintaining its homeostasis, every function is referring back to the self-correcting guidance of its DNA. Like a brilliant, self-knowing computer, DNA repairs itself if the code it contains gets damaged, using highly sophisticated mechanisms to detect errors that may creep into the code and correcting them before they cause further problems. Many geneticists say that the breakdown of DNA's precise self-repair mechanisms is what leads to the degeneration we call aging and to the cellular malfunctioning of diseases such as cancer. Ayur-Vedic interventions aim to enable DNA to express itself without impediment, without the errors that could lead to degeneration and malfunctioning. By approaching medicine from a level of life deeper than DNA, Ayur-Veda can help organize the incredibly complex task of error-free repair, reducing the millions of operations in your bodymind to a few basic metabolic principles that, when in balance, support healthiness from the "ground state" up.

### Creating Your Bodymind:
### Inside the Pre-DNA World

The unified field gives rise to all the structures of nature that we call the material world. But in between the unified field and the material world lies what neurophysiologist Candace Pert describes as "the non-material substrate which guides the flow of information." This is the pre-DNA world.

We know that every bit of material—every fingerprint, every robin's egg—has its own integrity and its own individualized patterns. The process of making such specialized matter out of the unified field requires certain kinds of transformations that are known in physics as "wave transformations." These emerging energy fields or patterns are the pre-DNA impulses, the subtle governing laws that give rise to your most essential individuality, structuring the basis for how you think and feel, how you look, how you grow, and how you stay alive.

In Ayur-Vedic terms, these patterns are called "modes of intelligence" or *doshas* (doe-shuhs). Doshas are the expressions of nature that occur precisely at the junction point between consciousness and matter. As Dr. Pert proposes, if we are to understand how to be truly healthy, "We need to start thinking about how consciousness can be projected into various parts of the body."

Maharishi Ayur-Veda offers an elegant description of how to do exactly this. It allows you to understand how this nonmaterial substrate flows into the physical material of your body and into your feeling and thought processes. It provides knowledge of how a few essential elements and principles construct the entire creation and give rise to the differences in individual bodymind constitutions. And, most significant, it enables you to experience pure consciousness itself.

## How the Five Elements of Nature Become "Our Bodies, Our Cells"

The five Ayur-Vedic *mahabhutas* (muh-hah-bhoo-tuhs) or elements from which we are created are known to us as earth, water, fire, air, and space. But these five mahabhutas provide more than the material aspects of life, more than the earth in our gardens and the breeze in the trees, more than the 50 percent water of which women's adult bodies consist. These elements also contain the deeper laws of nature which created them. In their intelligent but nonmaterial form they are best envisioned as substance (earth), liquidity (water), transformation (fire), mobility (air), and what is called in Vedic terms *akasha* (uh-kah-shuh), or space. We can envision akasha as that which surrounds matter, similar to what sculptors and architects call "negative space": the setting for the sculpture or the building, even if unnoticed, or, as the poet Edna St. Vincent Millay described it, "the fifth essence."

From these five mahabhutas arise the doshas, the three fundamental psychophysiological principles that manifest in all of nature and result in your individual bodymind. These are not unfamiliar to Western scientists. In fact, according to physicist John Hagelin, quantum physicists have identified five fundamental quantum-mechanical "spin types" of elemental particles, which recombine to form three "superfields" which can be equated with the five mahabhutas giving rise to the three doshas.[2]

Essentially, air and space give rise to *Vata* (vah-tuh) dosha, which is responsible for movement; in nature, Vata is best represented by wind. Fire and water give rise to *Pitta* (pih-tuh) dosha, which is responsible for metabolism, represented in the natural world by the sun. Earth and water give rise to *Kapha* (kuh-fuh) dosha, which is responsible for structure, represented in nature both as earth and as the ocean tides in relation to the moon.

Doshas are present in all aspects of life; they are expressed in the intelligence that is responsible for our digestion, for example, and in all the other processes and structures of our bodies; they are also the guiding principles of inner organization that enable us to digest food at the same time as we are running a marathon race. So when we consider the doshas, we are not simply looking at the bricks and mortar of the body, or even at the DNA blueprint. We are looking at the *collective inner thinking* of every worker at the construction site, at the intelligence guiding the development of every cell, the "inner blueprint" of the blueprint.

Like gravity and other principles of nature that we experience but can't "see," the doshas are powerful underlying forces determining our health, our appearance, even our personalities. We can regard the doshas both as philosophical ground rules for our bodymind and as practical, built-in physiological computer programs. Often, however, the doshas get out of balance and do not function optimally, and in time these dosha imbalances can cause us to experience ill health. Ayur-Veda identifies what we call illnesses as the result of imbalances in the doshas.

Our individual dosha programs align us with the various expressions of the elements in all aspects of creation. In this way, some of us might represent the element of fire more fully in our physiology and embody qualities more like the sun, heat, energy, and intensity. Others might express the element of air more completely and remind our friends and families of qualities of wind—breeziness, quickness, and changeability. Or some of us may present great solidity and represent in our personality qualities of the adobe—the strength, stability, and serenity of water and earth together. And depending on which doshas are most lively in each, we can pick out, among our family and friends, those with a predominantly fire nature, an air nature, or an earth nature.

## The Doshas and Constitutional Types

The Ayur-Vedic health system identifies the specific physical and psychological differences you see in individuals in terms of the predominance of one or more doshas. These make up your *constitutional* type. Physical appearance (whether you are thin, solid, dark, or pale), mental characteristics (whether you are quick-witted, thoughtful, or have a good memory), emotional characteristics (high-strung, temperamental, calm, Type A, or Type B), and social characteristics (talkative, loyal, or generous) can be identified within the dosha framework. In addition, your preferences for various foods, movies, friends, and types of weather, housing, and even vacation spots can all be understood in terms of which dosha(s) are predominant in your constitution.

Given the same life event, say, taking an exam, each of us will respond with differing physiological reactions to this potentially emotionally stressful event. In one recent study, some students taking an exam experienced a quickening heartbeat, while others taking the same exam perspired. This result is explained by the doshas: The former were most likely Vata types and the latter Pitta types; the Kapha types may not have become noticeably anxious at all.

As you will see later in greater detail, your constitutional type will also *predispose you to certain types of illnesses.* It's necessary to remember, however, that although one dosha may predominate, we each have three doshas and all three are active at every moment. So in a larger sense, identifying with one or the other dosha is limiting, particularly if we are healthy. But if we are ill or want to prevent illness, knowledge of the specific doshas and how they are balanced within our bodymind becomes very useful.

## The Functions of the Three Doshas

In medical terms, the doshas are the basic metabolic principles governing your entire psychophysiological structure and processes. Each dosha acts independently and cooperatively with the others. The Vata principle conducts movement and guides the flow of information and matter, creating the basis for orderliness within every part of you. It organizes nervous system activity and moves nourishment around and in and out of cells and throughout the entire bodymind. Vata is thus responsible for chewing, swallowing, and peristalsis, the movement of food from your mouth to your stomach and through the digestive tract. It is also associated with your mind, emotions, respiratory tract, circulation, and organs of elimination, as well as your bones and sexual organs. These are the sites where symptoms most often occur if things get out of balance or become overstimulated and out of control owing to excess Vata (i.e., excess quickness, air, lightness). Vata imbalance is thus associated with disorders related to overactivity of the nervous system, including emotional fear and a rapid heartbeat; an overabundance of air or dryness, whether in the joints or in the bowels; and mental "spaciness."

The Kapha principle commands the building of your structural body—your tissues, bones, strength, and lubrication, supporting cohesiveness and strength on every level. Kapha puts you on firm ground, giving you "a leg to stand on," quite literally. It is specifically associated with mucus and fluid production; it shows up most actively in your stomach, lungs, lymph system, mouth, and joints. When out of balance, it affects your body's ability to deal with excess fluids. Because of this, Kapha is responsible for water retention, heaviness, lethargy, and any kind of congestion.

The Pitta principle can be likened to a go-between for Vata and Kapha. It conducts the transformations of energy and heat production; it metabolizes food into activity; it keeps you "hot" on the trail, one-pointed, whether in focused thought or in unwavering pursuit of a particular relationship or career goal. Pitta is specifically associated with your digestion, the digestive enzymes that convert food into energy, and with your hormonal system, heart, blood, liver, intestines, spleen, eyes, and skin. It is the body's "cooking system," and any kind of inflammation caused by excessive "heat," such as skin eruptions, peptic ulcers, emotional irritability, or a flaring temper is associated with an overly active (or imbalanced) Pitta dosha.

### The Ayur-Vedic Bodymind Identification System

Everyone has all three doshas in different combinations—active to varying degrees at all times. But each of us has a relative predominance of one or two doshas or, in rarer instances, an equal balance among all three. Ayur-Veda delineates seven different constitutional or psychophysiological bodymind types into which you would fit: These are Vata, Pitta, Kapha, Vata-Pitta (or Pitta-Vata), Pitta-Kapha (or Kapha-Pitta), Vata-Kapha (or Kapha-Vata), and Vata-Pitta-Kapha.

Our constitutional bodymind type indicates what our individual nature is intended to be. This basic constitutionality is also known as one's *prakriti* (pruh-krih-tee), which is observable at birth. Each of us is thus born with a different activity level for each of the doshas, identified as our own particular psychophysiological makeup and resulting in differing patterns of sleep, eating, digestion, personality, interactions with others, sensitivity to noise and other stimulation, and so forth.

Most parents of more than one child will have noticed that one baby can appear quite differently constituted from another. The Ayur-Vedic descriptions of prakriti offer a complete picture of why this is so from a physical as well as a psychological perspective. Vata-dominant babies startle easily, have irregular bowel movements, and are extra sensitive to wet diapers, noise, or a cool draft. They laugh and cry more readily, are more interactive with others, and tend to wake up easily and sleep less than the other two types.

Kapha-dominant babies tend to be heavy, to have big bones, to put on weight easily, to be more reserved, to have regular bowels, not to be particularly sensitive, to cry infrequently, and to sleep longer and often through the night.

Pitta-dominant babies have hearty appetites, focus intently on objects, are sensitive to sun and light, become irritable, are easily frustrated, especially when hungry, and tend to be more prone to diaper rashes and/or eczema.

The dosha patterns represent innate predominance which tends to persist throughout life. As a result, some people are naturally quicker physically and mentally and have more nervous energy, while others are naturally more purposeful and calm. However, none of the doshas should be thought of as better or worse than the others, anymore than the sun is to be thought of as better than the wind or the moon. If your doshas are in balance, you will be healthy in mind, emotion, and body, no matter which dosha predominates. If your doshas are out of balance, you will notice physical, mental, and emotional symptoms that are "dosha-specific."

Even though we have not found a more precise and comprehensive psychophysical description of human constitution than this identification system of Ayur-Veda, such classification is not unknown in modern medicine. The endomorph, ectomorph, and mesomorph types are analogous to the doshic body types, but go no further than muscular-skeletal description.

There have also been a few studies designed to classify and identify physical types in terms of mental types. Cardiologist/

internist Caroline Thomas and psychiatrist Barbara Betz, for example, tracked the physical and mental health of 1,000 Johns Hopkins Medical School students for thirty years in order to correlate any connections between personality traits and health disorders over the long term.[3] They divided the students into three "temperament" categories at the outset. The first group, the Alphas, were "cautious, steady, self-reliant, slow to adapt and non-adventurous." The second group, the Betas, were "lively, spontaneous, clever and flexible." The third group, the Gammas, "tended toward extremes—sometimes they were overly cautious, other times heedless and tyrannical. . . ." The researchers observed that the temperament of an individual may be the essential contributor to illness and concluded that the temperament "is the underlying core of the self." In terms of the doshas, it is likely that the first group was Kapha, the second, healthy Vata, and the third, Pitta—but somewhat out of balance.

Now, it's your opportunity to figure out which of the doshas are most fully expressed in your psychophysiology. The following self-assessment questionnaire will help to identify your prakriti and determine which of the doshas are more active in you. This is a necessarily simplified evaluation, meant to give a brief overall assessment of your bodymind type, but obviously not meant to fully evaluate your health.

When you are assessing yourself, remember to *consider each question in terms of the general patterns of your entire life, not just how you may have been feeling lately.*

### DETERMINING YOUR BODYMIND CONSTITUTION

Please evaluate your constitutional traits as you've observed them throughout your lifetime, using the following rating system and putting a number in each blank:

0 = Describes me not at all
1 = Describes me a little
2 = Describes me quite well
3 = Describes me almost perfectly

| | VATA | PITTA | KAPHA |
|---|---|---|---|
| 1. My hair texture tends to be | ____ dry, curly, full of body | ____ straight, fine | ____ thick, wavy, shiny |
| 2. My hair color is | ____ medium or light brown | ____ blond or reddish tone or early gray | ____ dark brown, black |
| 3. My skin tends to be | ____ on the dry side | ____ delicate, sensitive | ____ oily, smooth |
| 4. My complexion (when compared with others of my race) is | ____ darker | ____ more reddish, freckled | ____ lighter |
| 5. Compared with others of my height, I have | ____ smaller bones | ____ average-size bones | ____ larger bones |
| 6. My weight is | ____ below average, I don't gain easily | ____ average | ____ above average, I gain easily |
| 7. My energy level | ____ tends to fluctuate, to come in waves | ____ is moderate or high, can push myself too hard | ____ is steady |
| 8. Regarding temperature, I | ____ dislike cold; am comfortable in the heat | ____ dislike heat; perspire easily; thrive in winter | ____ dislike damp cold, tolerate extremes well |
| 9. My typical hunger level | ____ can vary from excessive to no interest in food | ____ is intense; I need regular meals | ____ is usually low but can be emotionally driven |

10. I prefer my food/drink    _____ warm, moist, oily    _____ cold    _____ warm, dry

11. I generally eat    _____ quickly    _____ moderately fast    _____ slowly

12. My sleep is most often    _____ interrupted, light    _____ sound, moderate    _____ deep, long; I am slow to awaken

13. My dreams more often include    _____ flying, looking down at the ground, mountains, chase scenes    _____ fire, waterfalls, battles    _____ oceans, clouds

14. My resting pulse rate (beats per minute)

| | | |
|---|---|---|
| women | _____ 80–100 | _____ 70–80 | _____ 60–70 |
| men | _____70–90 | _____60–70 | _____50–60 |

15. My sexual interest is    _____ strong when romantically involved, low to moderate otherwise    _____ moderate to strong    _____ slow to awaken, but sustained; generally strong

16. I am most sensitive to    _____ noise    _____ bright light    _____ strong odors

17. My emotional moods indicate that I    _____ change easily, am very reponsive    _____ am quick-tempered, intense    _____ am even-tempered, slow to anger

18. My general
    reaction to
    stress is
    ____ anxious,
    fearful
    ____ irritated
    ____ mostly calm

19. With regard to
    money, I
    ____ am easy and
    impulsive
    ____ am careful,
    but I spend
    ____ tend to save,
    accumulate

20. Regarding my
    way of
    learning, I
    ____ learn
    quickly,
    enjoy more
    than one
    thing at a
    time, can
    lose focus
    ____ focus
    sharply,
    discriminate,
    finish what I
    start
    ____ take my
    time, tend
    to be
    methodical

21. I learn new
    material best
    by
    ____ listening to
    a speaker
    ____ reading or
    using visual
    aids
    ____ associating
    it with
    another
    memory

22. My memory is
    ____ best in the
    short term
    ____ good overall
    ____ best in the
    long term

23. My way of
    speaking is
    ____ quick and
    often
    imaginative
    or excessive
    ____ clear,
    precise,
    detailed,
    well-organized
    ____ soothing,
    rich, with
    moments of
    silence

24. If there were
    one trait to
    best describe
    me, it would
    be
    ____ vivacious
    ____ determined
    ____ easygoing

25. Regarding my
    relationships, I
    ____ easily adapt
    to different
    kinds of
    people
    ____ often
    choose
    friends on
    the basis
    of their
    values
    ____ am slow to
    make new
    friends but
    forever loyal

26. My family and ____ settled ____ tolerant ____ enthusiastic
    friends might
    prefer me to
    be more

27. This ____ indecisive ____ annoyed ____ sleepy
    evaluation
    made me feel

|  | VATA | PITTA | KAPHA |
|---|---|---|---|
| TOTALS: | _____ | _____ | _____ |

*Assessing Your Score*

If one column total is 15 or more points higher than the others, this is clearly your dominant constitutional type—Vata, Pitta, or Kapha. If two of the column totals are 0–15 points apart, you are a dual-dosha constitutional type: Vata-Pitta (or Pitta-Vata), Pitta-Kapha (or Kapha-Pitta), or Vata-Kapha (or Kapha-Vata). And if all three column totals are within 0–10 points of each other, you are a tri-dosha constitutional type.

Now let's consider what all this means in terms of your physical, mental, and emotional health.

## Predominant Vata Dosha: Light, Airy, Creative

Standing on a mountaintop, feeling the softness of the air and the expansiveness of the space around you, you are tuning into Vata (or Vayu [*vy*-oo], the wind). This may produce a sensation of exhilaration and blissful lightness; this is the experience of your Vata dosha.

Vata is the air and space principle, which represents the bodily functions concerned with movement and controls movement in our minds and bodies. Vata is also associated with lightness, quickness, dryness, subtlety, thinness, roughness, and coldness.

The Vata woman is blessed with a kind of lightness and flexibility; in its healthy state, Vata is expressed as joy, creativity, and exuberance. Think of Mother Teresa, Lily Tomlin, or Diana Ross.

In imbalance or excess, Vata can manifest as an emotional state of fearfulness, worry, insomnia, vertigo, and loneliness or emptiness. With too much Vata, you may have "butterflies in the stomach"—a feeling of flutteriness, of too much space. Or it can be physically expressed as dryness, whether in skin, nails, colon, bowels (constipation), nose, in the joints due to drying up of the synovial fluid (leading to osteoarthritis), in bone (leading to osteoporosis). An imbalance of Vata is also associated with other conditions such as endometriosis, poor digestion, flatulence, sciatica, lightheadedness, dizziness and lack of coordination, or a general sense of not being grounded.

In many ways, we are a Vata culture: rootless, upwardly or downwardly mobile, transitory. If an entire city can have a Vata imbalance, it would have to be New York, where millions of people, suspended in tall towers in the air, are looking for ways to get grounded and balance their Vata.

A woman with Vata dosha predominant has an abundance of quick energy, especially in the morning, but may tire easily later in the day. She is often very funny and charming, interrupts the conversation and then forgets what she wanted to say, but you forgive her because you know it's totally unintentional. Because a Vata woman often will be first to open up in a relationship, she appreciates the support of a loyal mate and loyal friends. And even though she loves to travel, she is at her best when a sense of permanency at home and at work are available to settle her restlessness.

For Vata, above all the doshas, it's extremely important to be regular in life, to compensate for a relative lack of stability in the body's functioning. To pacify Vata disturbances, we need four main things: rest, regularity, oleation (oil), and warmth. A Vata type may feel most comfortable and happy with soft, warmhearted people and sleep most comfortably on a soft bed. Vata types do best when they stay near the ground. They also enjoy water, preferably warm water. Generally, as we get older, our Vata tends to increase, making us feel drier, colder, and less tolerant of dry, cold winters, no matter which dosha has predominated earlier in life. Older people in general really do best in warm climates, especially near water. Consequently, there's an Ayur-Vedic reason for the migration of older people to California and Florida in the United States and to the warmer coasts of nearly every country where it is cold.

## Predominant Pitta Dosha: Clear, Fiery, Vibrant

You are at the beach. You run into the ocean. The water combined with the sun's heat produces the sensation of intensity, vibrancy, being fully and passionately alive. You are experiencing your Pitta dosha. In terms of the bodymind, Pitta serves as an energy interface, a kind of heat press or transformer that conducts the information flow associated with Vata dosha into the physical structure associated with Kapha.

In physiological terms, Pitta represents bodily functions concerned with metabolism, particularly digestion. The qualities associated with Pitta are heat, acidity, oiliness, sharpness, and fluidity. Excessive hunger and thirst are characteristic of an imbalanced Pitta. A Pitta-dominant woman is intense, but the intensity, unlike Vata, is focused, more like laser light. This produces a sharp mind, clear, direct speech and, if imbalanced, sometimes a sharp tongue. In its healthy state, Pitta is decisive, efficient, well-spoken, passionate, and hungry for life. In its less healthy state, Pitta can show up as a bad temper, annoyance, heartburn, stress-associated heart attacks, peptic ulcers, colitis, acne, rashes, early graying, and excessive hot flashes during menopause.

A Pitta woman is often courageous, clearheaded, and successful. But her internal mixture of water and fire also can produce a boiling over, an eruption of irritability or anger. These characteristics may be found in a personality that is also impatient, hotheaded, and opinionated even if controlled. Perhaps no woman today epitomizes the essence of Pitta more than former British prime minister Margaret Thatcher. Then there are Katharine Hepburn, Whoopi Goldberg, Connie Chung, and Hillary Rodham Clinton, to name just a few.

Seasonal biological rhythms often affect people's moods and conduct. During the summer, Pitta is obviously most prevalent, and hot weather tends to trigger aggressive behavior. According to statistics from the Des Moines, Iowa, Police Department, 30 percent more violent crimes are committed during the summer than during the winter. Researcher Craig Anderson at the University of Missouri found that as far back as the 1880s, "Hot temperatures have produced increases in aggressive motives and tendencies." But, he concluded, there are no studies as yet that attribute the rise to physiological factors.[4] From an Ayur-Vedic vantage point, summertime aggression and rising crime rates are not so enigmatic when understood as a nationwide Pitta imbalance.

Pitta women therefore thrive best with some cooling influences in the summer, both emotionally and environmentally. They love open windows even in winter and in cooler climates, and ski vacations can make them very happy. They like meals on time—they will not forget that it is lunchtime, as a Vata woman might. In fact, Pitta women can become a bit obsessive and fanatic about a lot of things. For this reason, they enjoy being around the tolerance of Kapha and the lightness of Vata for emotional comfort. But the Pitta woman is often the most successful woman: She is clear, focused, and gets things done. Pitta is associated with the years of adulthood through late middle age, the years when women of all body types are generally most active and productive. During the "Pitta" years, a woman with Pitta predominant can become so focused on achieving, whether at home or at another workplace, that she may need to schedule "down time" so she doesn't overtax herself.

## Predominant Kapha Dosha: Serene, Earthy, Wise

You are in a silent cave, enveloped by the softness of the cool earth. It is protective, it is deeply soothing, it feels like the womb of Mother Nature herself nurturing you. You are experiencing your Kapha dosha, "liquid, lovable, and wise."

Kapha represents the supporting structure of the body, earth, and also administers its lubrication, water. Kapha is also cohesive. If Kapha isn't active enough in your physiology, you may have the experience of feeling that you're not grounded. With too much Vata and not enough Kapha, you may have the feeling of becoming "unglued." With too much Pitta and not enough Kapha, you feel overheated, your blood pressure may become too high; you need Kapha's cooling, stabilizing influence. Kapha creates strong bones, strong teeth, and the capability of storing energy, which may result in well-proportioned, heavier bodies. The Kapha woman is often voluptuous, with beautiful large eyes, lustrous hair, and a serenity that attracts all of us. Oprah Winfrey, Sophia Loren, and Barbara Bush are examples of women with an abundance of Kapha, although they each have a good deal of Pitta as well. Earthly delights appealing to the senses of taste and smell, such as good food, appeal strongly to Kapha women. As Mrs. Bush once remarked, in comparing herself to Nancy Reagan (a Vata-Pitta): "The difference between Nancy and me is—and it's a sad one on my part—she didn't eat when she worried. Not me. I eat my way right through a crisis."[5]

Kapha, in its healthy state, is strong, long-lived, calm, Mother Earthly, forgiving, sweet-spoken, deliberate, able to hold on to money and friends. The Kapha-dominant woman is unflappable, stable, and profoundly loyal, a genuine comforter. In its less healthy state, Kapha manifests in the form of sinus problems, asthma, diabetes, and chest colds. The Kapha-dominant woman can become congested in any part of her body, especially in the lungs; she may also retain water and be susceptible to edema. She can likewise be "congested" in her personality and become complacent, heavy-hearted, greedy, and unwilling to move. Whereas a Vata woman may have her head in the clouds, the Kapha woman may become ostrichlike and bury her head in the sand, avoiding change.

Kapha-dominant women also can become somewhat lethargic and are more likely than Vatas or Pittas to become "couch potatoes." They need to participate in a regular exercise program. They also tend to require smaller quantities of food, which they have the advantage (and disadvantage) of storing so well. They may need to find opportunities for change, to consciously break old behavior and thought patterns to stay balanced. Kaphas benefit most from movement, dance, and travel, as well as from a warm, dry climate, stimulating activity, exciting friends, and occasionally a good alarm clock.

## Dual-Dosha Constitutional Types

As you may have noticed from your self-assessment, two doshas can be almost equal in predominance. If this is true for you, this makes you a dual-dosha type; you have qualities of two doshas lively in you, sometimes simultaneously, but often at different times. A Vata-Pitta woman may thus feel both expansive and highly focused; she may be spontaneous and original at times and clear and discriminating at others. Or, if both doshas are out of balance, she may feel too cold in the winter and too hot in the summer, whereas a more Vata woman may not mind the summer heat at all and a more Pitta woman feel quite comfortable in the cold weather.

If there's imbalance, a Vata-Pitta woman may push too hard to achieve and cause a Vata disorder resulting in anxiety, insomnia, and/or constipation. Her anxiety may thus diminish her enjoyment of her success. But when she is functioning in a healthy state, a Vata-Pitta women can combine the virtues of imaginative Vata with the clarity and discipline of Pitta to be a most creatively productive woman.

A Kapha-Pitta or Pitta-Kapha woman, on the other hand, has the blessing of the constitutional strength of Kapha along with the fire of Pitta to enable her to be dynamic as well as self-contained. She has Kapha's stability and Pitta's intensity. With a sharp Pitta intellect and Kapha's patience and ability to sustain attention to a task, her managerial skills are often excellent. But when out of balance, she can be a bit arrogant as well as egotistical, and often altogether too serious, lacking the humor and lightness of Vata.

A Vata-Kapha or Kapha-Vata woman has the benefit of opposites: the easygoing Kapha nature and the dynamism of Vata. This enables her to be expansive and yet stable. Free of the discriminating qualities of Pitta, she is often nonjudgmental and therefore gets along well with a variety of people. She may at times spend her money impulsively (Vata) and at other times become a deliberate saver (Kapha). She may not have to deal with the Kapha tendency toward heaviness, either in body or mind. Nor will she be overly anxious, although the potential combination of fear and lethargy may make for some procrastination and/or indecisiveness. The openness of Vata combined with the emotional depth of Kapha may make her vulnerable and easily hurt in relationships, especially if lacking the feistiness of Pitta. Since neither dosha does well in the cold, the Vata-Kapha woman may need more time in the sunshine than anyone else.

The "tridosha" woman—a Vata-Pitta-Kapha—is rare: In some

cases, she may have all three doshas fairly equally distributed but there may be imbalance in each, leading to more potential illnesses. But in general, when all three doshas are equally awake from birth on, your bodymind is more predisposed to maintaining balance in all three doshas, giving you excellent health. Environmental factors can influence any of us, however, so keeping up a healthy life-style if you are tridosha is of course essential.

## Imbalanced Doshas: The Precursor to Illness

As we noted earlier, women are often frustrated by the inability of the modern medical approach to diagnose their complaints because "pre-disease" conditions are not classifiable or treatable by the techniques of modern medicine. But they *are* easily explained and treatable when one understands how the doshas function. We are predisposed to developing what Ayur-Veda terms an "imbalance" in the dosha that is strongest in our constitution, because the qualities of that dosha are already highly active in our bodyminds.

The underactivity or overactivity of a specific dosha or doshas beyond that required by an individual for balanced physiological functioning is called *vikriti* (vih-krih-tee). Vikriti is an unnatural accumulation of one or more of the three doshas that is inappropriate for your particular body type. This could occur, for example, during a particular season associated with the dosha you have most lively. If you are Pitta-predominant, you may notice imbalanced Pitta at the end of summer and experience this time of year with discomfort and irritability. If Vata or Kapha predominates, you may more likely accumulate excess Vata or Kapha and feel most uncomfortable and imbalanced during the cold weather.

To better understand this principle, let's look closely at one example of dosha imbalance.

Vata is the most subtle and most easily influenced (least stable) of the doshas, so it is most quickly set out of balance. Moreover, Vata is the dosha that rules movement and thus carries the other doshas through the bodymind. When Vata is imbalanced, its disturbed course also will disturb the other doshas sooner or later. Vata also regulates the functioning of your intellect and nervous system: Any mental or emotional stress often affects Vata dosha first. As a result, most stress-related symptoms—anxiety, insomnia, weakness, fatigue, lack of mental clarity, loss of appetite, and general aches and pains—involve an imbalance in Vata dosha alone or with other imbalances.

Because Vata is sensitive and subtle, a woman of Vata constitution tends to be more sensitive and subtle, physically, mentally, and emotionally. When balanced, this heightened sensitivity will express itself beneficially in many areas of her life; perhaps she'll have an uncanny ability to intuitively size up a person or situation, or an artistic depth and flair, or she'll be a deeply sensitive and understanding mother and/or an astute businesswoman. But if these qualities become unbalanced, she may experience being very uncomfortable in extremes of temperature, she may overreact to outbursts of anger or hostility from others, or she may feel increased sensitivity to the effects of sleep deprivation or unsuitable food.

Most Vata-related disorders or diseases develop as a result of specific long-term life-style habits that increase the various qualities of Vata dosha. For example, insomnia, a classic Vata disorder (though occasionally due to a Pitta imbalance), is more or less the result of overactivity and irregular rest and sleep routines. A nighttime vigil increases Vata, primarily because of its asynchrony with universal cycles and circadian rhythms, while regularity and attunement with these cycles calm Vata.

Women who suffer from insomnia often consider themselves "night people" and may stay up until the early hours of the morning. This habit of staying up late tends to increase Vata as a whole and overenergizes an insomniac's nervous system so that sleep doesn't come easily when she does go to bed, or when she tries to go to bed earlier the next night.

If she feels deep fatigue the next day, the Vata-imbalanced woman will often turn to coffee, cola, or tea to experience her characteristic energy level. However, this serves only to create a deeper wave of fatigue a few hours later, the desire for another cup, and an eventual addictive habit. In addition, because caffeine is a stimulant, it speeds up the nervous system and metabolism and naturally increases already speedy Vata. After a day of caffeine, a restful sleep is even less likely. To turn this situation around, Ayur-Veda recommends a specific eating and rest program (see next chapter) that can alleviate the root cause, the Vata disorder. Note that we've looked at Vata imbalance here, but we can apply the same considerations to understanding Pitta and Kapha imbalances as well.

## Treatment of Imbalanced Doshas

Because Ayur-Veda is oriented to the person and not to the disease, the distinction between health and illness is understood as the distinction between balanced and imbalanced doshas, whether the symptoms describe a life-threatening situation or a superficial concern. Recognizing how the doshas are organized within your bodymind can aid tremendously in determining treatment beyond any primary or composite symptoms. As there are many qualities associated with each dosha, and each dosha governs a multitude of bodily functions, one imbalanced dosha can lead to a variety of physical and mental symptoms. By the same token, when measures are applied to balance a particular dosha, a number of problems may disappear at the same time.

The purpose of Ayur-Vedic treatment is basically to "remind" each dosha to do its proper job. Two main principles of treatment apply here:

1) The principle of treatment through natural balancing based on similarities and opposites
2) The principle of treating the "many in one": treating one cause to alleviate many conditions

### Natural Balancing of Similarities and Opposites

Ayur-Vedic treatment focuses on the balance of similar and opposite qualities, which are either reduced or increased depending on imbalances. Here's how it works: You may have created a Vata imbalance by irregular eating habits, rushing, mental overloading, or lack of adequate rest; or a Pitta imbalance by too much sun, too much alcohol, too much focused mental work, visual strain, or eating too much hot and spicy food; or a Kapha imbalance by not exercising enough, overeating, lack of mental stimulation, or too much exposure to a damp, cold climate. Specific eating regimes and other daily recommendations are thus prescribed on the basis of particular doshic qualities that are either excessive or inactive. The dual purpose is to calm down an overactive dosha or enliven a dormant one.

There are two principles at work: The first is *samanya* (suh-mahn-yuh), the "principle of balance of similarities," which states that any quality outside us increases the like quality inside us. Sudden motion is thus more likely to affect a Vata person than either of the other two doshas because quick movements share similar qualities with the nervous-system energy of Vata. Pittas are generally far more aware of summer heat and cannot tolerate it well; they also feel more Pitta qualities rising in the presence of another hot-tempered person. If the weather is very cold or a lot of cold foods are offered at a buffet, or if they interact with a "coldhearted" person, Vata and Kapha types will tend to notice an increase in Vata and/or Kapha doshas, because they are themselves cool.

Second is *vishesha* (vih-shay-shuh), the "principle of balance of opposites," which means that qualities *contrary* to the qualities of a specific dosha will tend to mollify, soothe, or balance that dosha. In the case of Vata, warm, friendly people soothe the imbalances and warm the heart, and the warm, moist air at the ocean on a summer's day leaves the skin smooth and soft. When your mind is relaxed and peaceful, Vata dosha is calmed and balanced. For Pitta, the cool, easy-going balance of Kapha and the quicksilver light-heartedness of Vata in people, places, and things balances the heat and irritability of Pitta; you'll find that hiking in the forests and other cooling activities such as windsurfing feel good to you. In the case of imbalanced Kapha, the dry wit of Vata, the focused warmth of Pitta, or ideally the dry heat of the desert balances and enlivens any heaviness and dampness you may feel.

### The "Many-in-One" Treatment

The first signs of dosha imbalance are usually fairly mild, since the disturbance in the bodymind's functioning has not yet reached the stage of a nameable disease. So Ayur-Vedic treatment is mild as well and, unlike most other medical treatment, extremely enjoyable. Yet it is simultaneously beneficial and practical; by treating the underlying cause as a dosha imbalance, one avenue of treatment can take care of an entire panoply of symptoms.

This is a revolutionary treatment approach. As we've discussed, in conventional medicine, a patient may see a variety of specialists for a variety of seemingly unrelated ailments without real identification of an underlying cause. Because Ayur-Veda recognizes individual differences, it allows for a range of physical and behavioral well-being and/or illness, which depend on individual constitutional type. For example, two patients with hypertension might receive different diagnoses of the central cause of their seemingly similar conditions, based not on the kind of disease but on the underlying imbalance that caused it. The imbalance may also be responsible for a number of other, less severe conditions, and fortunately, Ayur-Veda can detect and affect subtle symptoms as easily as more obvious ones. The glory of Ayur-Veda is that it offers not only the knowledge of medicine but the deeper knowledge of life itself as an expression of natural law.

## The Diagnosis and Treatment of Imbalance: Three Clinical Examples of Vata, Pitta, and Kapha

### A STORY OF VATA

*As she began to approach age forty, Janet realized that it was time to pay more attention to her health. As a clinical psychologist, she had devoted many years to her training, and later to caring for her patients. Now her own mind and body were demanding attention.*

*Although Janet always had been a "worrier," now she was not only worried, but fatigued and depressed. Psychotherapy and antidepressants had helped her mood considerably, but a series of troubling physical symptoms remained.*

*A lifelong tendency toward constipation had become so problematic that she needed laxatives to have a normal bowel movement. Her digestion was poor, with constant gas, bloating, and heaviness after eating. She suffered from vari-*

*ous aches and pains, particularly tension headaches. More-
over, she had lost twelve pounds over the past year, had not
had a menstrual period in five months, and was concerned
about her decreased libido.*

*When Janet first came for an Ayur-Vedic evaluation, she
weighed only 90 pounds, which was extremely light even for
her petite frame. Her physical exam was normal except for
her low body weight. In modern medical terms there was
nothing physically "wrong" with her health. In Ayur-Vedic
terms, however, she was suffering from a multitude of Vata-
related symptoms. Primarily a Vata constitutional type,
Janet was particularly susceptible to the Vata-aggravating effects of long hours, irregular and rushed meals, and lots of
intense mental and emotional work, of which she had had
plenty in her ten years of training and private practice.*

*Given an understanding of the characteristics of her con-
stitutional type, and the knowledge of how to balance Vata
through measures such as changing her schedule (allowing
more time for meals, sleep, and relaxation), going on a Vata-
pacifying diet program, and giving herself a daily oil massage, Janet set out to recover her health again. Within two
months she reported, "Normalcy has returned.... I am feeling happier, much more balanced, free of my former mood
swings, and I definitely have more energy."*

*After eight months, she had gained ten pounds back and
her periods had resumed. Elimination and digestion were no
longer problematic, and she reported "feeling great." One
year later, after having also begun to practice the stress-
reducing Transcendental Meditation technique, Janet finds
she now feels balanced in body and mind, without tranquilizers or antidepressants; moreover, only if she has an extended break in her routine does she suffer temporarily from
any of her previous symptoms. She writes, "I feel so fortu-
nate to have found this Ayur-Vedic approach to my health.
For me, it has been a treasure; so gentle yet powerful."*

# KNOWLEDGE

## A STORY OF PITTA

*Karen, an energetic, successful CPA, at age fifty was an acknowledged hard-driving, intensely focused "Type A," although at times she felt perhaps she should slow down a bit. She had always enjoyed relatively good health except for an annoying problem with hypoglycemia, which had forced her to be careful about eating too many sweets, which she nonetheless craved, and to require frequent snacks, especially when she was exercising.*

*Then she began to experience recurring pain. Without warning, for minutes or even hours at a time, she would feel a searing pain in her abdomen, in her chest, and sometimes in her back. Her initial medical diagnostic workup was inconclusive. However, the bouts of pain continued to occur every few weeks over the next year and a half. One night, the pain was so severe that her husband drove her to the emergency room, determined that he wouldn't take her home until they found out what was wrong.*

*Several hours later, the verdict was that she had more than ten large stones in her gallbladder, blocking the common bile duct. Her doctors strongly urged her to undergo immediate surgery. At that point there really seemed no choice, the pain was too great and was not expected to go away on its own.*

*Four days after the surgery, while still in the hospital, Karen was sharply awakened from a deep sleep: Unbelievably, the pain was back. This time it did not last, however; after further tests, it was decided that yet another gallstone had been passed. She was discharged from the hospital a few days later, but did not recover as quickly as she had expected. Two weeks later, she was still weak, with pains in her stomach and severe aching in her arms and legs. Her appetite was low, and in general she felt quite ill. She decided to go for an Ayur-Vedic evaluation.*

*At her evaluation, it was clear that Karen had a predominantly Pitta constitution, and that both Pitta and Vata were quite out of balance. In particular, Ranjaka Pitta, a more*

**83**

*specific level of Pitta that functions in the liver and gallbladder, was severely disturbed, accounting for both her long-term problem with hypoglycemia and her current problems with the biliary tract. Due to the disturbance in Pitta, her digestion had remained poor even after the gallstones were removed; hence her persistent low appetite. The weakness and aching joints and muscles were a side effect of her poor digestion, caused by the accumulation of improperly digested food.*

*Karen learned that her gallbladder problem was an imbalance primarily in Pitta dosha, which governs digestion and metabolism, and that to rebalance Pitta, she would need to make adjustments not only in her diet but also in her entire life-style. Her innate drive and energy, characteristic of a Pitta constitution, had driven her not only to career success but also to a state of psychophysiologic imbalance. She was given a Pitta-pacifying diet, specialized herbs, recommendations for how to improve her overall digestion, and guidelines on how to balance the doshas as part of each aspect of her daily routine. It was also suggested that she learn the Transcendental Meditation technique to reduce her stress level and to promote a smoother, more intimate connection between her mind and body.*

*Three weeks later Karen elatedly called to report how much better she was feeling. She had been following each of the recommendations, and she had made some other changes on her own: "I've really changed my workaholic-style schedule. I quit working late at night and am no longer booked every minute. I'm taking time for my daily oil massage and tub bath, which both feel wonderful. TM has me feeling settled and happy within, in both my mind and body. My energy seems strong and steady. Moreover, I can play two hours of tennis without even thinking about my blood sugar."*

The biggest change Karen made was to "change her mind," by changing her deepest intention for what she wanted for herself. As a well-organized Pitta woman, when she put her determined mind and focused energy on healing and re-creating balance, she made quick progress. But it was her heightened self-awareness that essentially enabled Karen to undergo a real shift in her personal priorities; even those changes she wasn't planning to make, such as rearranging her schedule to accommodate her health needs, happened easily, like second nature.

### A STORY OF KAPHA

*Laura, a forty-three-year-old chemist, was working for the U.S. government when she first sought out Ayur-Vedic treatment. After being transferred to a well-publicized "sick" (toxic) building, Laura had begun to suffer from intense sinus headaches, congestion, and even mild asthma. Her energy was lower than ever, and particularly while in the building, she suffered from lethargy, sleepiness, poor ability to concentrate, and reduced mental clarity. Her digestion was sluggish, her stools loose, and she had gained extra pounds that she just couldn't lose. She needed nine or more hours of sleep at night and still could barely drag herself out of bed in the morning. She had also become very depressed.*

*Her Ayur-Vedic examination made it clear that Laura was experiencing a Kapha imbalance. Although triggered by environmental toxins, Laura's specific reactive symptoms were also a reflection of her innate Kapha constitution and a lifelong tendency to develop Kapha-type imbalances.*

*Laura's Ayur-Vedic treatment consisted of a Kapha-reducing program to eliminate accumulated toxins stored in her bodymind. She began a Kapha-pacifying diet and increased her intake of fluids, particularly plain hot water. This alone made an immediate impact on her digestion and reduced her sinus congestion. In addition she began to practice TM daily to reduce mental stress, which was expressing itself in the form of a chronic Kapha-type depression— lethargy, low energy, oversleeping, and weight gain. She found that she could now make it through the day without a headache, and was increasingly clear, focused, and productive, even in the same building environment.*

*In the spring, when she ordinarily became more debili-*

*tated by her symptoms during "Kapha season," she under-
went Ayur-Vedic "Panchakarma" (puhn-chuh-kahr-muh), a
series of treatments to promote elimination of excess waste
and balance the doshas. With these treatments, she experienced an increase of energy in the springtime, and improvement of all her symptoms for the first time in years. Now,
although she still has to watch her diet and be alert to keeping Kapha balanced, Laura reports that she is leading a far
more comfortable life, no longer debilitated by the depression, headaches, and fatigue.*

## The Simplicity of Healing Based on the Balance Principles

From an Ayur-Vedic perspective, severe disease is the result of severe imbalance: The disruption in the doshas creates the disruption
in the cells and tissues leading to symptomology. Whether considering the molecular, structural, visceral, mental, or emotional levels, Ayur-Veda conceives of our health as grounded in *dosha
patterns*. The doshas quietly and elegantly organize our bodymind,
like traffic patterns that may seem random when we are driving
within them but when seen from an airplane are noticeably structured as organized patterns of avenues and streets (except perhaps
in Boston). In this way, the Ayur-Vedic concept of balance and imbalance serves to help us make the needed adjustments to keep on
track.

Because Ayur-Veda extends beyond symptoms to the deeper
structures within one's bodymind, a disease is never identified as
solely physical, mental, or emotional. The balance within our
doshas will determine the quality of all aspects of who we are, including our way of speaking, our sensitivity to the remarks of others, our tendency to be affected by the sun, our appetite for sugar,
or the effect of our premenstrual symptoms.

Using individualized Ayur-Vedic methodology with regard to
food, for example, the Vata-imbalanced individual, according to
samanya, or the principle of similarities, is going to have adverse
reactions to foods that further aggravate Vata: cold foods, caffeine,
raw vegetables, and dried beans, among others. Similarly, those of

us with a Pitta imbalance may overreact to spicy and acidic foods; Kapha-imbalanced people may need to avoid certain mucus-producing dairy products, sweets, and so forth.

You can use the following Dosha Qualities Chart to identify your predominant doshas(s) and the balances and imbalances you may be experiencing. In addition, you will be able to see some examples of what may be causing the imbalanced dosha in your life. Then you'll know what to reduce or avoid in order to rebalance the dosha.

## DOSHA QUALITIES CHART

| | EFFECT OF BALANCED DOSHA | SYMPTOMS OF IMBALANCED DOSHA | CAUSES OF IMBALANCED DOSHA |
|---|---|---|---|
| VATA | Exhilaration<br>Mind clear<br>  and alert<br>Perfect<br>  functioning of<br>  bowels and<br>  urinary tract<br>Proper formation<br>  of all bodily<br>  tissues<br>Sound sleep<br>Excellent vitality<br>  and immunity | Rough, dry skin<br>Weight loss<br>Pain<br>Anxiety<br>Restlessness<br>Worry<br>Constipation<br>Joint pain<br>Weakness<br>Decreased<br>  concentration<br>Insomnia | Excessive exercise<br>Wakefulness<br>  (staying up late,<br>  not enough<br>  rest)<br>Excessive raw<br>  foods<br>Suppression of<br>  natural urges<br>Cold<br>  overexposure<br>Overwork<br>Fear, grief, worry<br>Agitation<br>Fasting<br>Pungent,<br>  astringent, and<br>  bitter foods<br>Late autumn and<br>  winter (Nov.–<br>  Feb.) |

| PITTA | Lustrous complexion | Excessive body heat | Anger |
|---|---|---|---|
| | Contentment | Inflammation | Strong sunshine |
| | Perfect digestion | Skin diseases, rashes | Burning sensations |
| | Softness of body | Heartburn | Fasting |
| | Heat and thirst mechanisms balanced | Peptic ulcer | Wine, vinegar, alcohol |
| | Strong intellect | Excessive sweating | Pungent, sour, or salty foods |
| | | Excessive thirst | Late summer and autumn (July–Oct.) |
| | | Excessive hunger | |
| | | Frequent aggressiveness, irritability | |
| | | Diarrhea | |
| | | | |
| KAPHA | Strength | Pale complexion | Sleep during daytime |
| | Normal joints | Coldness | Lack of exercise |
| | Stability of mind | Lethargy | Heavy food |
| | Dignity | Excessive sleep | Sweet, sour, or salty foods |
| | Affectionate and forgiving nature | Dullness | Milk products |
| | Strong and well-proportioned body | Asthma, bronchitis, colds, allergies | Spring and early summer (March–June) |
| | Courage | Excessive weight gain | |
| | Vitality | Yeast infections | |
| | | Lack of motivation | |

## The Senses and the Doshas

Each of the doshas is most influenced by specific senses based on the five elements. Vata is associated with touch and hearing, Pitta with sight and taste, and Kapha with taste and smell.

Because Vata types are generally sensitive to sound, they need a quiet place to sleep or study and can be easily soothed by the right piece of music. They also are the most reactive to touch, are particular about clothing textures, and can benefit deeply from a loving hug or a body massage.

Pitta types are sensitive to light, take in visual information in great detail, and respond happily to pleasing surroundings and food suited to their body type. A sweet, creamy dessert can soothe them into a relaxed and easygoing frame of mind.

Kapha types are often most sensitive to taste and smell, which stir memory and emotion (by virtue of associated pathways in the brain). They therefore tend to be driven to eat more for emotional comfort than by actual hunger. Kaphas thrive on a diet rich in delicious flavors, satisfying their sensual nature. A Kapha diet also provides appropriate spices and lighter foods, which encourage sharper digestion. Aroma therapy can offer a simple and effective approach for keeping Kapha types balanced.

For a basic approach to balancing your doshas, identify your predominant doshic imbalance(s) from the list of characteristic symptoms. Then follow the suggestions for your dosha(s) given below. You'll get more details in the following chapter.

### VATA

1. Follow a regular routine, with set times for meals, sleep, and rising. Pay attention to getting enough rest.

2. Favor warm, cooked foods and avoid cold foods and drinks and large amounts of salads and raw vegetables. If your diet is very low in fat, try adding a bit more oil.

3. Give yourself an *abhyanga* (ah-bhyun-guh), a warm sesame oil massage, daily before your morning shower or bath (see chapter 12 for instructions).

### PITTA

1. Be sure your meals are on time, particularly your noon meal.

2. Avoid hot spices, tomatoes, vinegar, alcohol, refined sugar, and other acidic or pungent foods in your diet.

3. Give yourself plenty of time to get where you need to go and avoid overscheduling and overworking.

KAPHA

1. You need a regular exercise program. Pick whatever exercise you like, and do it for as long as necessary each day to feel invigorated.

2. Avoid oversleeping, especially daytime napping. Get up by 6:00 A.M. to feel lighter and more energetic all day.

3. Eat a diet richer in vegetables, fruits, and legumes, and lighter on sweets, meat, dairy products, and fatty foods.

## The Ayur-Vedic Physician and Dosha Balancing

If you need further guidance, there are Maharishi Ayur-Veda physicians throughout the world trained to identify even the subtlest dosha imbalance. They can provide ways to reawaken the self-referral, self-repair program within your bodymind and can recommend specific approaches to help rebalance the doshas. Ayur-Veda enables both doctor and patient to understand the origin of symptoms from the deepest levels of psychophysiology and produce a cure directly based on that subtle awareness. Even when the physician uses Western technology to diagnose and treat, Ayur-Veda further offers a more individualized program for each patient.

Here are a few of the medical principles based on the doshas for you to be aware of if you want to educate yourself or your Western-trained physician.

In general, a Vata-dominant woman will tend to be more sensitive to medication, so the doctor may want to try a lower dose to make sure she can tolerate it. She may also be more sensitive to the demands of surgery and need to structure a careful postoperative recovery program.

A Pitta type has more of a tendency to be allergic, and is more prone to a rash or inflammation, so the physician could help her identify possible allergic reactions. A Pitta-dominant type is more susceptible to a duodenal ulcer and thus more in need of an intervention to help her slow down. Following an illness, the Pitta woman may be impatient to be up and about and get back to her routine, so an Ayur-Vedic physician will often recommend more structured periods of rest to counteract the Pitta tendency to overdo it too soon.

A Kapha type may be more susceptible to postsurgical depression and/or lethargy than the other doshas, so an Ayur-Vedic doctor can help identify drugs, foods, or activities to decrease these conditions. Kapha-dominant types do, however, usually have a stable physiological structure and often have the easiest recovery from surgery.

Let's turn now to the simple, practical ways that Maharishi Ayur-Veda provides for each of us to balance our doshas—the best eating, sleep, and exercise approaches to keep our bodyminds functioning smoothly daily, weekly, monthly, yearly, and throughout a long, long lifetime of effortless good health.

# Chapter 4

### ❀

# BALANCE

## In the Best of All Possible Health: The Maharishi Ayur-Veda Eating, Sleeping, and Exercise Programs

*One whose physiology is in balance*
*and whose body, mind and senses*
*remain full of bliss,*
*is called a healthy person.*

Shushruta Samhita

Maharishi Ayur-Veda offers very specific and simple programs for reorganizing three of the daily life experiences on which your health most fully depends:

1. Eating
2. Sleeping
3. Exercise

### Ingesting and Digesting

Every interaction with your environment is a form of ingestion requiring some kind of digestion. Whether you ingest a mystery novel, a romantic conversation, or a strawberry ice cream cone, each experience realigns your bodymind in one direction or another. The better you digest, in every sense of the word, the less stress you place on your psychophysiology. Eating is one form of ingestion/digestion, but it involves far more than food. As you start to consider all the ways that Ayur-Veda strengthens and reinforces your digestive capabilities, it's good to keep in mind the primary reason for eating à la Ayur-Veda: to become fully happy and satisfied, not by decreasing the pleasureable activity of eating but by increasing the even more pleasureable production of happiness through a balanced physiology.

Ayur-Vedic doctors, known from ancient times as *vaidyas* (vaidyuhs) prescribe food as the first preventive medicine. Each patient's individual psychophysiology is taken into account and the patient is offered knowledge of *ahara* (ah-ha-ruh), which means proper diet. According to the Ayur-Vedic texts, ahara should (1) purify your physiology, leading to (2) a strong mind promoting clear thinking, which then produces (3) useful activity, which leads to (4) the fulfillment of your desires. In this way, a good eating routine can bring you the greatest happiness and satisfaction in life.

The first consideration is why we as adults have to learn to eat properly again. What happened to our innate ability to eat right?

### How Innocent Eating Habits Become Artificial

In our early infancy, all of us knew how to eat perfectly, innocently attuned to nature's guidance. As babies we automatically chose foods that would provide us with all the necessary nutrients for our growth, if our parents encouraged us to do so.

But many parents—even goodhearted, intelligent parents—have a poor understanding of what their children should eat. The result is the development of unhealthy eating desires and habits, which can significantly overwhelm, through constant reinforcement, a child's natural impulses. This often leads to a lifetime pattern of improper diet, improper eating habits and, in some cases, a distortion of the meaning and purpose of food.

Chronic overweight, digestive difficulties, anorexia nervosa, bulimia, and a host of other results of unnatural eating are especially apparent in the lives of women. This may happen because women's bodies are more harshly judged by nonhealth criteria in our culture and because women seem to have a more constant affiliation with food, whether because of role expectations, a natural affinity, or some combination of both.

This "artificial" intelligence, based on years of unhealthy eating, has overridden our biological intelligence so many times that our built-in cues—genuine hunger signals, sensitive taste buds, and inner knowledge of satiety—are quite remote. What is needed is a means to get back to the way we would eat if we were still innocent, to reawaken our natural biological intelligence to help us overcome the conditioning that has led many of us to such poor eating habits. We need to remember how to listen to what our bodies are telling us about the most desirable kinds of nourishment.

## Ayur-Vedic Eating: Returning Your Body to Its Owner

You may not want to believe that what you eat has anything to do with your stiff, inflamed hip joint. Or with your congested lungs. Or with both at once. But it does. And you may not want to know that what you eat has something to do with why you are bored at work or why you had an argument with your spouse. But it does. The integrative health principles of Ayur-Veda clarify these connections and allow you to pursue better eating habits.

Because it can reestablish within your bodymind the knowledge of innocent nourishment, Ayur-Veda can overcome a lifetime of bad eating habits and help you change to a healthier way of eating *without a struggle.* By regaining your rightful connection with the natural resource of your inner biological intelligence, you never again have to rely on unnatural means of weight loss such as powdered supplements or crash dieting, which only weaken you and distance you further from self-knowledge by adding yet another layer of artifice to nutritional habits.

Attaining a healthful balance in eating happens when you reattune to your body's signals and learn to respect those signals. That's all it takes to remain healthy and at a good personal weight. Once you are attuned to this inner menu, you can fearlessly go to restaurants with your friends and not suffer from either a desperate state of deprivation or from out-of-control desire.

## The Four Main Ayur-Vedic Nutritional Insights

*1. Diet is a therapeutic modality.* It is every bit as important as other medical treatments. It is the central means for balancing the doshas. Eating the right foods, in the right amounts, at the right time, in the right way, can do more to prevent disease and retard aging than almost anything else. Maharishi Ayur-Veda looks at proper diet as a way of imbibing concentrated packets of intelligence of nature to keep the bodymind well organized and on course.

*2. How we digest food is more important than what we eat.* Western nutrition has put a great deal of attention on what to put into our mouths and stomachs, but almost none on what happens afterward. Although proper diet is extremely important in Ayur-Veda, good digestion is even more essential. The best diet in the world is useless and even harmful, if poorly digested.

*3. Different people need different foods.* Western nutritional recommendations tend to be universal, for example, everyone needs x grams of protein per day, no one should eat too much fat or too many sweets, and so on.[1] Ayur-Veda may discourage fat for one patient and recommend it for another.

*4. The taste of food is nutritionally important, not merely an "extra."* It's fascinating that we maintain good taste in art and good taste in music but we don't uphold good taste in our food choices! Studies on animals have shown that they choose foods that supply nutritional elements they lack; their choice is based on their sense of taste and smell, the two senses interacting closely. Healthy babies also spontaneously choose foods that supply the kind of nourishment they need on the basis of taste.

Ayur-Veda has examined carefully the connection between taste and nutrition and recognizes that taste has a health-producing effect. It uses this knowledge as a basis for dietary recommendations. *Rasa* (rah-suh), which means taste, is the first part of the word *rasayanas* (ruh-sah-yuh-nuhs), herbal compounds that Ayur-Vedic physicians prescribe for balancing various aspects of the doshas.

This taste approach is more comprehensive yet easier to apply to daily life than counting calories, proteins, and vitamins. Each "taste group" has a different balancing physiological effect. Most

**95**

American meals overemphasize what Ayur-Veda calls the "sweet" and "salty" taste groups and underrepresent the "bitter" or "astringent" tastes. Over time, this discrepancy may increase the Kapha imbalances of overweight that are so common in most Western societies.

We'll consider the first two Ayur-Vedic nutritional insights on health and digestion in later chapters. For now, let's explore the specifics of dosha-balancing eating on the basis of taste.

## The Tastes and Qualities of Food

These are two characteristics by which food is classified in its effect on the doshas: taste and quality.

### TASTES (RASAS)

We are most familiar with three main tastes in our culture: sweet, sour, and salty. These three tastes tend to balance Vata, and may be a natural balancing factor in our diet, especially with a typical Vata-imbalanced life-style. These three tastes also favor the increase of Kapha and may be at least partly responsible for the national tendency toward unhealthy overweight and arteriosclerosis.

Ayur-Veda describes three additional tastes with which we are less familiar but which are equally important in a balanced diet: pungent (hot, spicy), bitter, and astringent.

For an ideal menu of nutrients to balance the doshas, a sample of all six tastes should be included in each meal, or at least in each day's diet as a whole. Obviously, not all tastes will be desired in equal amounts. But leaving out any one of the six tastes can lead to any number of cravings. Since our national diet does not readily provide or promote half of the six tastes, these cravings tend to persist, setting up an unhealthy cycle of overeating and improper nourishment.

Taking in all six tastes helps eliminate cravings. Cravings are often born out of the skewing of your usual diet toward sweet, sour, and salty. This tendency is usually resolved by adding foods with pungent, bitter, and astringent tastes. When you begin to have meals, especially lunch, that include the six tastes, you will probably notice that your later afternoon and nighttime cravings subside. Once the taste requirements are taken care of, most of us are cured of the munchies and the desire to keep snacking on one thing after another throughout the afternoon and evening, never feeling completely satisfied.

What gives each food its characteristic taste? Attributes of molecular structures create specific tastes and smells: In Ayur-Veda, each molecular structure reflects its "elemental" composition in terms of the five basic elements—air, earth, water, fire, and space (akasha)—identified in the previous chapter. Specific combinations of two of each of the elements make up the six Ayur-Vedic tastes as follows:

> air and earth: astringent
> space and air: bitter
> air and fire: pungent
> fire and water: salty
> earth and fire: sour
> water and earth: sweet

As you may remember, dual combinations of the elements also make up the three doshas. Applying the principle of balancing through opposites, which we considered in chapter 3, certain tastes are found to balance each of the doshas.

### VATA AND KAPHA

Vata's space and air are opposite to Kapha's water and earth and are balanced by an opposite trio of tastes:

Sweet, sour, salty: balances Vata, aggravates Kapha
Pungent, bitter, astringent: balances Kapha, aggravates Vata

### PITTA

Pitta has its own unique combination of balancing tastes.

> Sweet, bitter, astringent: balances Pitta
> Pungent, sour, salty: aggravates Pitta

### Some Examples of the Six Tastes

Sweet: Sugar, milk, butter, ghee, rice, breads, pasta, grains
Sour: Yogurt, lemon, grapefruit, aged cheese
Salty: Salt
Pungent: Hot, spicy food, jalapeño peppers, ginger root,
 cayenne
Bitter: Spinach, other green leafy vegetables, turmeric,
 horseradish
Astringent: Dried beans, lentils, dhals (pea or bean soups and
 purées), green leafy vegetables

#### QUALITIES (ATTRIBUTES)

There are twenty Ayur-Vedic attributes of foods in all, but six of them are of greatest importance:

> Heavy, light
> Oily, dry
> Cold, warm

The six attributes, like the tastes, balance through their opposites:

> Qualities of *heavy, oily, warm* balance *Vata.*
> Qualities of *light, dry, warm* balance *Kapha.*
> Qualities of *heavy, oily, cold* balance *Pitta.*

### The Maharishi Ayur-Veda Eating Program

*Without proper diet, medicines are of no use,*
*With proper diet, medicines are of no need.*

Ayur-Vedic proverb

Ayur-Veda provides knowledge of how to eat according to your constitutional type and to eliminate imbalances in the doshas. As we've discussed, most inappropriate eating is caused and accompanied by dosha imbalances; these are gently corrected through favoring those foods and drinks that are best suited to you and truly satisfy you. Ayur-Vedic menu-planning and food preparation are easy when you follow these simple guidelines.

As we saw in Chapter 3, two principles govern balance in your bodymind: increase and decrease. Remember that Samanya is the intake of anything outside the body that is similar to something within the body, causing it to increase; and vishesha is anything taken from outside that is dissimilar from something within the body, causing it to decrease. These two principles come into play when you are choosing food. You either add or subtract foods to increase something you have too little of, or you add or subtract foods to decrease something you have too much of. Specific disorders can be alleviated with an eating program to pacify or balance the primary dosha that is out of balance.

To make food choices, you can rely on your natural, spontaneous desires, your bodymind's way of expressing what it needs to achieve balance. For example, few balanced Pitta types will claim an attraction to hot, spicy foods, but they are notorious for having a "sweet tooth." Kapha types, on the other hand, when their doshas are pretty much in balance, tend to crave spicy foods and often don't have a strong affinity for sweets. A balanced Vata type is most likely to favor sour or salty foods, such as yogurt, pickles, or cheese. So one of the first principles of food selection in Ayur-Veda is to "eat what you like."

BUT, the choice has to be innocent. As we've considered, we've all been influenced more or less by family eating habits, the media, the medical community, and other outside sources and have largely intellectualized and emotionalized our eating. What we think we like has for the most part become separated from what we need nutritionally, and thus our hunger signals can send us reaching for the wrong thing—brownies or potato chips, which are not universally wrong choices, unless they don't satisfy our nutritional hunger. Here are three suggestions to help you get your eating habits "back to innocence," in order of importance:

1. Follow an eating program appropriate to any current doshic imbalances (vikriti). You can both participate in the Eating Program provided in chapter 5 and follow one of the dosha-balancing programs presented later in this chapter.

**99**

2. Modify your eating program according to the seasons and your living environment.

3. Follow an eating program appropriate to your body type (prakriti).

### Choosing Dosha-Specific Foods

You can also start to learn about the qualities of each food and how they relate to the doshas. For example, apples are considered sweet, astringent, light, rough, and cool and therefore increase Vata, decrease Pitta, and are good for Kapha. Bananas are sweet, smooth, and heavy and therefore increase Kapha, slightly increase Pitta, and decrease Vata. Among the grains, wheat is considered sweet, cold, unctuous, and heavy; rice is cold, sweet, and light; corn is dry, hot, light, and slightly astringent; and barley is described as cold, dry, light, sweet, and astringent. Think about how each type of grain would increase or decrease each dosha. Soon you'll be identifying food qualities with ease.

The eating programs listed below include foods whose tastes and qualities help to balance or pacify each dosha. In choosing which program is best suited for you, consider these three factors:

*1. Your predominant dosha imbalance.* If you related strongly to signs or symptoms of a particular doshic imbalance, then follow the program to balance that dosha. If a doctor trained in Maharishi Ayur-Veda has recently recommended a specific eating program for you, follow that one. Three general eating programs are given later in this chapter. However, it's important to note that following a dosha-balancing diet is not a substitute for medical diagnosis and treatment.

*2. The current season and your environment.* Adjust your dosha eating program to the season. For example, in Kapha season, even Vata types would do well to decrease their intake of oily, heavy foods such as cheese, fried foods, etc.

You also want to balance your environmental conditions with your food choices. Food reflects the quality of the environment in which it was grown. Foods grown in deserts tend to be light in their qualities, while foods grown in moist areas tend to be heavier in their qualities. If you live in a cold, moist environment, you should favor light, dry, warm, hot food. And if you live in a dry, hot environment, you'll want to balance it with cold and oily foods.

3. *Your underlying constitutional type.* If you are basically healthy and constitutionally dominant in one dosha, then follow the program that is balancing for that dosha. If you are a combination type, go with the dosha that is stronger, or the program that includes more of the types of foods you are naturally drawn to.

IMPORTANT NOTE: One of the biggest mistakes is worrying that you might make one. Don't get rigid and ignore the pleasure of eating and the real blessing of food. Your connection to the process of being nourished and an underlying sense of fulfillment is always more significant than anything you eat.

## Making Eating Choices from Deeper Inside Than Your Mouth

Listen to your bodymind with the idea that it will tell you exactly what you need to eat. You'll be surprised that much of the time you won't be hungry at all. This inner knowledge may conflict with a louder demand from your intellect proclaiming that you most definitely want some chocolate candy. So settle back and wait, listening to your body on an even deeper level. If you aren't hungry, you might not notice any particular desires for food. An entirely different desire might come up, perhaps to read, see a friend, or go for a walk.

Wanting more and more in life is natural, but we should be careful not to try to fulfill other desires through feeding ourselves with food when we can enjoy more bliss and more happiness via other experiences and other senses than taste.

You'll know if you are genuinely and innocently hungry by listening closely: If you are truly hungry, your body will often present you with a specific desire. Let's say it's for something sweet, and you think of a juicy peach. But you also think of chocolate candy. If you can freely choose, favor the peach. This is a sweet that has more "intelligence" in it than chocolate candy; it is sweet yet it also has good nutritional value and gives your bodymind far less opportunity to create *ama* (ah-muh), impurities and blockages that prevent perfect health. So it will ultimately satisfy you more, beyond your taste buds and stomach. It will give your digestive processes a better chance to produce *ojas* (o-juhs), the vital substance that creates balance and health, which will bring you bliss, a deeper and far more long-lasting pleasure than the happiness you may have learned to associate with a piece of chocolate candy. Neuropharmacologist Sarah Liebowitz says, "Our emotional life and state of mind will be affected by every bite we eat."[2] Highly processed foods, packaged foods, leftovers, deep-fried foods, as well as alcohol, caffeinated drinks, carbonated drinks, and chocolate are best left out of your regular eating regime for optimal health. If you are a junk-food junkie and find the idea of giving up your favorite foods daunting or depressing, then don't think in terms of giving them up. Rather, make a point of *adding* more vegetables, whole grains, fruits, and fresh juices in your daily diet, and start to follow some of the digestion guidelines to reduce ama and promote ojas. By focusing on *adding things that are good for you* rather than taking away things that are not, changes in the direction of healthier food choices will occur automatically and be maintained effortlessly.

Within a few weeks, you'll probably find that your tastes have changed, and you do not crave sweets or salty chips or chocolate (or whatever) nearly so strongly. If you aren't ready to say good-bye to them, however, you won't. If you can make a choice, choose with hindsight; that is, choose what you would like to have chosen looking back from the imagined future. When you're really in doubt, try and keep to the ultimate choice maxim: Choose the highest—the best, the healthiest—first.

### Ayur-Vedic Food Preparation

Ayur-Veda gives us a wonderful insight into the preparation of food. We all can attest to the difference between foods prepared by friends and foods that are bought in fast-food stands or eaten in certain intense, noisy restaurants. The difference between home-cooked meals and restaurant meals often has less to do with the kind and quality of the food and more to do with the loving attention of the cook and the environment, both surrounding the preparation of the food and surrounding the intake of the food.

Ayur-Veda suggests more than cleanliness in the kitchen; it recommends that the cook preparing the food be happy, strong, and healthy. The cook sees to it that a calm, pleasant, and pure atmosphere prevails during the preparation; sweet words and nonhurried activities promote the best atmosphere for preparing food.

### Food Digestion

*Agni* (uh-gnee), the "digestive fire," is the process that is responsible not only for the digestion of our food in the gastrointestinal tract but also for all the transformations of metabolism and assimilation. All tissues have their "flame," their metabolic principles; it is agni that transforms one tissue to the next, as we'll discover in the next chapter.

There are essentially four states of agni: (1) *sama* (sah-muh), or balanced, agni; (2) *manda* (muhn-duh), or diminished, agni; (3) *tikshna* (teek-shnuh), or overabundant, agni; and (4) *vishama* (vih-shuh-muh), or irregular, agni. Manda agni is often the result of a Kapha imbalance. Tikshna agni, where there is persistent hunger, is generally the result of Pitta imbalance. Most people who have ulcers in an early stage experience the subtle burning and overactivity of Pitta in their digestive tract. Vishama agni occurs in conjunction with wide fluctuations in appetite and digestive capacities and is usually a sign of Vata imbalance.

A normal functioning agni leads to lightness in your bodymind an hour or two after a meal, regular bowel movements in the mornings, regular urination, normal burping, and a normal sensation of thirst. Sama or balanced agni results in energy and interest in your work and other activities, a feeling of mental clarity, and a sense of cheerfulness.

#### SOME SUGGESTIONS TO DIGEST

1. Eating the heaviest meal around noon is a good idea because this is the time of day when the agni in your physiology and in the environment is strongest.

**103**

2. Generally, the later you eat, the lighter you eat.

3. Breakfast is really only necessary if you have a very strenuous physical job, or if you are uncomfortable skipping breakfast. For most of us, a cup of warm milk or a glass of fruit juice is sufficient.

4. If you are ill or under a great deal of mental or emotional stress, the gastric fire isn't as strong as usual; your diet should reflect the situation and be lighter, since your digestive tract will not be able to optimally digest the heavier foods.

### A WORD ABOUT FASTING

The gentlest form of fasting in Ayur-Veda is to take in only liquids, which can include juices, soups, and puréed vegetables. A partial fast can include eating a regular lunch and having liquids for the evening and morning meals. If you fast, be sure to take in plenty of noncarbonated, decaffeinated fluids and avoid strenuous activity. This gentle kind of fasting promotes lightness in your physiology and can stimulate the agni. It also upholds clarity in your senses and thoughts, increases energy, and promotes inner silence. People who have Kapha imbalances and/or overweight problems might consider fasting on liquids regularly, perhaps one day a week. Individual needs will vary, and the most important thing to go by is how comfortable you feel.

After you stop fasting, follow a light, non-oily diet on the first day, slowly increasing the heaviness of your foods. We don't recommend fasting for longer than twenty-four hours without a physician's guidance.

### Three General Ayur-Vedic Eating Programs

The dosha-balancing programs outlined below can provide general guidelines if you have identified signs of a particular doshic imbalance.

Overall, Vata types and those with Vata dosha imbalances should enjoy regular meals and avoid more than one-day light fasting.

### FOODS TO FAVOR

These foods are best suited for Vata. Try to choose them over the foods in the "Reduce" section.

| | |
|---|---|
| General | Warm foods and drinks, unctuous (oily) food, food with predominantly sweet, sour, and salty tastes |
| Grains | Rice, wheat |
| Dairy | All dairy products |
| Sweeteners | Natural whole cane sugar, molasses, honey |
| Oils | All oils |
| Fruits | Sweet fruits, grapes, cherries, peaches, melons, avocado, coconut, bananas, sweet oranges, sweet pineapples, sweet plums, sweet berries, mangoes, fresh figs, dates, apricots, stewed fruits |
| Vegetables | Well-cooked vegetables, beets, carrots, asparagus, cucumber, sweet potatoes |
| Nuts | All nuts |
| Spices | Black pepper (in small quantity), cinnamon, cardamom, cumin, ginger, salt, clove, mustard seeds |
| Animal foods (for nonvegetarians) | Chicken, turkey, seafood |

### FOODS TO REDUCE

The following foods taken in large quantities are not as suitable for Vata. They are best avoided or reduced in quantity and frequency.

General          Dry goods, cold or iced foods and drinks, foods having predominantly pungent, bitter, or astringent tastes

Grains           Barley, corn, millet, buckwheat, rye, oats

Fruits            Dried fruits, apple, pear, pomegranate, cranberry (apples and pears acceptable if cooked)

Vegetables     Avoid raw vegetables. Potato, brussel sprouts, broccoli, cabbage, peas, cauliflower, lettuce, spinach, bean sprouts, zucchini, and celery may be eaten in small or moderate quantities, but should always be well-cooked.

Beans           All beans should be avoided except for dhal, green beans, and tofu.

Animal foods   Beef
(for nonvegetarians)

### The Overall Vata Food Principle:
**Favor sweet, sour, salty, heavy, unctuous, hot foods and avoid pungent, bitter, astringent, light, dry, cold foods.**

### PITTA-PACIFYING DIET

#### FOODS TO FAVOR

These foods are most suitable for Pitta. Choose them when possible over the foods in the "Reduce" section.

General          Cool foods and drinks, foods with predominantly sweet, bitter, and astringent tastes

Grains           Wheat, oats, barley, white rice

Dairy           Milk, butter, ghee

Sweeteners    Any natural sweetener except honey and molasses

Oils             Olive, sunflower

| | |
|---|---|
| Fruits | Sweet fruits, grapes, cherries, melons, avocado, coconut, sweet oranges, sweet pineapple, sweet plums, mangoes, pears, pomegranates |
| Vegetables | Asparagus, pumpkin, cucumber, potato, broccoli, cauliflower, celery, lettuce, zucchini, okra, sweet potato, beans, green beans |
| Spices | Coriander, cinnamon, cardamom, fennel, black pepper (small quantity) |
| Animal foods (for nonvegetarians) | Chicken, turkey, egg white |

### FOODS TO REDUCE

Large quantities of the following foods are not as good for Pitta. When possible, they should either be avoided or their intake reduced in quantity and frequency.

| | |
|---|---|
| General | Foods with predominantly pungent (hot and spicy), sour, and salty tastes; foods and drinks with warming properties |
| Dairy | Yogurt, cheese, sour cream, cultured buttermilk |
| Sweeteners | Honey, molasses, refined white sugar |
| Oils | Almond, sesame, corn |
| Grains | Corn, millet, rye, brown rice |
| Fruits | Grapefruit, sour oranges, sour pineapple, sour plums, papayas, persimmons, olives |
| Vegetables | Hot peppers, radish, tomatoes, beets, onion, garlic, spinach |
| Spices | Ginger, cumin, fenugreek, clove, celery seeds, salt, cayenne pepper, mustard seed |
| Nuts | Cashews, sesame seeds, peanuts |
| Animal foods (for nonvegetairans) | Beef, seafood (shellfish especially), egg yolk |

*The Overall Pitta Food Principle:*
*Favor sweet, bitter, astringent, cold, heavy, and*
*unctuous foods and avoid pungent, sour, salty, hot,*
*light, and dry foods.*

## KAPHA-PACIFYING DIET

### FOODS TO FAVOR

These foods are best for Kapha. Choose them when possible over foods in the "Reduce" section.

| | |
|---|---|
| General | Lighter diet, dry foods, warm foods and drinks, foods with predominantly pungent, bitter, and astringent tastes |
| Grains | Barley, corn, millet, buckwheat, rye |
| Dairy | Low-fat milk |
| Sweeteners | Honey |
| Fruits | Apples, pears, pomegranates, cranberries, persimmons |
| Vegetables | Radish, asparagus, eggplant, green leafy vegetables, beets, broccoli, potato, cabbage, carrot, cauliflower, pumpkin, lettuce, celery, sprouts |
| Spices | All spices except salt |
| Beans | All beans except tofu |
| Animal foods (for nonvegetarians) | Chicken, turkey |

### FOODS TO REDUCE

Large quantities of the following foods are not as good for you. They should either be avoided or their intake reduced in quantity and frequency.

| General | Unctuous (oily) foods, cold or iced foods and drinks, foods having predominantly sweet, sour, and salty tastes |
|---|---|
| Grains | Large quantities of wheat, rice, or oats |
| Dairy | Cheese, yogurt, buttermilk, cream, butter |
| Sweeteners | All sweeteners except honey |
| Fruits | Sweet fruits, grapes, bananas, avocado, coconut, dates, figs, pineapple, watermelon, papaya |
| Vegetables | Tomato, cucumber, sweet potato, zucchini |
| Spices | Salt |
| Nuts | All nuts |
| Animal foods (for nonvegetarians) | Seafood, beef, pork |

***The Overall Kapha Food Principle:***
***Favor pungent, bitter, astringent, light, dry, and hot***
***foods and avoid sweet, sour, salty, heavy,***
***unctuous, and cold foods.***

## Recommendations for All Doshas

### SEVEN PRINCIPLES

1. Yogurt, cheese, cottage cheese, and cultured buttermilk should be avoided after sunset.

2. It's better not to heat honey or cook with it.

3. Avoid ice-cold beverages and foods, as they interfere with digestion.

4. Food should always be fresh and of the best possible quality. Avoid leftovers if you can.

5. Food is best if warm and well-cooked.

6. Food should be pleasing to the nose and the eye as well as the palate.

7. Food prepared by a happy and contented cook in a

pleasant environment will have the best influence on your health.

Drinking or sipping hot water is an important Ayur-Vedic addition to your daily eating and digestion program. As the ancient texts state, "Waters are the medicines for everything; may they act as medicine to thee." Boiled water has properties that balance all three doshas. The boiling process imbues the liquid with the air qualities of Vata; the liquidity of the water is Kapha; and the heat is Pitta. For the last reason, those with Pitta dosha predominant should not drink it too hot. Drink hot or warm water with and after meals and sip it throughout the day for reducing ama and keeping the digestive system in good working order. Take as much as you want at any given time; just a few sips at a time is fine.

### TWELVE WAYS TO PRODUCE BLISS WHILE EATING

1. Eat in a quiet, restful atmosphere, so you can really taste and digest the food while eating.

2. Other sensory experiences of sight, sound, touch, and smell associated with the food will all contribute to the feeling of satiety and decrease the chances of overeating.

3. Always sit to eat.

4. One way to settle down and feel deeply nourished by the food is to say a grace before the meal.

5. If at all possible, eat at approximately the same times each day.

6. Eat your food hot or at least warm. The digestive enzymes in the stomach and in the mouth were designed to perform best within certain pH (acid-alkalinity) and temperature ranges. Warm food maximizes the efficiency of the digestive enzymes. Cooking foods also tends to bring out flavors that uncooked foods may not have and thus enhances the pleasure.

7. Try not to work, read, or watch TV during meals. You want to avoid dividing your mind and body when you are eating. For example, if you eat popcorn while watching a movie, you rarely notice that you've eaten a bucketful, some-

thing you'd certainly notice and rarely do if you ate it quietly with your attention on nothing else.

The daughter of a famous artist was asked what was the most important thing in her father's life. She replied, "Eating an apple, when he's eating an apple." Try your own eating awareness experience with an apple. First feel the apple in your hands, the smooth skin, noting its coolness and the subtle color variations in the skin. Smell the apple, then cut it into thin, delicious slices, noticing the bright color of the apple and savoring each slice on your tongue. Chew it slowly and swallow it without distraction. Try eating this way as much as you can during meals.

8. Try not to eat too quickly or too slowly.

9. Eat to about three-fourths of your capacity. To judge whether or not you are eating about the right amount of food, you should have a feeling of lightness in your body an hour or two after a meal. Otherwise, the quality and quantity of food should be reevaluated. You might want to try some lighter foods.

10. Avoid having a meal until the previous meal has been digested. Allow three to six hours between meals. You'll know if you are experiencing true hunger, not just emotional or intellectual desire for food, and have fully digested the previous meal if there is some lightness in your body and a clear physical sensation of hunger that originates in the upper abdomen. In this way, we know that we are not overeating and/or extinguishing our agni.

11. Water or juice is fine with all meals. Milk is best with toast, cereals, or sweet-tasting foods and is not so good with full meals that include the other tastes.

12. In general, each meal (or your total daily meals) should be balanced to include all six tastes. Or you may want to choose tastes according to your constitutional type and your particular physiological needs.

1. The nature of the food
2. The method of processing
3. Combining different foods
4. The quantity of food
5. The place where you eat your meal
6. How much time you take to eat
7. The overall environment
8. How you digest your food
9. The quality of your awareness while you eat

## The Doshas and the Twenty-Four-Hour Sleep-Wake Cycle

The key to being in tune with the sleep-wake cycle, like the key to eating, is balance. All the organs and glands of our human physiology, along with everything else in nature, function in cycles of rest and activity. Whether we remember it or not, our individual bodyminds are tuned in to collective environmental rhythms, and our sleep-wake cycle follows the circadian rhythm arising from the rotation of the earth on its polar axis.

The seasonal changes reflect and affect the three doshas in ourselves and in all of nature as do the shifts from night to dawn, day to dusk, and dusk to night. Each period is characterized by an increase of activity in one of the three doshas. In the past few years, researchers have learned that the time when a person is most likely to have a heart attack or a stroke is around 9:00 A.M., for at that time blood platelets are more likely to clot and this can cause clogging in the arteries and capillaries. Modern medicine has no explanation for this, but Ayur-Veda observes that this is a Kapha time of day, when clogging and clotting, signs of Kapha, are most in evidence. Eventually, the onset of any illness may be correlated with each of these Ayur-Vedic dosha times:

Vata time: 2:00 to 6:00 A.M. and 2:00 to 6:00 P.M.
Kapha time: 6:00 to 10:00 A.M. and 6:00 to 10:00 P.M.
Pitta time: 10:00 A.M. to 2:00 P.M. and 10:00 P.M. to 2:00 A.M.

## Fatigue and the Doshas

Most of us living in Vata-aggravated times and nations get less sleep than we need. According to sleep disorder specialist William Dement, M.D., at the U.S. National Commission on Sleep Disorder Research, it seems to have become a sign of stoic resolve in an overly active society to get by on only a few hours of sleep, and then to feel guilty about getting a full night's sleep. As a result, reports Dement in a 1992 study, over 40 million Americans suffer from chronic sleep disorders and another 20 million have sleeping problems.

By understanding the influence of the circadian rhythms on the doshas, we might develop better therapies for sleep disorders. But, more important, we can immediately adopt routines that help prevent such disorders in the first place.

Your own individual physiology does make a difference in the amount of sleep you need, but there are also general characteristics to consider. By about the age of sixty, most of us (around 80 percent) find that we are waking up more often throughout the night and awakening earlier in the morning. Ayur-Veda reminds us that we become more Vata as we age and therefore will sleep fewer hours, in true Vata fashion. While most of us require about eight hours in our twenties, we only need about six hours on average in our fifties.

## The Ayur-Vedic Bedtime Program

According to Ayur-Veda, the ideal sleep routine calls for arising during Vata time and retiring during Kapha time. The dosha "principle of similarity"—samanya—is at work here: The quality present at the start of an activity tends to influence the activity throughout its duration. Therefore, if you start the day during the time of Vata, associated with alertness, creativity, and action, you will have more energy, creativity, and alertness during the day and will accomplish more with less effort.

Few of us are in the habit of arising before 6:00 A.M. and may not be able to immediately verify this by our own experience.

However, most of us have slept late, well into Kapha time, and may well have noticed that when we get up late, having slept even more than usual, we feel groggy and somewhat lethargic all day. This is because by lying in bed for several hours in the Kapha time of slowness and stasis, the bodymind becomes permeated by these qualities, and a "lazy-day feeling" results.

You may feel a bit grumpy if awakened before your sleep cycle is complete: The more you sleep, the more Kapha you enliven. This could increase the chances for lethargy and depression. Some studies have shown that depressed patients who are put on a sleep cycle that begins at around 6:00 P.M. and ends at about 2:00 A.M. (Vata time), experience marked improvement in symptoms of depression, which is generally sustained if they adhere to that schedule.

The secret to getting up early is, of course, getting to bed early. "Bedtime" is a phrase you may not have used since childhood, except in relation to your own children. But in Ayur-Veda, choosing the precise time of day to sleep is a powerful technique for creating balance in the doshas. You may find that around 9:00 or 9:30 P.M., you start to feel sleepy. It's a time to relax with a good book, the paper, or a favorite TV show. But if you stay up past 10:00 P.M., into Pitta time, you usually get a "second wind"; your mind perks up and it's off for another hour or more of activity. If you went to bed at that first sign of sleepiness, you would most likely fall asleep quickly, during Kapha time. Retiring during Kapha time is ideal because the deep, calm influence of Kapha dosha predominates in your bodymind. Sleep tends to come quickly, is sound and restful, and is therefore more health-producing. As a matter of fact, many people discover that when they start going to bed regularly before 10:00 P.M., they require less sleep than they do with a later bedtime.

In addition, Ayur-Veda suggests that sleeping during Pitta time (10:00 P.M. to 2:00 A.M.) is important for digestion and assimilation; staying awake during this time tends to oppose this essential process of metabolism. Staying up past 10:00 P.M. also increases the likelihood of food cravings, as metabolism and hunger levels rise with the increase of Pitta. Skin problems also are Pitta-related and may improve if you go to bed before Pitta time.

Some women find going to bed early to be incompatible with

their work schedule, their family's schedule, their social lives, or even with what they perceive to be their unique biorhythms: "I'm a night person," some of us will say. This is often a Vata-Pitta woman, perhaps an artist, writer, or entertainer, who finds she "comes alive" at night, during Vata and Pitta times, and feels dull and dragged out during the day. This usually results from a long-term pattern of staying up late, which aggravates Vata and Pitta, and sleeping late to compensate, which aggravates Kapha and leads to feeling tired all day. If you are this type of woman, trust that you can feel just as peppy and creative during the Vata and Pitta times of the morning and afternoon. If you start to go to bed before evening Pitta time, you can find you are remarkably creative and productive when you start your day during early-morning Vata time.

Many of us work in the evenings or on a night shift or are required to change our sleep times around because of our jobs. If you are in such situations, you will need to take special care to keep Vata balanced through other Ayur-Vedic measures, such as the Vata-balancing eating program, daily massage, warm baths, and plenty of rest and recuperation when you're not at work.

Of course, there will always be plenty of exceptions to these "good times" of rest. Life is, after all, not for the purpose of routines, but for greater happiness, enjoyment, and fulfillment. The idea is to help your bodymind establish a healthy pattern: If your usual schedule is one of balance, one that keeps your immunity strong and bodymind resilient, then you will do yourself no harm by an occasional late night or two. But if your established rest pattern relies on late night for entertainment or for catching up on work, your health is being jeopardized, and your priorities probably need some rearranging.

When making any major change in your life-style, the Maharishi Ayur-Vedic guideline is always to do so gradually and comfortably. So, if you're in the habit of going to bed at 1:00 or 2:00 A.M., make midnight your bedtime goal for a month or so. As midnight starts to feel natural, shift your bedtime to 11:00 or 11:30 P.M., and so on. Most women find that because they feel so much better in the morning when they go to bed earlier, these changes are very easy. And the jarring experience of being awakened by an alarm clock becomes unnecessary, as your body starts naturally waking up at the appropriate time, in tune with nature's wake-up calls like the birds (or with the city's wake-up calls like the trucks . . .).

It's not unusual for many of us to start skipping our morning cup of coffee, because we feel so alert and energetic with this routine. We discover a new freedom from fatigue, from that never-ending feeling of "If I can just get through the day, I can catch up tonight."

## Seasonal Changes and Ayur-Vedic Routines

We've seen how to begin to adjust your daily routines to take advantage of the biological cycles in nature, which are also present in your bodymind. These simple adjustments are vital for maintaining your health and longevity. The study of biological rhythms, a fledgling field in Western medicine, is a precise and sophisticated discipline in Ayur-Veda medicine, specifically addressing health issues in terms of the link between human life and the changing environment, as both are expressed in your biochemistry.

Consider, for example, the hormone cortisol, which regulates your body's metabolism and serves as an essential stress-resisting chemical. Without it, almost any activity would overwhelm you. Your body's production of cortisol has a twenty-four-hour cycle that corresponds to a daily pattern in nature. Your adrenocortical glands secrete it maximally during the early morning, around 6:00 A.M., and minimally in the late afternoon, when nature is preparing to rest.

Thousands of natural cycles in your psychophysiology synchronize with the larger environment. Just as nature orchestrates daily and monthly cycles of rest and activity, of nourishment and purification in every aspect of life, so there are cycles within your bodymind that are timed to the seasonal cycles as well. The seasons thus serve as more than a clothing guide: they are a primary "health" rhythm in our lives.

The three main Ayur-Vedic seasonal cycles are

> Kapha season: mid-February to mid-June
> Pitta season: mid-June to mid-October
> Vata season: mid-October to mid-February

Although regional weather patterns may modify seasonal qualities to a certain degree, or alter the time periods somewhat for each season, basically these dosha seasons apply throughout the Northern hemisphere. In some areas, such as Hawaii or Southern California, Pitta season lasts most of the year, while in Alaska, it's either Vata or Kapha season nearly year-round. Even in these areas, however, there is at least a subtle shift in the seasons that is noticeable to those who live there. The dosha effects of the weather also can change dramatically, even in a single day; there can be sudden shifts from a hot, humid day (Pitta), to a cool, windy evening (Vata), frequently following a late afternoon thunderstorm (Kapha).

From an Ayur-Vedic perspective, changes in diet and routine to accommodate your bodymind responses to the changing seasons are just as natural as putting on an extra sweater on an autumn day, or reaching for a hat before going out into 110° noonday sun during an Arizona summer. You can become aware of seasonal health for a simple, easy way to understand and ingest some of nature's best medicine.

### KAPHA SEASON
#### (MID-FEBRUARY TO MID-JUNE)

Kapha season brings Kapha bodymind awareness. Quite simply, we get "spring fever," that kind of sweet "lie-on-the-grass-and-soak-up-the-sun" feeling, as our bodies seek to melt away the Kapha heaviness and coldness that has accumulated during a cool, damp winter. Often spring allergies flare up during Kapha season, as well as colds, pneumonia, bronchitis, and other conditions indicative of excess Kapha. We may start to feel that it's time to let go of our winter insulation which may have crept up around our hips and waistlines.

The effects of the season on your bodymind can also be understood in terms of the principle of opposites—vishesha—we considered earlier. Kapha's slow, static, heavy, oily, cold nature is opposed by quick, moving, light, dry, and warm qualities. You can benefit from increased exercise and lightening up your diet. For everyone, regardless of body type, the Kapha season is a good time to keep active and to increase exercise. Spring sunshine brings the feeling of "warm at last," so getting out and enjoying the spring sun, especially in the morning, is a good Kapha balancer. Treat signs of "spring fever" with an earlier bedtime, rather than an afternoon nap or "sleeping in": Daytime sleep and sleeping late in the morning increases Kapha.

You can adjust your eating routine, regardless of body type, to suit the Kapha season. Spicier, lighter, and drier foods, toasted or baked, are preferable to fried and oily, heavy foods.

The most Kapha-producing food to consume during Kapha season is ice cream. What could be more Kapha-increasing than an ice-cold, rich, creamy, sweet dessert? So avoiding it is ideal if you have excess Kapha. If you have a propensity for colds, asthma, bronchitis, or allergies at all, you will probably notice improvement, perhaps dramatic, if you reduce your intake of ice cream and other cold foods and drinks. If you are a strong Kapha type, you should definitely avoid ice cream and will benefit from following the Kapha-pacifying diet at this time of year.

## PITTA SEASON
### (MID-JUNE TO MID-OCTOBER)

Pitta season brings its natural heat and is a favorite season for Vata and Kapha types who must cope with their own qualities of cold along with the cold weather the rest of the year. But for Pitta types, the heat is on in more ways than one: They start longing for the coolness of the mountains with the first summer breeze. Everyone, not just Pitta types, can remain healthier during Pitta season by engaging in cooling activities, especially enjoying the water, which becomes more appealing now. But with the increase in outdoor activities, it's also important to guard against too much sun exposure, to which Pitta types within all races are particularly sensitive. Sunbathing is unhealthy for Pitta, because it increases the risk of skin cancer, which is already greater for Pitta types or for those with a Pitta imbalance.

However, ten minutes a day of early-morning sun is good for your health, from the Ayur-Vedic perspective. Try to avoid unnecessary exposure during the Pitta time of the day, between 10:00 A.M. and 2:00 P.M., when the sun's rays are most direct. And do any exercise during the cooler Kapha times—in early morning or evening: A great Pitta-balancing form of exercise is evening walking, especially in the moonlight, in the woods, or in the mountains.

During Pitta season, all dosha types can include more fresh fruits, especially juicy, cooling ones like melons or mangoes. Even when it's very hot, however, it's still preferable to avoid iced or cold beverages with meals, owing to their dampening effect on the digestive fire, the internal "cooker," which is also naturally set lower in the summer. Those who are strongly Vata or Kapha, or have weak digestion, will benefit by continuing to favor warm foods and drinks even in the summer. Pittas should not overdo spicy foods and should also take care not to overload on tomatoes, even those delicious ones fresh from the garden. Shellfish should similarly be eaten sparingly.

If too much Pitta accumulates during the summer, skin problems, urinary tract infections, and other inflammatory conditions tend to flare up by September, along with some irritability.

## VATA SEASON
### (MID-OCTOBER TO MID-FEBRUARY)

The first cool breaths of autumn winds blowing through leaves of changing colors can bring a refreshing reprieve from the heat of the Pitta season. Entering Vata season, however, calls for special attention to diet and daily routine for all body types, in order to keep Vata from increasing too much. Vata is associated with a rise in colds and flus, especially at the start and end of Vata season, early fall and early spring.

You may find that your sleep becomes lighter, your skin drier, and your bowels less regular at the onset of Vata season. This can be counteracted by increasing the amount of oils in your diet, doing a daily oil massage, and making sure that you go to bed during Kapha time. Following your natural desire for warm soups, hot casseroles, and hot drinks during Vata season will increase internal body heat and keep Vata pacified and your digestive fire strong.

Cold drafts on your head and neck area increase any vulnerability to Vata- and Kapha-related illness such as cold, flu, cough, etc. So during Vata season, you need to keep the head area in particular protected from the cold when going outdoors after an indoor workout, or while engaging in outdoor winter activities. (Yes, many of our mothers were Ayur-Vedically correct!)

The change of seasons is brought along by the movement of Vata dosha, and therefore Vata tends to increase temporarily *between* seasons. Moving Vata stirs up any accumulated ama collected from the previous season, which is why colds, for example, are so common at the change of the seasons. Eating a little less than usual, avoiding cold foods and drinks, as well as rich desserts, cheese, ice cream, and other heavy, hard-to-digest foods, and drinking hot water frequently will help keep your digestive fire and immune system strong and less vulnerable to a cold virus. With a little extra attention to getting rest and eating well at these times, Vata will stay balanced, and there will be less tendency to get sick.

Now let's turn to another daily life health program for which Ayur-Veda has some specific guidelines to help us maximize health and minimize the aging process.

## Exercise Based on Ayur-Vedic Principles

Exercise can fulfill two fundamental health-giving purposes, according to Ayur-Veda, to eliminate ama from the bodymind and to promote greater mind-body coordination. Its main purpose is not simply to "work out" your muscles or even your cardiovascular system. Muscular strength is only a very limited aspect of health, and exercise is only one factor affecting cardiovascular health. Exercise is most valuable when it serves to strengthen the connection between consciousness and your physiology, structuring health at a very fundamental level.

Therefore, the real key is to learn to exercise in a way that not only strengthens your body but also enhances its intelligence, orderliness, and all other qualities that underlie good health. This can happen when exercise becomes a medium through which your mind's attention becomes self-referral, creating a healthy, integrating feedback loop between mind and body. When this feedback loop is functioning well, exercise is not only safe and health-promoting but also blissful. This is the basis for the experience many athletes describe as being "in the zone," when time seems to slow down and even stop and their every move seems to be effortlessly and perfectly executed.

The Ayur-Vedic principles of exercise that follow are general, but, like all the Ayur-Vedic programs, the exercise principles support a customized approach to health based on individual doshas.

## THE THREE MAIN MAHARISHI AYUR-VEDIC EXERCISE PRINCIPLES

### 1. EXERCISE ACCORDING TO YOUR BODYMIND TYPE

If you are a Vata type, you inherently need less vigorous exercise. Regular daily exercise, yes, but not too strenuous. With your more delicate bone and joint structure, you would do well to choose brisk walking, hiking, swimming, or bicycling over more jarring activities such as jogging. Because of a natural enthusiasm for life and a love of movement, women with a predominantly Vata constitution tend to overdo physical activity, especially dance or aerobics, which they often love. Therefore, if you are Vata, be particularly alert to signs of increasing Vata dosha, such as shortness of breath, weakness in the muscles, or other signs of fatigue. Even before these signs occur, it's a good idea to rest, or some further imbalance in Vata may result.

Pitta-type women are often athletic, with moderate builds and good innate stamina, and can benefit from whatever exercise they enjoy. They generally love competitive sports or goal-oriented body-building, distance running, etc. If you are Pitta-predominant, the most important caveat is "Don't strain." If you are like most Pittas, you like to push yourself, and this tendency can make exercise a time when stress is accumulated rather than eliminated. You can be especially prone to overheating, dehydration, and sunstroke, so you'll find cooling exercise such as water sports (with sun protection) and winter sports particularly soothing and balancing.

Kapha types are the least likely to seek out exercise, because of their slower, more sedentary tendencies, but they are usually most in need of it. Kapha women may thus require the added incentive of joining a health club or enrolling in a regular dance or aerobics class. But because they have strong, well-lubricated joints and greater body mass, Kapha women can usually benefit from just about any kind of exercise. And because they have a generous proportion of muscle, they are especially good at endurance sports, such as distance rowing, running, and swimming. If you are a Kapha type, you can exercise to the point of "working up a good sweat," which is good for your specific bodymind, whereas it often signals overheating for Pitta or overexertion for Vata. It promotes the removal of excess fluid from your body and mobilizes congestion from your tissues, two conditions to which a Kapha type is prone.

### 2. EXERCISE IN ACCORD WITH DAILY DOSHA CYCLES

From the Ayur-Vedic viewpoint, the best time of the day for exercise is in the morning during Kapha time. If you exercise at this time, you counteract any Kapha tendencies and wake up your body. Kapha time is also the least likely time to disturb Vata and Pitta doshas, which are often too energetic and may become aggravated through exercising. It's best not to exercise during Pitta time (10:00 A.M. to 2:00 P.M.), in order not to interfere with digestion of the noon meal. If you exercise during Vata time in the later afternoon, 2:00 to 6:00 P.M., be sure you feel rested, as you may be opposing the natural tendency of your body to rest after the day's activity. A 15-minute easy walk in the evening after dinner is excellent for promoting proper digestion of the evening meal, when Kapha dosha is again most dominant.

### 3. EXERCISE ACCORDING TO YOUR BODYMIND RESPONSE AT THAT MOMENT

As we've seen, no particular exercise or amount of exercise is right for all the doshas; in this same way, no particular exercise or amount of exercise is right for any one person *all the time.* Because Ayur-Veda is a customized medical system, it can help you tune in to how your body changes hour by hour, day by day. As your body changes, so does its tolerance for exercise. Try not to exercise according to how much you think you ought to, or according to some arbitrary goal you have set. Consider how you feel at the moment. If you have a chance to learn the Ayur-Vedic technique of self–pulse assessment (see chapter 12), you can learn to monitor your physiology accurately at any time.

You can also use your heart rate to monitor your bodymind. Professional athletes are often instructed to take their pulses in the morning before arising. If the rate is ten or more beats above the usual, this means that some extra activity is going on in the body, perhaps fighting an infection, indicating that more rest is needed that day. Ayur-Vedically, an increased heart rate reflects an increase in Vata dosha, which is best counteracted by rest.

Of course, you don't have to take your heart rate every morning to be tuned in to your body; you can listen and not push beyond the point of comfort. This will keep you in a self-referral mode and help you avoid exercise that produces ill health. Pain or discomfort are signals that your awareness has lost connection with your body to the point of incurring damage. When you keep your mind and attention finely tuned, you maximize not only the cardiovascular and muscular benefits but strengthen the mind-body-integrating value of exercise.

### THREE OBVIOUS BUT NONETHELESS IMPORTANT EXERCISE CONSIDERATIONS

*1. Try not to exercise around mealtimes.* It is best to avoid vigorous exercise half an hour before a meal and one-and-a-half to two hours after a meal, so you aren't opposing the metabolism of digestion.

*2. Try not to exercise before sleep.* Exercise generally enlivens Vata dosha and is therefore less desirable before you want to sleep, although a short walk in the evening can be helpful for insomnia. It's better to prepare for sleep with the "sleep" dosha, Kapha, and save exercise for when you want to awaken daytime Kapha.

*3. Exercise with attention to your menstrual cycle.* During your monthly period, exercise should be much lighter than usual for all doshas; easy walking is best (see chapter 9).

### BODYMIND INTEGRATION THROUGH ASANAS

Another Ayur-Vedic approach to developing interconnectedness of mind and body is through the gentle waves of movement and rest

**123**

found in *asanas* (ah-sa-nuhs), which are a form of yoga exercise. Asanas are a sequence of comfortably held positions to stretch your body as you breathe. Asanas promote balance in the doshas, reduce stress, and enhance the connectedness of consciousness within your psychophysiology. They enable you to re-create a bodymind memory of full flow in a body that may sometimes feel like a static pond. They provide integrating movement that can be done as a prelude or warmup before more vigorous exercise, or independently, as part of a daily routine. This physical stretching, when combined with self-referral awareness, serves to dissolve stress. You may find yourself walking with more energy, breathing more fully, and feeling lighter, more integrated, and more joyful throughout your daily activities. You can learn the asanas at a Maharishi Ayur-Veda Health Center or through specific programs at a Transcendental Meditation Center.

In the meantime, we highly recommend the following home stretching program called *surya namaskar* (soo-ryuh nuh-muh-skahr), which means "salutation to the sun." It combines movement and breath, and it stretches the muscles and works all the joints simultaneously. The stretches are done in silence without music or talking, so you can keep your awareness comfortably on each movement.

### Surya Namaskar

1. The optimal time to perform this stretching exercise is in the morning before breakfast. If you are practicing the TM Program and/or are doing the asanas, this exercise should be done before both. If you want to do this exercise at other times of the day, it is best to do so at least half an hour prior to meals or at least three hours after meals.

2. See the diagram, which illustrates one full cycle of this yoga exercise.

3. A maximum of twelve cycles per exercise session is advised. The minimum depends on your level of comfort and enjoyment.

4. There are two "equestrian" positions per cycle. Alternate knees during each cycle, keeping the knee in a straight line with the foot, not pulled forward at an angle. You may

1. Salutation Position

*Normal, restful breathing*

2. Raised Arms Position

*Inhale*

3. Hand to Foot Position

*Exhale*

4. Equestrian Position

*Inhale*

5. Mountain Position

*Exhale*

6. Eight Limbs Position

*No breathing, then . . .*

7. Cobra Position

*Inhale*

8. Mountain Position

*Exhale*

9. Equestrian Position

*Inhale*

10. Hand to Foot Position

*Exhale*

11. Raised Arms Position

*Inhale*

12. Salutation Position

*Normal, restful breathing*

*Surya Namaskar* (Salutation to the Sun)

only be able to rest on your fingertips in this position, which is fine.

5. Hold each position for about five seconds. The one exception to this is the sixth position, which is held only momentarily.

6. Please note the breathing patterns recommended for surya namaskar. The inhale or exhale begins as you start to move into each new position. If you finish inhaling or exhaling before the end of the five-second "hold" period, then maintain the breath until the inhale or exhale of the next position starts.

7. As you assume the twelfth position, exhale for five seconds. If you continue into another cycle, breathe normally (as desired) for five seconds in Position 1 before moving into Position 2.

8. After completing the last cycle, lie down on your back, arms at your sides, palms facing up, for two minutes.

### THE EASE OF EXERCISE

An exercise and fitness program based on Maharishi Ayur-Veda principles has been developed with the help of Dr. John Douillard, a sports chiropractor, a former professional triathlete, and director of the Invincible Athlete Program.

The main rule for Ayur-Vedic exercise is this: *Be easy and do not strain.* In general, says Dr. Douillard, we should exercise to about half of our capacity (not to the 70- to 80-percent capacity currently popular). If you can just barely survive an hour and a half of vigorous tennis, then forty-five minutes should be your time for now: Increased stamina will come as you continue to play for forty-five minutes on a regular basis.

Exercise should be done while breathing through your nose, unless there is some nasal blockage. The Ayur-Vedic rule is not to exert yourself beyond the point that you need to breathe through your mouth. This is the simplest indicator point of oxygen debt, telling you that your muscles require oxygen that is not being provided. To exercise beyond this point will create stress, age the body, and defeat the purpose of exercise. As you continue to exercise only up to the point of needing to breathe through your mouth, you'll soon be breathing and working out far more effi-ciently, exercising effectively but with a comfortable, stress-free physiology. We can and must learn to do at 130 heartbeats per min-ute what you are used to doing at 175 beats per minute; it's a far healthier route to go, increasing your cardiovascular efficiency and strength while maintaining balance and comfort without strain.

### SUGGESTIONS FOR AEROBIC WORKOUTS

If you do an at-home aerobic exercise program or go to an aerobics class, here are some suggestions[3] to help you avoid aging as you ex-ercise:

1. Do at least a ten-minute gentle warmup, keeping your heart rate under 100 *before* you do any stretching. This warms up your muscles.

2. Do some stretching before the aerobic workout.

3. Take your heart rate about every ten to fifteen minutes. If you are under thirty, keep your heart rate under 150. If you are over thirty, keep your heart rate under 130, or you are aging your body.

4. Breathe primarily through your nose throughout the workout. Unless you have a nasal problem, you are working too hard if you can't get enough air. This is all the information you need to decide to slow down.

5. Don't talk while you work out. You want your body and mind to be perfectly in tune with each other for maximum benefit and integration.

6. Keep your attention on three things: (1) your breathing, (2) your form, and (3) your level of bliss. Self-referral questions such as "How am I feeling right now?" can help you determine whether your bodymind is enjoying and flowing with or work-ing against the workout. The goal is to feel good throughout the session.

7. Take at least ten minutes to cool down. Stretch every part of your body that you've worked out and then lie down on your back and rest silently for at least two minutes. Take your heart rate afterward. It should be well under 100.

In the following chapter we'll discuss how your tissues and cells are organized to keep you healthy; how imbalances in the doshas can lead to illness; and how Ayur-Veda can help you create balance in your doshas and help provide a more profound experience of vibrant health than you may have ever imagined.

# Chapter 5

### INTELLIGENCE

## Facilitating the Flow
## of Biological Intelligence
## to Restore Our Health

*If you always remember the real nature of things,
you get rid of misery and illness.*

Charaka Samhita

Dr. Louis W. Sullivan, former U.S. Secretary of Health and Human Services, observed that "Americans today are taking a more active interest in their health than ever before. They are coming to realize the influence that they themselves have on their own health destinies and overall health status of the nation." He pointed out that because medical care alone will not eliminate the devastating impact of chronic disease, it is crucial that we build a "culture of character" in our population—a culture of thinking and being that actively promotes responsible behavior and life-styles that are maximally conducive to good health.

Some think we can overdo it. We now have a societal preoccupation with being healthy, writes John Poppy, to the point of "medicalizing enjoyment," of doing things such as jogging simply because they are good for our health. But doing enjoyable things for our health may be one of the best societal preoccupations we could have. We desperately need this kind of national attention on health, because, as David Sobel, M.D., a specialist in preventive medicine, reports, "Virtually everyone over the age of fifty has one or more chronic diseases—arthritis, cardiovascular disease, cancer, high blood pressure, whatever—to some degree." Dr. Suresh Rattan, a molecular gerontologist, concurs: "At fifty, just when we have learned how to live, just when we are finally ready to give something back to society, we start to fall apart . . . such a waste!"

So we find ourselves about to enter the twenty-first century with a collective goal of wanting good health and working hard to have it, yet finding ourselves becoming sick. It would seem that we should be able to eliminate illnesses and fulfill our national desire for health. But first, we have to rethink what prevents us from fulfilling this desire.

## Stress: The Common Factor in Illness

In modern medical thinking, the term that best describes impediments to normal psychophysiological functioning is *stress*. Stress can be defined as any event or condition that produces imbalance in your bodymind, causing it to have to adapt in order to restore balance, often inappropriately gearing it up for an illusory battle. A variety of illnesses are currently grouped under the heading "stress-related."

Stress is not endemic to any particular culture nowadays, but is associated with high-paced living the world over. In Japan, for example, a nation noted for the unique longevity of its citizenry, a new stress-related condition, *karoshi*, is defined as "early death from overwork." But does the work or the reaction of the person to the work bring this about? We know that more people die of heart attacks on Monday morning at 9:00 A.M. than at any other time of the week. The idea of work and what it represents to us may be more lethal than work itself. The conclusion is that stress may be internally or externally created, but it's how you *respond* to it that matters. One of your friends may go to a loud concert and come away frazzled with jangled nerves, whereas another friend is ready and eager to go again the next night.

We are now learning to handle stress from the inside. The concept of "managing stress" has emerged today in reference to life-style programs designed to provide respite from modern life. They include aerobic exercise, a healthy diet, and other bodymind technologies that result in an increased sense of well-being and are designed to reduce the risk of falling ill from stress-related diseases such as hypertension.

Stress also has a specific *medical* meaning. It identifies a common quality of illness itself, hidden and unseen as long as each disease, with its own list of symptoms and treatments, is analyzed separately. This is at once a very new and very old realization.

For years within the Western medical profession, all illnesses were considered separate and distinct in cause and condition. It seems unbelievable, with what we now know, that we are still relying on this approach. Public and private funding for health research and treatment continues to be allocated "by disease," whether to the cancer wing of a hospital or to a national disease foundation, whether cystic fibrosis, arthritis, diabetes, or sickle cell anemia. But wouldn't we be doing a better job if we found out not only the distinguishing characteristics of each disease but also what diseases have *in common?*

Dr. Hans Selye, who originated the term "stress," recalls the time when he was a young medical student making the rounds of the various parts of a hospital that was typically organized by kinds of illnesses: "I saw people who were sick with this disease and sick with that disease. There was something about it that was in the back of my mind and I couldn't quite place it. They had something in common that nobody had identified." One day, as Selye was walking down a corridor, he suddenly thought, "Of course, they're all sick and they all *look* sick. And there's something they share— some kind of 'stress' that goes beyond the particulars of what they're sick with." Selye's great discovery was that underlying all illness, there is something that overrides the distinctions between illnesses and refers to an overall lack of functioning.

Modern medicine has incorporated some of Selye's thinking and softened a few of its hard, categorical definitions. Doctors acknowledge that when we can eliminate the effects of stress from our daily functioning, we can establish far better conditions for healing, regardless of what organ or process is primarily involved.

Maharishi Ayur-Veda goes much further and deeper, identifying a stress disorder in our physiology that is associated with and underlies all disease, and proposing that disease, *any* disease, takes hold when a person loses touch with the innermost level of consciousness, with nature's inner program, with a most potent source of "internal" medicine. Diseases thus represent episodes of disorder in biological systems that normally function in an orderly way. Disease results when part of the bodymind "forgets" the experience of wholeness on which its smooth, integrated functioning ultimately depends.

This separation of the part from the whole is identified in Maharishi Ayur-Veda as the real cause of sickness. In its most obvious consequence, it is the malignant tumor that has decided to grow on its own, without regard for the rest of the body. Or it can express itself as an extreme mind and body separation, such as happens with anorexia nervosa. When a sixteen-year-old girl weighing seventy pounds looks in the mirror and sees her emaciated profile as "fat," her way of seeing has started to act like a distorting mirror in an amusement park. She has lost touch with her own being and doesn't even realize that she is sick. This occurs when the body and mind are most separated, and the concept of "bodymind" as a single expression of life has fallen apart.

### Who or What Is Responsible for Disease?

How does disease happen to us individually? What is our own role in the bringing about of disease? In a *Boston Globe* article, Linda Weltner recalls a sick friend asking the question, "How can I understand the presence of this illness in my life?" While it's natural to question the "why" of an illness, the answer ought not to occasion a psychological rehashing of all one's stressful, life-damaging feelings, thoughts, and actions. Research indicates that this kind of negative self-analysis or "advice" from well-meaning friends and family is not helpful. No matter what the circumstances, it's hardly useful to hear, "Michelle brought this on herself." What *is* helpful is unconditional love and support, both toward ourselves and from our friends. In a study conducted at UCLA, researchers found that the best contributions family or friends could make to a cancer patient's recovery were love, support, calm concern, and mainly "just being there."[1]

For those of us who have been seriously ill or been around someone who is, we are well aware that this *loving attention* is a very real medicine. It is important to keep remembering this, whether we are the sick individual or whether we are tending a sick person. When one is very ill, simply getting out of bed can be the equivalent of climbing Mount Everest. Acknowledging the huge amount of energy, risk, and mental and emotional stamina—the courage to be ill and to want to get well—is the most healing and loving thing we can do for ourselves or for our friends.

But when we get sick, many of us *do* wonder, "Did I give myself this disease for a reason?" The answer will vary according to our private belief systems. Some of us will feel we did contribute to the process and may feel a sense of control and inner reorganization as a result; some of us will most definitely feel we did not. As the poet Audre Lorde wrote, "[Although] I do believe I have aided my body in fighting cancer . . . , I totally reject the idea that we are responsible."

To be told to think positively, to be told to rethink your illness, is not in keeping with the understanding of unified field healing in which your body and mind are *already* united and interdependent. Our thoughts, emotions, and physical experiences are already joined at the deepest levels of our bodymind. Anger, depression, joy, and elation, according to this model, all have their own physiologies and are merely fluctuations in the bodymind field. And this is what the latest PNI research recognizes as well.

While we may not be responsible for our diseases, we are responsible for our health. As an essential prevention system, Maharishi Ayur-Veda enables us to understand and enliven the connection between consciousness and health. What do we mean by this connection? Usually when we talk about our body, we mean our physical body, but underlying our physical body are the more subtle levels of our functioning: our ego, our intellect, our mind, and our emotions. And underlying those aspects of awareness is your self in its universal consciousness. Your physical body takes direction from these deeper levels of your bodymind, recreating and transforming itself depending on your emotions, desires, ideas, notions, beliefs, and intellect (which themselves reflect a deeper union with the unified field).

This understanding helps clarify some confusion in recent

bodymind healing techniques: We don't repair the immune system or any other bodymind system simply with a thought. The thought has to be connected to a field of healing, to an underlying field of consciousness. Positive thinking that does not go deep into a person's physiology and awaken this self-healing field is not going to change cellular functioning. When we enliven our resource of consciousness, we help our bodymind to remember its own intelligence, its own healing nature, to effortlessly maintain and promote the balancing of our doshas. This gives us a whole new vision of illness, with regard to diagnosis and treatment. It helps us to recognize that disease is not something separate from us, or something that is simply out of our control, or something that only the medical profession can attend to.

Sometimes, however, we may need further assistance from a physician. This doesn't mean we have "failed" in our responsibility to ourselves; we are simply taking whatever additional steps may be necessary to allow our physiology to regain the memory of its own good health. The healing process is always an inner one: It is consciousness transforming itself, returning the bodymind back to itself, restoring it to its original nature.

## Allowing Self-Healing

As modern medicine is beginning to realize at last, only the bodymind can really repair itself. At best, a physician may help create the conditions for healing, and this applies even to specific medical procedures. If, for example, a urinary tract infection is treated with a typical (sulfa-type) antibiotic, the antibiotic does not actually kill the bacteria; it merely slows its growth so that the body's defenses can catch up and get rid of infection more quickly. Many antibiotics work in this way, inhibiting growth rather than actually destroying the disease-causing organism: *It is the bodymind itself which is the healer, not the antibiotic.*

Many of us have intuitively understood that the majority of diseases and preconditions that doctors routinely treat via their prescription pads would eventually go away by themselves through innate healing mechanisms, if one's immune system were basically strong.

Some years ago, the *New England Journal of Medicine* published an article by its then editor, Dr. Franz Ingelfinger, in which he encouraged physicians and patients alike to have more confidence in their own impeccably designed healing systems. He observed that perhaps 80 percent of all patients have either self-limiting illnesses (which will eventually go away on their own) or illnesses that modern medicine can't cure. He further observed (and research has since corroborated) that of the remaining 20 percent, around half are dramatically helped and around half are misdiagnosed or just have "bad luck." So even with the most advanced drug and surgical technologies, our bodies are still required to respond and work in concert with these strategies to effect the healing response.

Often, the drugs and surgery may not be necessary at all. Simple changes in our daily lives are all that may be required. We know, for instance, that a significant percentage of all cancers are directly linked to what we eat. The exciting research conducted by Dr. Dean Ornish at the University of California at San Francisco and published in the British medical journal *Lancet* found that *changes in life-style alone* (a routine consisting of a low-fat vegetarian diet, little alcohol, and no caffeine, along with yoga exercises and stress-management techniques including meditation) reversed the damage caused by cardiovascular heart disease in as little as twelve months, with *no* recourse to drugs or surgery.

Other studies have demonstrated that a meditation practice alone can have dramatic effects on health. Research psychologist David Orme-Johnson and his colleagues found that the rate of hospital admissions for cardiovascular disease was 87 percent lower for practitioners of the Transcendental Meditation technique than for those in a matched sample of nonmeditators over a five-year period.[2] (Additional longitudinal studies have shown that regular practitioners of the TM technique have a significant lowering of unhealthy cholesterol levels over time, as compared to a matched control group eating the same diet, corroborating other studies that indicate that decreasing stress leads to more normal levels of cholesterol in the blood).[3]

The underlying reason why these programs work is a simple one: *We are reestablishing healthy functioning when we give our bodymind an opportunity to reset itself.*

So the real work of the physician and/or healer is to bring us back to ourselves. As Dr. Albert Schweitzer pointed out decades ago, "Each patient carries his own doctor inside him. They come to us not knowing that cure. We are at our best when we give the doctor who resides within each patient the chance to go to work."[4] This self-healer within the bodymind is the doctor within us. True health exists, we are reminded, when nature is allowed to be itself. Once we take our awareness inward to this internal healer, it's the most natural thing in the world to be well and keep well.

Moreover, the experience of this self-healing aspect of medicine brings the realization that a disease is not separate from our body nor something that happens *to* our body; rather, it *is* our body, albeit a body that has become progressively out of balance. But because the body has a high biological IQ, it can also remember how to heal itself.

As most of us realize, ideal medicine does not cure disease, it prevents it from arising in the first place. Prevention has to start before a person first becomes aware of subtle imbalances or disturbances, whether they are physical, mental, or emotional. Before we are actually aware that we are sick, a great deal already has gone awry in the bodymind. If the disturbances continue for too long, a disease will become apparent, whether it's arthritis or manic-depression or colon cancer, depending on our history and our dosha imbalances. But it's really not wise to wait until an illness gets a name before treating the condition that is causing it.

Ayur-Veda gives us a different outlook on illness. In modern medicine, once we identify a disease by name, the temptation is to push the illness outside ourselves. By categorizing people by the diseases they manifest (cancer patients, heart patients, or AIDS patients), the reasons why a particular individual has that particular set of symptoms are disregarded. And we end up wondering why one person gets heart disease and another person with an almost identical history does not. In Ayur-Vedic terms, the focus is not on the disease category, but rather on the imbalances within the individual's bodymind that create symptoms. From the modern medical perspective, one person with tonsillitis is like another person with tonsillitis. From the Ayur-Vedic perspective, these patients may have symptoms of tonsillitis for very different reasons. The emphasis in Ayur-Veda is not only on treating the symptoms, but on getting the individual's system back into balance and eliminating the cause of the symptoms.

## The Lost Connection

Maharishi Ayur-Veda sees disease originating as a result of the breakdown of the bodymind's own integrity based on its loss of contact with the unified field. We don't really catch a flu; our immune system breaks down and only then is a flu bug "catchable." But before the immune system can break down, the connection between nature's program and the body has been weakened.

For thousands of years, Ayur-Veda has recognized and tested this "missing link" between health and disease, locating its origins first in the separation from inner intelligence, leading to behavioral problems such as wrong choices in diet, daily routine, and lifestyle. This can lead to an imbalance in the doshas, resulting in weakened digestion and excess wastes accumulating in the tissues. The entire process from health to disease is both sequential and simultaneous.

Rather than focus on the wide variety of diseases that may develop, Ayur-Veda focuses on two main processes: *How the body's balance is maintained and how the body's balance breaks down.* It is these processes which lay the groundwork for health or disease in the first place and provide the knowledge and conditions for healing. As a result, Ayur-Vedic routines and treatment programs for various illnesses sound far more alike than different, particularly since they generally focus on balancing the doshas and eliminating the blocks to such balance.

Now we're going to explore more deeply the two essential situations that Ayur-Veda addresses, imbalance and balance. First we'll delve into what can happen when we lose the connection to our biological intelligence within, leading to specific causes of imbalance that set us on a course of illness. Then we'll look at what good health is and how it ought to feel; what you experience when you remember wholeness and your intimate connection with nature's intelligence.

## The Origins of Illness: The Metabolic Breakdown

The Ayur-Vedic tradition has long understood the key role of metabolism in the sickness-health continuum. Modern medical researchers are now beginning to reach similar conclusions. In a recent article published in the *Journal of the American Medical Association* entitled "When Does Diabetes Start?" an endocrinologist from the Johns Hopkins University School of Medicine commented on research that indicates that adult-onset diabetes is not merely a disease of high blood sugar with attendant long-term effects on the other body tissues. Rather, the high blood sugar previously considered the "cause" of the other problems associated with diabetes is really only one symptom of a deeper, underlying metabolic disturbance of both sugar and fat, signs of which are evident long before the blood sugar is clinically high enough to be classified as diabetes. In other words, diabetes doesn't suddenly appear in full-blown form for unknown reasons. It is a fairly late road sign along a path that medical research can now identify as a long-term, gradual disturbance in digestion and metabolism.

Findings such as these are highly significant for anyone who is ill or has the preconditions for illness, because they enable both the individual and the medical profession to take preventive measures before a disease manifests in a serious, life-threatening way. Ayur-Veda allows us to identify the antecedent conditions of disease as they manifest, allowing us to understand how we can be "a little sick" or "not totally well," and still be treated effectively.

Ayur-Veda's focus on dosha-specific prevention and sequential cure begins with our digestive processes. Although most of us give little thought to our digestion—unless we've overdone holiday feasting or succumbed to a gastrointestinal flu—the process of eating, digesting, metabolizing, and eliminating are the most fundamental physiological activities that support our health on a day-to-day basis. The most important daily task of your body is its own re-creation, and the energy and building blocks for that reconstruction are supplied most consistently by the food you eat, and more subtly by the "food" you eat mentally and emotionally—by what you read, whom you fall in love with, how you feel about your job, and so forth.

No matter what you take in, physically, mentally, or emotionally, you go through a similar process of digestion. It is the task of your bodymind to break these experiences and substances down completely, absorb them efficiently, metabolize them properly, and eliminate the resultant wastes effectively. Otherwise, what happens?

On the gross physical level, we might get up in the morning, look in the mirror, and discover a tongue with a thick coating on it. This is a tongue that did not just suck on a Tums. So we may wonder, "What's that?" Or we may wake up feeling stiff everywhere, particularly in our joints, neck, and spine and feel as though we had run a marathon the day before. The trouble is that we didn't—but we do perhaps recall having eaten several big meals. Or we awaken feeling heavily congested, even though it's the middle of summer and no flu is going around at the moment. By Western medical standards, there's nothing really wrong here. By Ayur-Vedic standards, we are showing specific and important preconditions of illness that could take root in a more serious way. Primarily, we are showing clear signs of digestive disorders: A coated tongue, muscle and joint pain, and congestion are all the results (depending on our doshas) of improperly digested food. So, too, are other symptoms such as gas, constipation, frequent loose stools, skin rashes, and loss of appetite. But what do we do with this information?

Like modern medicine itself, until very recently, few of us have paid much attention to subtle manifestations of digestive disorders that are not yet an ulcer, a tumor, or an obstructing gallstone. And so it may feel strangely new to ask what happens when food is not processed properly and wastes not eliminated completely. Ayur-Veda encourages us to ask such questions because it considers the consequences of inefficient digestion to be a primary physical cause of disease, readying us for the development of illnesses such as cancer, cardiovascular disease, arthritis, and menstrual disorders. So let's take a closer look at the Ayur-Vedic description of how digestive and metabolic pre-illness occurs.

## The Illusion of Separation: The Ultimate Source of Disease

Maharishi Ayur-Veda tracks the ultimate source of disease back to the mind's illusory separation from nature's intelligence. When the mind is well connected to consciousness, the body is fully nurtured. Just as a slight intention in your mind can move your arms through the air against gravity, so your mind is perfectly capable of regulating all aspects of the body's movement and chemistry in ever subtler and more complex ways at every moment. But this is not simply your own personal thinking. It is your biological intelligence at work, and the more you are in tune with this harmonizing resource, the more naturally and spontaneously healthy you are. When every cell in your body remembers the reality of underlying wholeness and knows itself to be invincible, then you are perfectly healthy.

How did we lose this experience of wholeness and invincibility in the first place? Maharishi Ayur-Veda describes the process of this loss as *pragya aparadh* (pruh-gyah-uh-puh-rahd), "the mistake of the intellect." The mistake occurs when the intelligence in any given aspect of our psychophysiology becomes so absorbed in its own small individual life that it loses sight of the unity underlying its existence. Without its biological intelligence fully operative, one part of the body can get partially or entirely disconnected from the whole, because the good health of each and every cell relies on the unrestricted exchange of information with every other cell.

For example, a tumor cell seems to concern itself with its own life and forgets its connection with the rest of the body: Its mistake is that it sees itself only as separate. Cut off from the knowledge of how it's supposed to behave in the context of the entire system, oblivious, perhaps due to defects in its DNA, to the shared cellular knowledge of eons of learning, the tumor begins to act out of concert with the collective good and takes off on a path of noxious growth, spreading destruction. (It's interesting that the word "malignancy" comes from *malign* which means "to speak ill of others." In the case of a tumor, there is a certain inappropriate egotism and a going against the needs of the other cells; a tumor cell thought might thus be, "Who cares about the rest of the body? I'm going to reproduce, become powerful, and take over.") The only way to correct this mistake is for the cell to remember its true nature.

We can further understand the consequences of the mistake of the intellect by seeing how it manifests in our daily lives as stress.

### The Essential Cause of Stress: Restricted Vision

According to the findings of psychologist Richard Lazarus and his colleagues at the University of California at Berkeley, the negative health-related symptoms of stress come more from the chronic, cumulative effects of everyday hassles, the wear and tear of daily life, than from the major life traumas, such as the death of a loved one. Furthermore, these hassles affect us all differently. This means that how we deal with them is far more important to our health than the events themselves.[5]

We can easily observe that what may be stressful for one person may be exhilarating for another. To an adventurous pilot, the wild bumps and sudden drops of her single engine plane are challenging and exciting, but to the average airplane traveler, turbulence usually creates some anxiety. Who we are and what we bring to an experience are far more significant than the experience itself. When our perspective is limited, everything can seem overwhelming and stress can dominate our awareness. But the situation can just as easily change. We may fret over an inconvenience in our weekend schedule or bemoan the loss of an investment, but the moment we stop to count our blessings, we adopt a broader perspective, and the stress we had been focusing on immediately recedes.

Maharishi Ayur-Veda helps us to recognize that if our awareness could be infinitely expanded to the unified field underlying all the changes in our lives, no event would be stressful. Our physiology would be so healthy and strong that even apparently stressful experiences would bounce off us without leaving much of an impression. Not that we would respond inappropriately; in fact, we'd probably respond even more appropriately without the accompanying fear.

Thus, we would spontaneously possess the knack of seeing all our life experiences in a bigger and perhaps more positive light, realizing that whatever is happening to us at the moment serves some beneficial purpose, if we are able to recognize it and work with it.

Imagine a large construction site surrounded by a big plywood barrier with some small peepholes. Looking down at the site through one of the tiny peepholes, you can only see a few workers and a small part of the work area. You might believe that this small area is the whole building site. But when the barrier is taken down, you realize that although your small view is still there in its entirety, you now see the full setting, the whole enterprise. The group of workers you saw before is still doing the same thing—but is no longer the dominant focus of your awareness.

The fundamental factor in prevention and healing lies not in restriction but in expansion, in expanding your bodymind awareness to overcome pragya aparadh and thereby to open yourself to a wider range of possibilities. This applies to any of the interactions between body, mind, and emotions.

## Ama: Blockages to Health

It could be clogged arteries, the loneliness of a closed heart, arthritic immobilization, writer's block, or what is called cellulite. Or it can even be a doubting thought, such as "I'll never be able to . . ." It can result in a universe of skepticism, where one feels bound and restricted. Ayur-Veda calls the cause of these conditions *ama*, that which builds up in the body and prevents our connection with the unified field, disallowing smooth psychological or physical functioning. Its opposite qualities are superfluidity, lightness, and flexibility built on a foundation of deep stability. No matter where or how it manifests, ama is characterized by the many consequences of poor digestion of food or experience, the unnecessary baggage that can slow down or completely impede any aspect of our psychophysiological experiences. Like carbon buildup in an automobile, ama buildup is not a good thing. It can occur anytime when our awareness is not fully established in the unified field of consciousness.

The concept of ama helps us visualize the process of illness as a series of obstructions to our full psychophysiological function-ing. Accumulated ama eventually results in a breakdown in the body's homeostatic (balancing) mechanisms, leading to aging and to disease, whether primarily identified as physical, mental, or emotional. It may initially block our arteries, our mental acuity, our eyesight, our hearing, or restrict our ability to experience and express love, happiness, satisfaction, optimism, bliss, or any of the other mental and emotional correlates of good health and longevity.

Improperly digested food particles are the principal reason for the buildup of physical ama—any toxin or waste not utilizable by the body as food. But while poorly digested food is the principle source of ama, it has several other causes: Excesses of *any* by-products of metabolism that build up in our bodies because of overproduction or underelimination are also a type of ama. These excesses might include uric acid causing gouty arthritis or certain components of bile, a kind of "sludge" that forms gallstones or "bad" cholesterol.

The major problem with bodily ama lies in its propensity to in-crease in the body's tissues over time. This leads to several difficul-ties. The primary effect is blockage. Just as an accumulation of shoes, suitcases, and boxes in the front hallway can block our pas-sage to and from home, so ama particles block the dynamic flow of functioning, whether in the digestive track or in the communi-cation channels between brain cells, or anywhere else in our psychophysiology. This can occur on the deepest level of the bodymind, where ama can block the flow of biological intelligence itself, the steps of knowledge required to organize the cellular me-tabolism that re-creates body tissues.

Moreover, the buildup of ama can provoke the onset of any number of illnesses by blocking the minute channels through which nutrients, oxygen-rich blood, hormones, and immune cells flow to cleanse and revitalize every cell of the body. When ama ac-cumulates, even a few small areas of bodymind functioning can start to receive a smaller and less adequate share of this nutritional bathing. They can then begin to weaken in a stagnant pool of met-abolic wastes, cut off from the body's cleanup crews, such as the macrophages of the immune system. The overload of fat or fluid that forms as a variety of cysts, or excess secretions of mucus expressed as allergies, may be the result of a Kapha imbalance. An inflammatory reaction might result from a Pitta imbalance and show up as rheumatoid arthritis or any of the various autoimmune disorders such as common forms of hyperthyroidism, colitis, or systemic lupus erythematosis—or as more vague disorders, such as skin rashes. If ama blocks joint movement and the production of synovial fluid, it may be the result of a Vata imbalance, which can cause cracking joints, neck pain, the chronic aches and pain of fibromyalgias, or the loss of cartilage and overproduced bone growth at the joints, resulting in osteoarthritis.

Toxic chemicals such as certain nitrates, drugs, pollutants, pesticides, cigarette smoke, alcohol, and preservatives ingested through our air, water, food, medical therapies, or bad habits can also get stored in the bodily tissues as a form of ama. These chemicals often lead to the overproduction of "free radicals," molecules in our blood that can cause any number of serious illnesses.

### Ama, AGEs, and Free Radicals

The complications of diabetes provide a good example of the concept of ama. One of the recent studies on the mechanism of long-term complications of diabetes indicates that the excess glucose that builds up in the blood and tissues of diabetics has a direct and damaging effect on various bodily tissues. Dr. Anthony Cerami and his colleagues at the Rockefeller University Medical Biochemistry Laboratory have been working for years to discover just how this excess sugar can destroy tissue and accelerate the aging process. They have found that a chemical reaction takes place between sugar and protein molecules, resulting in "sticky" particles called AGEs (advanced glycosylation endproducts). These AGEs stick to the surrounding protein molecules (the building blocks of a number of important body tissues), binding them into an abnormal, latticelike structure in a process called "cross-linking." Cross-linking has been found to create conditions for aging, including accelerating arterioschlerosis (hardening of the arteries), dimming vision through cataract formation, damaging kidneys and lungs, and tightening the tendons that connect muscles to bones, causing stiffness and lack of flexibility. Studies in bacteria already have shown that even DNA can be damaged by AGEs, laying the groundwork for mutations that could result in various forms of cancer.

If we look at this discovery from an Ayur-Vedic perspective, excess glucose is clearly a form of ama (an excess metabolic by-product not being used or eliminated properly by the body) that results from improper digestion and metabolism, accumulates in the tissues of the body, and causes formation of sticky AGE substances, which cause disease or degeneration in the surrounding tissues.

Another common pathway for many ama-associated illnesses is the generation of *free radicals*, which are chemically unstable molecules, usually derivatives of oxygen molecules. When free radicals are produced too fast, the body is unable to break them down chemically, causing the destruction of nearby tissues. Some of this damage occurs as the result of our exposure to the sun, pesticides, air pollution, chemotherapy, radiation, processed foods, certain drugs, and cigarette smoke.

Free radicals are not ordinarily inappropriately destructive; they are part of the natural metabolism of the body, being generated from the food we eat and the oxygen we breathe. As long as one's body can quickly neutralize the free radicals after they are formed, with the help of certain enzymes such as "superoxide dismutase" (or SOD), which we all have, then no harm is done. If free radical generation gets out of hand, however, perhaps owing to an over-abundance of toxins or an overactive immune system, then tissue damage starts to occur. Eventually this will influence the process of disease and accelerate the aging process. Indeed, medical researchers now believe that an overwhelming majority of diseases, as well as the aging process itself, involve excessive free radical generation in some way: Current research studies are finding a link between too many free radicals and heart disease and cancer.

So how do we keep free radicals on the healthiest path?

A fundamental principle in Ayur-Vedic healing is that nature provides an antidote or balancing factor for any imbalance that may occur. This certainly applies in the case of free radicals: Many naturally occurring foods have been found to contain substances that have "antioxidant" or free-radical-neutralizing properties: Whole grains, fresh fruit, and vegetables keep us healthy because they are rich in antioxidants. At present, researchers at several medical institutions are currently studying the effects of an Ayur-Vedic herb compound called *Maharishi Amrit Kalash* (uhm-riht-kuh-luhsh), or MAK, which has been formulated from ancient Ayur-Vedic prescriptions. Japanese immunologist Yukie Niwa, a renowned authority on free radical generation and antioxidant treatment, conducted research on MAK as a scavenger of free radicals.[6] He found MAK to be more effective than any of 500 other known free-radical scavengers previously studied. It also was found to be nontoxic. These preliminary results have been repeated by researchers at Loyola University.[7] The research on free-radical scavenging and Ayur-Veda has really just gotten under way, but it may have important implications for reducing coronary artery disease, cancer, and aging. (See chapter 12 for the results of other research on MAK.)

## Overcoming Separation, Stress, and Ama

The internally toxic effects of life experiences, emotions, interpersonal interactions, thoughts, and addictions that are experienced as clearly negative also result in ama. These damaging mental and emotional states generally produce simultaneously damaging physical correlates (toxins) in the body, such as excess acid in the stomach, excess adrenaline, or imbalanced neurotransmitters. If not metabolized and eliminated, or if our bodymind is chronically bathed in a biochemistry of fear, hate, aggression, or stress, we may well experience the toxicity of physical ama, along with a kind of "mental" ama that resides in the memory banks of our brains. This mental ama can result in the perpetuation of negative emotions and negative responses in a number of behaviorally repetitive situations throughout our lives.

At every moment, whether we are sound asleep, or dreaming of medieval castles, talking with a friend on the phone, driving through rush-hour traffic, eating a meal, or doing several things at once, we are continually molding, restructuring, and reordering our physiology. Almost all the current research on mind-body medicine is verifying this commonsense observation, which has been grossly ignored and misunderstood in the West for centuries. We are now, however, beginning to recognize and accept, both as patients and doctors, that consciousness *creates* our psychophysiology.

The logical consequence of this understanding is that disease in your body reflects what is going on in your mind, at least to some degree, because bodies and minds are not separate from each other. Ama in our nervous systems thus represents the biochemical imprint of incompletely "digested" or unresolved mental or emotional experiences. Almost all mental and emotional difficulties we face are the results of poorly learned patterns of behavior and interaction. Therapy of whatever kind generally must address the issues of unlearning and relearning. As reported in the *American Journal of Psychiatry,* even a computer program that teaches depressed patients how to "unlearn" their pessimistic responses to rejection and other life defeats was found by University of Wisconsin researchers to work as well as therapy with a therapist.[8]

Maharishi Ayur-Veda offers a sophisticated and elegant model of how changing brain patterns can change behavior. Rather than work through the cognitive processes, we can enjoy a process such as Transcendental Meditation, an easily-learned mental technique that quiets down the mind and deeply rests the body, giving us a way to transcend the reasoning brain and experience a direct hookup with our own physiology. What can this do for us? In a word, it can dissolve stress effectively and help us develop a better-functioning bodymind, thereby adding high-quality years to our lives, well beyond what many of us might expect, given our genetic backgrounds, our carcinogenic environments, our chronological age, or whatever appears to limit us.

A recent study attests to the ability of individuals to systematically ingest this mental "longevity factor" directly through the practice of TM.[9] At Harvard University, research psychologists Charles Alexander and Ellen Langer and their colleagues evaluated the effects of three different self-development programs on elderly nursing-home patients (with an average age of 81 years). Most strikingly, 100 percent of the TM group subjects were alive three years after the program began, in contrast to the lower survival rates for the other treatment groups and controls and to the 62.5 percent survival rate for others in the population pool from where the subjects were drawn. Moreover, the subjects practicing TM showed significant improvement on three measures of cognitive flexibility compared with controls and subjects in other treatment groups, and had significantly lower systolic blood pressure. The authors concluded that "changes in state of consciousness . . . through specific mental techniques can indeed mediate substantive improvements in the health . . . of the elderly." They also noted that *the benefits resulted from a self-referential technique rather than an external program* and that "the great advantage of practicing a self-referential mental technique is that it opens the possibility of empowerment from within." From the perspective of Ayur-Veda, the subjects were fully in touch with a real basis of healing. The resulting bodymind changes were apparently far more significant than any psychological feeling, emerging as a substantive measure of cellular invincibility. The strengthening of the bodymind from deep within permeated the entire cell system.

We've explored how the primary cause of disease is understood to be the bodymind's separation from the inner field of consciousness. Our bodyminds are fully set up to produce a substance called ojas. Ojas is the source, process, and product of that subtle shift in awareness that eliminates such separation.

### Ojas: The Product and Process of Perfect Health

Ojas is defined as the vital substance in the bodymind that both produces balance among Vata, Pitta, and Kapha and is itself produced when diet, digestion, behavior, and mental and emotional states are balanced and healthy. Ojas is most clearly observed on the skin of healthy people as the smoothness and "glow" of vibrant health. A person with good ojas has softness even in a firm body, good color, and a balanced personality. Although research on the physiology of health, as opposed to disease, is finally becoming more commonplace, ojas has not as yet been discovered by modern medical science. However, it is described at length in the ancient Ayur-Vedic texts as a quality of radiance, as a barely perceptible, milky, fine, oily substance. It is said to have properties that are exactly opposite from toxic substances such as alcohol and poison. Ojas permeates the whole body, giving it both strength and immunity, a property known as *bala* (bah-luh). Ojas is responsible for the integration and the nourishment of the physiology, as well as the mind and the intellect.

In a sense, the entire purpose of Ayur-Vedic knowledge is to support all our psychophysiological structures and functions in such a way so that ojas is constantly generated and maintained. All the Ayur-Vedic techniques for our body, mind, and behavior are designed to produce life-supporting ojas and eliminate ama. Whereas ama blocks the expression and flow of biological intelligence in our bodies, ojas facilitates it. When ojas is lively in our physiology, it spontaneously leads to balanced thought, speech, and action. According to the Ayur-Vedic literature, every little activity hurriedly done leads to the disintegration of ojas; every fully awake, conscious activity leads to its production. By creating a fully alert mind, ojas overcomes the mistake of the intellect, pragya aparadh, and creates the memory of wholeness. This is how the basis of sickness and suffering is eliminated.

Ojas has been described as both a "superfluid slide" which enables the transfer of knowledge from consciousness to matter and as a *semi*material substrate, as much consciousness as it is matter, a physical medium by which nature can most fully express herself in us. Ojas is thus both an end product and a process that increases our immunity, our bala, along with our bodymind strength, enabling us to move toward a long, disease-free life span. When ojas is fully operative, the individual has attained a state of perfect health. When ojas is fully depleted, immunity—the orderly intelligence, integrity, and homeostasis in the bodymind—is completely lost.

It doesn't really matter whether we think of ojas as an actual product or as a transformative process leading to homeostatic equilibrium and immune strength in the body. The value of understanding ojas is that it identifies a specific state of balance, of ideal functioning in the bodymind, in which all the tissues are being well nourished and maintained at their highest level of physiological efficiency, creating strong immunity and clarity, bliss and happiness. Ojas is thus a state (knower), a substance (known), and a process (knowing), described as the full flow of biological intelligence, linking together consciousness, intelligence, and matter.

## The Srotas: Channels for Ojas

In order to reach all the parts of your bodymind, ojas needs channels through which to flow. These channels, called *srotas* (sroe-tuhs), are the passageways of your body, the spaces encompassed by the blood vessels, capillaries, lymph circulation systems, and so forth. Ojas flows through the srotas, through all the gaps in the physiology. In fact, your entire body is full of srotas. We can think of srotas as channels for nature, for our biological intelligence. If there is an obstruction to the flow of biological intelligence—if some information doesn't arrive where it is needed—part of the body gets cut off from the whole, and this can lay the groundwork for disease: A carcinogen gets trapped in the breast glands, the immune cells cannot reach a virus lodged in the lung tissue, bacteria start to proliferate in the bladder, etc. A biology of disorder caused by blockages takes over the biology of orderliness.

Open srotas allow ojas to flow most easily and keep us at the peak of health. Ojas is the vitality in each srota, which is "seated in the gaps," according to the ancient texts. We feel best if we keep the "gaps" clean. *Panchakarma,* an Ayur-Vedic purification program, has as its main purpose the cleansing of the srotas to allow ojas to flow freely. Ayur-Vedic medicine is essentially organized to create conditions to enhance the production and flow of ojas to every corner of the bodymind through fully open srotas.

We can picture the process as a flow: Intelligence enters our physiology through ojas, and ojas flows through our physiology in srotas. Ama can of course block any of the srotas, so it is important to reduce the amount of ama, but it is of even *more* importance to increase the amount and strength of ojas in our physiology.

To summarize: The physiology of health, in Ayur-Vedic terms, can be basically understood in terms of a continuum. As we develop greater balance in the doshas and higher states of awareness, the amount of ama in our psychophysiology decreases and the amount of ojas increases.

## Bliss: The Experience of Ojas

The mental and emotional experience of ojas is described as bliss. The word "bliss" has a somewhat frivolous connotation in our culture, but in Ayur-Vedic terminology, it is used as a serious and profound description of a joyful, ecstatic yet serene experience associated with the feeling of total healthiness, created by the balancing effects of ojas in our psychophysiology.

Ayur-Vedic medicine is preparative as well as preventive: It prepares our physiology and our psychology for the experience of bliss. Since every cell is capable of manufacturing neuropeptides and can therefore transform every thought into matter, we become part of the process of determining our own biochemistry and are thus capable of creating our own state of bliss.

Bliss can be experienced as a melting feeling of universality, often based on an experience of sudden insight or knowledge whose subtlety is of such high quality and intensity that it can only be experienced as pure love. According to many of the spiritual and religious teachings throughout history, this is the state we were designed by nature to experience and live, a state of "heaven on earth," one we naturally gravitate toward with each new transformative journey we embark upon.

Maharishi Ayur-Veda describes the state of bliss as a real and consistent daily experience of psychophysiological integration. As you get rid of mental ama, as old memories (even nonconscious ones) and the residues of past emotional stress—the rejection, doubt, and disappointments of our lives—disappear, and as the physical wastes and toxins in our cells and tissues are fully eliminated, more and more of your true nature shines through. You become the person you were designed by nature to be—the most intelligent, loving, awake, creative, and happy individual you can imagine being and then some.

Now, in case you were wondering how you're doing in the ama and/or ojas department, here's a self-evaluation opportunity. Consider it an ama or ojas assessment, depending on whether the cup is half empty or half full . . .

**151**

## OJAS SELF-ASSESSMENT

0 = Describes me not at all
1 = Describes me occasionally
2 = Describes me most of the time
3 = Describes me almost perfectly

Circle the number that comes closest to your experience:

1. I wake up in the morning feeling limber, light, and subtle.    0   1   2   3
2. My tongue is pink and clear during the day.    0   1   2   3
3. I generally have a bowel movement on arising.    0   1   2   3
4. I feel satisfied after meals and don't need to continue to eat.    0   1   2   3
5. My abdomen feels comfortable after eating.    0   1   2   3
6. My digestive tract is generally free of gas.    0   1   2   3
7. I freely choose what I want to eat or drink without feeling driven by cravings.    0   1   2   3
8. I do not have any food allergies.    0   1   2   3
9. I rarely, if ever, get yeast infections.    0   1   2   3
10. My sinuses and nasal passages are clear and open.    0   1   2   3
11. My periods are regular and the flow is moderate.    0   1   2   3
12. I don't get menstrual cramps.    0   1   2   3
13. I don't experience symptoms of PMS.    0   1   2   3

(If you are going through or are past menopause, answer the next three questions instead of the previous three.)

11a. My menopause is (was) easy physically.    0   1   2   3
12a. I really do not (did not) get hot flashes.    0   1   2   3
13a. My menopause is (was) easy emotionally.    0   1   2   3

If you no longer have menstrual periods owing to surgery or other circumstances but have not yet reached menopause, either refer back to earlier menstrual experiences or skip questions and add 4 or 5 to final score.

14. In general, my skin is clear and smooth.    0   1   2   3

15. My joints move smoothly and easily without cracking.  0  1  2  3
16. My limbs feel light and agile.  0  1  2  3
17. I experience my emotions fully but am free of mood swings.  0  1  2  3
18. I can honestly say I feel happy almost all the time.  0  1  2  3
19. My mind is usually focused, clear, and sharp.  0  1  2  3
20. Although I can get angry, I don't usually lose my temper.  0  1  2  3
21. Even in the midst of winter, surrounded by sneezing people, I do not get colds, flus, or other such infections.  0  1  2  3
22. My breath is generally fresh.  0  1  2  3
23. I look younger than my chronological age.  0  1  2  3
24. I sleep well and feel rested in the morning.  0  1  2  3
25. I have good energy, and it is always steadily available.  0  1  2  3

SCORE _____

**60-75:** Very high level of Ojas. We congratulate you! Your bodymind responses indicate that you are in wonderful health and experiencing very few symptoms of ama.

**44-59:** High level of Ojas. You are doing very well in terms of your health. You can use any of the guidelines in this book for further prevention.

**28-43:** Average level of Ojas. Your health is good but be alert. Some additional attention to your daily life-style and habits will help to promote greater vitality and immunity. Consider the ama-reducing, ojas-increasing eating program in chapter 6, along with the other appropriate regimes.

**Below 28:** Low level of Ojas. You could benefit from some ama reduction and some ojas enhancement (see end of chapter 6). You will no doubt feel better if you pay more attention to your health habits and life-style and participate in the relevant programs presented in chapters 4, 7, and 12.

In the following chapter we examine the various ways we become sick physically, mentally, and emotionally and see how the Ayur-Vedic approaches call on levels of prevention and treatment that nourish the deepest kind of healing.

# Chapter 6

❀

# NOURISHMENT

## Creating the Transformations from Sickness to Health

*Imbalance of the dhatus is disease*
*which is known as unhappiness;*
*their balance is health*
*which is known as happiness.*

*The remedy of all disorders is*
*the balanced use*
*of knowledge, materials and time.*

Charaka Samhita

Disease is not simple; it originates from a complex interplay of genetic predisposition, social and environmental influences, diet and behavior, and the relative success of our bodymind in digesting these, and metabolizing and eliminating excess substances. The specific areas in which we may personally experience damaging effects depends to a large extent on our individual doshas, our family and personal histories, and our life-styles. The good news is that just about any of these preconditions can be overcome and even reversed. As we've seen, Dr. Dean Ornish's research on successfully reversing heart damage through dietary and stress reduction programs demonstrated the healthful results of unclogging the entire system, including the arteries.

Many of the well-known diseases involve the accumulation of metabolic wastes resulting from imbalanced digestion.

- Accumulated "bad" cholesterol paves the way for arteriosclerosis, stroke, and heart attack.
- Undigested fat can produce blockages leading to lipomas, cirrhosis of the liver, eye disease of hyperthyroidism, and obesity leading to other physical problems.
- Underutilized carbohydrates can cause diabetes and its myriad complications, including cardiovascular disease and cataracts.
- Excessive protein by-products can predispose us to gouty arthritis (urate crystals), osteoporosis, and conditions such as Alzheimer's disease.
- An overconcentration of minerals can create conditions such as kidney stones and many forms of arthritis.

It is noteworthy that many of the mysteries of illness that have baffled modern medicine can be solved by Ayur-Vedic diagnostic understanding and treatment approaches. We can look at two specific medical conditions—food allergies and autoimmune disease—as examples for recognizing the role of ama in disease.

### The Role of Ama in Food Allergies and Autoimmune Disease

An estimated 30 million Americans experience adverse reactions to certain foods, yet these allergies don't fall into the typical class of immune system disorders. As health writer Jane Brody noted in a *New York Times Magazine* article, "Among classically trained allergists, there is no agreement on how to categorize the various adverse reactions to food or how to diagnose them." Even the vast majority of holistic medical personnel, she writes, "diagnose allergies on the basis of tests whose validity has not been proved, and . . . prescribe . . . diets and vitamin and mineral supplements— virtually the same for every patient . . ."[1]

In Ayur-Vedic terms, food allergies may arise because we simply do not digest food properly. With the presence of ama, the body could mistake an innocuous nutritional molecule for a harmful invader known as an *antigen*. Or if digestion is malfunctioning, and food is not suitably broken down through digestion, the food molecule *is* a toxic substance, not recognizable as nutrition, and the body, in its wisdom, tries to eliminate it.

Just as hay fever is the consequence of the immune system mistaking ragweed pollen for something harmful, food allergies result when the immune system mounts a mistaken and unnecessary response to an antigen. This unnecessary immune system workout takes its toll on our overall health. Its symptoms often mimic those of a low-grade flu: fatigue, mental fogginess, gas, and occasional nausea or diarrhea.

People who have been treated with an elimination diet for food allergies tend to hold on to one misconception: that they are permanently allergic to the specific foods, and therefore must abstain from them indefinitely. This is hard for most of us to do if we are allergic to a large number of desirable foods, and in many cases it can result in an imbalanced and nutritionally poor diet. The Ayur-Vedic approach, however, suggests that once digestion is improved and food is consequently broken down into the proper simple molecules of sugar, protein, and fat that are recognized by the body as nutrition, no antibodies will form to react with the food at this point. The moral of the food allergy story is this: We are not really allergic to food, but only to the improperly digested end product of food. When that is (literally) eliminated, so is the food "allergy."

Another related ama-induced mechanism is involved in a group of illnesses referred to as autoimmune diseases. Here the immune system itself, which is usually our ally in fighting disease, actually seems to be *creating* disease. Autoimmune disorders can usually be controlled through drugs such as steroids, which suppress the immune system but can lead to a reduced resistance to infections and to other potential side effects in various organ systems in the body. Such drugs unfortunately never actually cure the disease, as symptoms usually reappear after the drugs are stopped.

The term "autoimmune" refers to the fact that certain disorders involving the immune system form antibodies against our own bodily tissues: In this sense, the body is attacking itself. Why should this occur? Since these are largely acquired diseases, the body is not being confused by its own genetic program. But there must be some underlying conditions that prompt this unnatural immune attack. Ayur-Veda contributes an important understanding here.

As we've seen, when ama accumulates in a joint or in the thyroid or in the lining of the intestines, it may set up an inflammatory reaction, because the immune cells arrive to devour and scavenge the waste particles. This inflammatory reaction involves free radicals, which if released in excess due to a heavy buildup of ama in these areas, may damage the adjacent tissue. The result is the joint pain and swelling of rheumatoid arthritis or the slow destruction of the thyroid gland, as in Hashimoto's thyroiditis (the most common cause of hypothyroidism, occurring mainly in women) or the intestinal inflammation of ulcerative colitis or Crohn's disease. It may be that, at some point in the battle against the chronic deposition of ama, the bodymind actually begins to mistake the adjacent tissues for foreign antigens and starts to form antibodies directly against the joint lining, or the thyroid tissue or the intestinal wall. In some cases, the immune system becomes so overstimulated that it even forms antibodies against its *own* antibodies, as occurs with the "rheumatoid factor" of arthritis.

Ayur-Vedic treatment focuses on eliminating ama. With the gradual elimination of ama from the tissues, the immune system begins to settle down and the symptoms begin to abate. With proper diet and routine, even recalcitrant cases of autoimmune disease in patients dependent on steroids and other immune-suppressant drugs can be improved and in some cases managed without steroids, once the ama condition is under control. (However, patients should not decrease or discontinue prescribed medications on their own on the basis of guidance given in this book. They should work in concert with their physicians, whether Ayur-Vedically trained or not, who may decrease their medications gradually as their symptoms abate with this program.)

Now let's turn to another level of the "why" of disease in order to understand more clearly how digestion and metabolic imbalance play a role in disease and aging, as described by the ancient Ayur-Vedic physiologists.

## The Transformation of Physiology Through Digestion

We know that nearly every disease state involves both internal and environmental factors, which lead to the "switching on" of a *disease* potential. Conversely, there also must be internal and environmental factors that can activate our *health* potential. Maharishi Ayur-Veda asserts that a blueprint for this road to psychophysiological invincibility lies within every human being, and any of us can fulfill our birthright if we can switch on this healthy mode of functioning. Here's how this activation of our health potential within the digestive and eliminative processes can occur.

When we eat, we are literally transforming packets of energy and intelligence into the creating of our bodies. In essence, we are transforming intelligence from one form to another, and that is why, in Ayur-Veda, the different levels of metabolism are referred to as transformations of consciousness.

The Ayur-Vedic sequence of digestion begins the instant you see, smell, or even think of eating. Your saliva, which contains the first set of digestive enzymes to begin the breakdown of carbohydrates, begins to flow. You take a bite. As the food enters your stomach, acids break the food down into simpler components; enzymes and digestive hormones are secreted by your stomach, pancreas, and small intestine, as the food flows into the intestines. From here, the nutrient fluid, called chyme, is absorbed across the intestinal lining and into your veins, which carry it to your liver. That's how it works to this point. If we were reviewing the commonly accepted medical theory of digestion, the process would now be considered complete. But Ayur-Veda considers this just the beginning. . . .

## How the Body Is Nourished and Nourishing: The Dhatus

Ayur-Veda describes seven tissues, which are called the *dhatus* (dhah-toos). Essentially, the dhatus are seven transformations of consciousness within the bodymind. Each dhatu has its own agni, its own metabolic process, known as dhatu agni, seven consecutive stages of enzymatic (biochemical) processing, which ultimately result in all the body tissues' receiving nourishment. The later stages of digestion depend on the prior ones, as one tissue level prepares the nutrients for use by the next level, and so on.

The end product of a well-functioning dhatu sequence is ojas, the finest product of digestion, experienced as vitality in your body and bliss in your mind. Ojas is ultimately what keeps Vata, Pitta, and Kapha in balance and the dhatus in sequence. As we've seen in chapter 5, ojas, which is as much consciousness as it is matter, is found at the junction between the two, produced throughout the whole bodymind and located at the deepest level of your psychophysiology.

The dhatus and ojas mutually sustain each other. In the following list, the seven dhatus are associated with various aspects of the body, but as you'll see later, they are also associated with mental and emotional processes.

1. *rasa* (ruh-suh)—blood plasma, lymph
2. *rakta* (ruhk-tuh)—red blood (hemoglobin, or oxygen-carrying component)
3. *mamsa* (mahn-suh)—muscle
4. *medha* (may-duh)—fat
5. *asthi* (uh-sthee)—bone
6. *majja* (muh-jah)—central nervous system and bone marrow
7. *shukra* (shoo-kruh)—ova and sperm

Each dhatu has its own set of enzymatic and metabolic processes—its *agni,* or fire—which essentially "cooks" the nutrients for assimilation and use by the next successive body tissue. But if any enzymatic step gets disrupted, the composition of the nutrient fluid becomes unsuitable for assimilation by the subsequent tissue and it turns into ama. The ama gets deposited in the surrounding circulatory channels or tissues, furthering the likelihood of more ama formation at this "stuck" level of metabolism with digestion of the next meal. This can cause any number of subsequent conditions that are troublesome and yet seem, from a Western point of view, to have little to do with digestion. Here is an example of one such situation.

### HOW OVEREXERCISING
### UNDERMINES METABOLISM

An example of the domino effect in dhatu transformation is demonstrated in women's physiologies by the intimate relationship between the fourth and fifth dhatus, medha and asthi. Medha dhatu and its metabolism actually includes much more than fat tissue; it includes all the activity of the hormones, reproductive and others. Asthi dhatu involves primarily the bone and cartilage and their metabolism.

It is now known that women athletes whose menstrual periods cease due to overconditioning lose calcium from their bones and frequently develop osteoporosis, even at a young age. This cessation of the menstrual period is attributed to the fact that the pituitary gland and the ovaries function normally only when there is certain minimum amount of total body fat. When the body fat of these athletes has fallen below that threshold, their hormone levels drop, and their periods stop. Since estrogen plays an important role in bone metabolism, the lack of estrogen can also lead to the loss of calcium from the bones and the development of osteoporosis.

In Ayur-Vedic terms, this situation illustrates of the principle of the sequential interdependence of the seven tissues in metabolizing. The overconditioned athlete develops her mamsa dhatu at the expense of medha, losing too much body fat proportionate to her weight. This results in a lack of proper hormonal balance (also a factor of medha dhatu), and a resultant lack of nourishment for asthi dhatu.

Let's take a look at some other women's health problems that to date are poorly understood by modern medicine, and whose origins Ayur-Veda attributes to dhatu imbalances.

### DHATU BLOCKAGE, FIBROCYSTIC BREAST
### CONDITIONS, AND BREAST CANCER

The three dhatu agnis most often associated with women's health disorders are rasa, medha, and asthi. Rasa dhatu represents the first level of digestion, wherein food gets transformed into microscopic nutrients, which are then carried throughout the body in the clear plasma portion of the blood. All the body tissues are nourished via the flow of rasa, which, through the blood plasma and lymphatic fluid, carries nutrients from the digestive tract, bathes the cells of the body with nutrient fluid, and carries off the wastes from metabolism. Like all our organs, the health and nourishment of the breasts, ovaries, and uterus are connected to the health of rasa dhatu.

Because of improper digestion, ama can accumulate in the tissues of the body. As a result, fibroid tumors of the uterus, ovarian cysts, and a fibrocystic condition in the breasts may develop. In the case of ovarian cysts, blocked channels result in the persistence of one or more fluid-filled cavities in the ovary, which in some cases may lead to abdominal pain. Fibroid tumors of the uterus can result in excess bleeding and other complications. Whereas these conditions are sometimes treated surgically in modern medical practice, they can be initially addressed through an Ayur-Vedic treatment program.

In fibrocystic breast syndrome, blockages can occur in the ducts, glands, and lymphatics of breast tissue, and uncomfortable cysts can form in the breasts when fluid accumulates. Fortunately, fibrocystic breast tissue is generally no more troublesome than that. And although it is not known exactly what role these processes play in cancer formation, breast specialist Susan Love, M.D., Director of the UCLA Breast Center, reminds us that any woman with fibrocystic disease does *not* have an increased risk of breast cancer.

So how do we get breast cancer? Although there is certainly some genetic predisposition, 80 percent of women who get breast cancer have *no* family history of it. Nor is there clear evidence that high-fat low-fiber diets directly cause breast cancer, but improper diet and other ama-creating factors do seem to play a role in increased risk.

One preliminary study—which bears mentioning because of its potential importance in the prevention of breast cancer, although its results need confirmation by further research—has implicated accumulated toxins in the breast as an increased risk factor for breast cancer. The study found that, among women having biopsies for removal and diagnosis of suspicious breast lumps, women whose lumps turned out to be cancerous had an average 50 percent higher level of carcinogenic chemicals in their breast fat as than those whose lumps were benign. This implies that exposure to pesticides and other pollutants in our food, water, and air may be contributing to the rising incidence of breast cancer in industrialized societies. Certainly this is a very important research area for women, since it offers another approach to prevention.[2]

According to Dr. Love, "It may be just that we're overnourished as a society, and that's what increases breast cancer risk." From an Ayur-Vedic standpoint, this makes sense. If we eat too much and digest poorly, it is more difficult for the bodymind to eliminate excess waste. Keeping the breasts healthy thus means not overdoing products that are difficult for us to digest or have no nutritional value, such as caffeinated beverages and chocolate, thereby avoiding ama buildup.

Ama appears to be a primary factor in the pathogenesis of every disease, and we need to take the right steps to combat it. Actually there are only three: first, to mobilize ama out of your tissues and open up your channels of circulation; second, to begin to digest food properly, so ama is not formed. (You'll find more specifics to help balance your doshas through the ama-reducing and ojas-increasing eating program at the end of this chapter.) Third, and most important, to remember that "bliss eliminates ama." The best medicine is quite simply to enjoy the people, places, and experiences that produce bliss in you.

### Ayur-Veda and Cancer

If we find out we have some form of cancer, the need to eliminate physical ama is accompanied by the further need to eliminate the emotional and mental ama caused by the *fear* of cancer, which has been said to be almost as debilitating as the disease itself. Some of the cancer fear should be dissipated by the knowledge that cancer is something every mind and body is dealing with in our carcinogenic world:

—*What would you do if your doctors told you that you had cancer?*

—*I would tell them they have cancer, too....*

# NOURISHMENT

We all have a little cancer. And once we know that, the thought of actually "getting cancer" is far less frightening. Carcinogens—cancer-causing agents—are everywhere. We inhale them, we eat them, we drink them, and we share them with our families and loved ones. The bodymind protects most of us from any serious outcome, but some of us will have a cancerous tumor form from these random cells. And while benign tumors are more or less respectful of nearby healthy tissues and stay self-contained, malignant tumors do not respect boundaries but behave wildly and inappropriately. These cancer cells do not heed the message to stop dividing the way normal cells do. Sometimes the growth is rapid; sometimes it is a "slow-dividing" cancer.

For many cancers, tumor formation may have taken as many as twenty or thirty years, and to reassert balance in the bodymind using non-invasive programs under these conditions would be too time-consuming. In this situation, Ayur-Veda recommends surgery if other interventions can't shrink the tumor quickly or easily. Surgery is a traditional Ayur-Vedic intervention when used respectfully: Ayur-Vedic physicians were the first to introduce the practice of surgery to the medical world thousands of years ago. However, since surgery is generally a Vata-increasing experience, it's best if we precede and follow it with a Vata-balancing program. If radiation or chemotherapy is required, then an overall recovery program to detoxify the body following these treatments is highly recommended.

*Following a seven-hour surgery for a malignant brain tumor, five-year-old Jenny recovered during a two-week stay within the settled atmosphere of a residential Maharishi Ayur-Vedic Health Center. There she received daily Panchakarma treatments, lots of good food, and lots of loving attention. She returned several more times during the next year and a half after each series of follow-up radiation treatments. Jenny's recovery, while difficult, was far more rapid than her doctors had expected.*

*Along with the physical recovery from the surgery and the side effects of the radiation such as hair loss and nausea, she also needed to eliminate the stressful fear and Vata imbalance that these intense experiences produced in her body, mind, and heart. She is now nine, is doing well at school, and is a happy girl who does not seem in the least traumatized physically or emotionally by her bout with cancer.*

An Ayur-Vedic physician helping patients deal with cancer can provide a useful program of treatments that is based on constitutional type, specific imbalances, and life-style considerations, which can also certainly include modern medical treatment intervention—surgery, radiation, chemotherapy, or all three. Any adverse bodymind reactions to these treatments can be addressed by Ayur-Vedic dosha-balancing programs. But restoring connection with the source of healing within remains the overall guiding principle and practice.

The creation of this reconnection is known as *smriti* (smrih-tee), or memory. The purpose of each Ayur-Vedic bodymind intervention is to refer each cell back to its true nature. The cell is given the opportunity to "remember" its proper function in a given psychophysiological process. Disorder in the form of cancer or another serious imbalance comes about when this sequential order is disturbed. Ayur-Vedic treatment focuses on arresting the disorder while correcting the improper sequence through the smriti, through reviving the cellular memory. The goal is a healthy nervous system functioning in perfect coherence such that consciousness is fully awake within us at all times, and no disorder can again arise in body or mind.

### The "Why" of Chronic Overweight: Fat Metabolism and Medha

One of the most familiar kinds of ama-induced disorders experienced by women is chronic or severe overweight.

It has been found that when a certain part of the hypothalamus is inoperative, we lose sensitivity to our own bodily signs of hunger such as low blood sugar and stomach contractions, and start to eat in response to less appropriate visual and social cues. According to neuroscientist Sarah Liebowitz at The Rockefeller University, our brain chemistry determines what we eat, how often, how much, and even how fast. She discovered that a certain region of the hypothalamus, the paraventricular nucleus (PVN), is primarily responsible for appetite control.

Maharishi Ayur-Veda offers another explanation of how and why chronic overweight occurs and provides us with a program to restore the memory of appropriate hunger signals.

When a woman discovers that she can no longer drop the extra ten pounds she gained in a few weeks the way she used to; or that as she approaches the age of forty, a few pounds gradually accumulate each year without a change in her eating habits; or that even though she is restricting calories, she has difficulty losing weight—these are all signs of ama blocking the metabolic system. Until the ama is removed, the metabolism remains imbalanced, resulting in the "yo-yo" effect (bouncing back to one's previous weight and higher soon after losing it), uncontrollable cravings, and a perpetuation of the deeper issues involved in unnourishing eating.

Becoming overweight mostly involves malfunctioning medha or fat metabolism. Blockage of metabolism at this level of transformation gives your body a feeling of being starved, leading initially to cravings, particularly for the quick energy of sweets, then to weight gain, and potentially to high cholesterol, and possibly diabetes. This type of weight gain is difficult to lose, even when carefully restricting calories, because your body is holding on to what it perceives as barely adequate, not excess, nourishment. As a result, you may experience what is known as "false" hunger, a *real* condition within the bodymind. According to Ayur-Veda, Pitta is increasing in an effort to burn up or metabolize the ama obstructing your contact with this inner field, and you are interpreting this increase in Pitta activity as hunger. Or you may still feel hungry and have deep cravings for more food even after a full meal. Or you may feel temporarily satisfied but then find yourself wandering around the kitchen an hour later, not exactly hungry but still not satisfied. This kind of hunger comes from the starving tissues, not from your stomach. Your body is indeed sending you a distress signal of hunger, but the solution is not to put more food in your mouth or stomach; it is to put more nourishment into the tissues through proper dhatu-transforming digestion.

In a most fundamental sense, our minds are far more involved in the eating process than we may want to believe. Our brain cells, not just our bodies, decide when we are thirsty, for example. The bodymind determines our blood sugar level and the amount of fat in our body. The reason we eat despite all intentions not to is that our bodymind is generally far less interested in how we look than in keeping us healthy.

So even if we think we want to weigh a certain amount, our brain may have a very different idea for an ideal bodyweight. Furthermore, a Vata-type bodymind is going to respond entirely differently than a Kapha type. And even though a Kapha constitutional type might be perfectly healthy even when heavy and her bodymind may be working perfectly, she may feel socially less healthy in a "thin"-oriented society.

Some overweight women *do* increase their risk for coronary disease. Dr. Joann Manson at Harvard Medical School found that women thirty to fifty-five who had been slim at the age of eighteen and had put on weight over the years were at greater risk than women who had been overweight at a younger age. From an Ayur-Vedic perspective, these were Vata and Pitta women, not Kapha-type women, who would also have been naturally somewhat heavy at eighteen.

On the other hand, research has indicated that gaining weight as you grow older is actually healthier than losing weight, as long as the gain is not excessive. The bottom line seems to be that if you recognize the normal weight gain that occurs as you grow older as a condition of health, and not as a conspiracy to keep you off the cover of *Vogue,* and pay attention to *digesting* and not *dieting,* you will feel and look better. You are much better off focusing on the elimination of *waste,* not on the elimination of *weight,* which is far less essential to your good health. By restoring healthy eliminative processes, you can structure healthy weight loss *automatically.* Let's examine how this process works.

Adult females have about twice the body fat of males: This is natural. But 25 percent of all American women between the ages of thirty-five and sixty-four weigh at least 30 percent more than is desirable for their health. The weight gain often associated with middle age in women actually has its start much earlier, as the gradual effects of poor eating habits, irregular routine, and stress result in ama accumulation and the steady undermining of the balance of carbohydrate and fat metabolism. A new study by the Centers for Disease Control has traced the start of weight gain back at least to one's mid-twenties: Women who are overweight at age twenty-five to thirty-four are more likely to have a major weight gain in the following ten-year period, and women of any age are twice as likely as men to experience a major weight gain (defined as a 20 percent or greater increase in body weight).

From the Ayur-Vedic perspective, an underlying tendency to gain weight is due to a gradually disrupted metabolism that, when corrected, can restore normal weight and health, without the usual side effects and misery of dieting and tissue starving.

*Carole S. is a thirty-eight-year-old lobbyist in Washington, D.C., the mother of three young children, and a woman who has battled excess weight since her teenage years. As a young adult she had achieved a fairly comfortable weight of 165 pounds. After her first child was born, she managed to lose most of the weight gained during pregnancy. However, after the birth of twins, she never was able to take off more than 20 of the pounds she gained during nursing. Added to the stress of raising a young family of three active baby boys, her concerns over her weight became overwhelming. After unsuccessful attempts to lose weight on her own through various methods, she enrolled in a popular diet program utilizing prepackaged foods and lost 60 pounds, regaining her previously hard-won trim figure. But some very uncomfortable problems took hold.*

*"Upon completing my diet," Carole recalls, "my metabolism was functioning at a very low level. My endocrine function was also very low and I had not had a period for many months. For two months, I starved myself on about 1,300 calories of regular food per day—and gained weight. At that point, I began to have rather dramatic food binges. Over the next eight months I regained 40 of the 60 pounds that I had lost, with no letup of the binges. I was feeling both physically and emotionally miserable.*

*"Finally, I began the program to eliminate ama. Within days, the binges stopped with no discomfort. I was suddenly able to eat normally—about one-quarter of what I had been consuming previously. Furthermore, for the first time in months I actually lost weight, instead of gaining, had my*

*first period in over a year, and experienced a deep feeling of
happiness in my body instead of the usual misery. It was a
tremendous relief and a tremendous surprise. I really didn't
believe I would ever have a normal appetite and a normalizing of my weight at the same time."*

### Fat Metabolism, Female Hormones, Heart Disease, and Diabetes

Ayur-Veda recognizes that fat metabolism, especially in women, is
intimately connected to our reproductive hormones, to blood sugar and cholesterol metabolism, to the health of our cardiovascular
system, and to the health of asthi, the next tissue after medha in
the sequence of dhatus.

We know that heart disease is the most frequent cause of death
in women over the age of sixty-five. Hormones and the eliminative
elements of the menstrual cycle itself (as we'll discuss in chapter 9)
do seem to protect premenopausal women. The relationship between fat metabolism, heart disease, and a woman's hormonal system is being established via research findings such as the following:

> 1. Before menopause, women have better cholesterol pro-
> files and one-seventh the rate of heart disease as men.
> 2. It takes ten years following menopause for women to
> lose this advantage.
> 3. No relationship has been found between cholesterol
> level and cardiovascular disease in women during the years be-
> fore menopause.
> 4. Changing the natural levels of hormones in women be-
> fore menopause, as has occurred in recent decades with the
> use of certain oral contraceptives, tends to *increase* the risks
> of strokes, blood clots, and other cardiovascular problems.
> 5. Female hormones help the liver to produce more "good"
> cholesterol.

There is also a well-established association between blood sugar
and fat metabolism in diabetes. Being overweight predisposes us to
develop adult onset diabetes, and diabetes involves abnormalities

in fat metabolism, specifically elevated blood cholesterol and tri-glyceride levels, which can lead to cardiovascular disease. The interrelationship between these metabolic pathways and a woman's hormonal system is illustrated by a condition called "gestational diabetes," a complication brought on by hormonal changes occurring during pregnancy. Generally the condition goes away after delivery, but women who develop this temporary form of diabetes during pregnancy are more likely to develop the more permanent condition later in life.

Hypothyroidism is another condition linked to a woman's hormonal system that involves fat metabolism, along with an elevation of lipid levels. Hypothyroidism is four times as common in women than men; irregularities in the menstrual cycle, PMS, and infertility have been associated with it.

In all these conditions, ama blockage or imbalance of metabolism at the level of medha can lead to weight gain, high cholesterol, and possibly diabetes and/or cardiovascular disease. Rather than focusing on treating each component with a specific drug, as modern medicine does, the Ayur-Vedic approach is to restore balance in metabolism by creating the conditions by which our bodies' mechanisms can effect a fundamental reversal. *Since the imbalance was caused by the gradual accumulation of ama, the systematic removal of ama from the tissues is intimately involved in a cure.*

### Freedom from Addiction: Eliminating Substance Abuse Through Ayur-Veda

Ama plays games with our minds as well as with our bodies. The process of addiction can be understood as a bodymind mix-up caused by ama-induced misinformation.

Our societal view of addiction is that an addicted individual is bound to one or more of a variety of initially pleasurable processes that are often harmful—physically, psychologically, and behaviorally. The idea that an addict can be both knowledgeable about the harm caused and still addicted has led to anti-abuse programs that generally focus either on substituting a lesser addiction for a greater one (such as methadone for heroin) or on creating a medium or culture of outer resources (such as the twelve-step programs) that arm the addict with a variety of psychological tools to first accept and then overcome the addiction.

While there are certain genetic predispositions to addiction—it was recently discovered, for example, that there is a gene for a tendency to alcoholism—there is no addiction that is solely physical and leaves out mind and emotions. For this reason, there are many predisposed children of alcoholics who do not become alcoholics. Essentially, addiction is a great example of a true bodymind illness: Over 50 percent of narcotics abusers have experienced major depression, and 87 percent have a known history of psychiatric disorders. From a psychological standpoint, all current treatment programs involve ways to replace the dependence on drugs or alcohol with social support and internalized self-referral qualities, such as higher self-esteem and greater independence. But addiction is structured at a much deeper level of bodymind functioning than the psychological. It is structured in every cell. To correct the distortion of addictive cells, we have to encourage the memory within cells to change their behavioral functioning.

Because the physical, mental, and emotional aspects of addiction are all part of the bodymind, the changes needed for a transformation to nonaddictive eating come from the deeper levels of bodymind functioning. This applies to all addictions. A food addict, for example, to some extent, is not eating more than she ought to—she's simply trying to eat enough. The hunger is very real, and therefore so is the addiction. But the overeating is not happening only because of some unresolved conflict from the past, although that pattern may be there as well. It is happening because the bodymind is reasonably searching for adequate satisfaction for the mind and heart, as well as for the body. What is being sought is the connection to consciousness, to something deeply nourishing. Once exposed to a more satisfying source of bliss, the less useful habit is automatically dropped.

Every genuinely effective technique to obliterate negative addictive behaviors must therefore promote the experience of bliss. Ridding the body of toxic materials, getting deep rest, and enjoying the support and attentiveness of loving family and friends can all certainly help move one in the right direction, but the deeper memory of how bliss itself feels must be reawakened. Ayur-Vedic intervention seeks to treat the addiction right at the gap where consciousness becomes matter, thereby correcting any underlying mistakes in physiological functioning, including those formed through genetic predisposition. The addiction disappears when the memory of bliss is restored.

Perhaps one of the most unnecessary addictive situations is that of the number of women who are "medically addicted," from taking legal drugs daily in large doses. Through the years, some doctors have allowed women to maintain a secret addiction, in keeping with a societal norm that prefers its female addicts (as well as its female AIDS patients) to remain invisible. Perhaps because of the greater responsibilities for family care assigned to women, a chemical dependency in a woman is perceived as more socially irresponsible than in a man. And because of the dangerous prenatal effects of such conditions as fetal alchohol syndrome, pregnant women who abuse chemicals are granted the least societal understanding. There is also less social and personal support for women who drink than for men who do so. Like heart disease, alchoholism has been thought of as a "man's" illness, although men and women drink for different reasons; women tend to drink in response to life crises.

Moreover, from a purely physiological standpoint, women have a tougher time with the physical effects of alcohol addiction: They are at a greater health disadvantage than men. Women seem to absorb about 30 percent more alcohol and get intoxicated more quickly than men who have taken in the same amount of alcohol, not only because of relative physical size, but because women have far smaller quantities of the protective enzyme alcohol dehydrogenase, which breaks down alcohol in the stomach.[3] This enzyme mitigates against the absorption of alcohol into the bloodstream. Women alcoholics tend to lack it entirely and can lose all gastric protection against alcohol absorption. As a result, women who drink rely more on the functioning of their livers for physiological protection, so their livers have to work harder. Similarly, some studies suggest that women metabolize nicotine more slowly than men; consequently, although they might smoke fewer cigarettes than men, they maintain the same level of nicotine in their bodies. In Ayur-Vedic terms, women addicts are thus often faced with an even greater ama and imbalance problem than men.

According to Maharishi Ayur-Veda, addiction means that our

bodymind is trying to balance itself, albeit in inappropriate ways, when it is no longer able to create its own nurturance or its own happiness. If we don't feel nurtured and happy, we rarely feel healthy. Unfortunately, many people try to achieve psychophysiological balance, nurturance, and happiness through food, drug, and alcohol abuse. But this ultimately becomes a direct route to further destroy the validity of the integrity of the bodymind.

Substance abuse and dependence occur when we attempt to create inner balance by bringing something from the outside into our bodies in order to fulfill our very natural desires for happiness, peace, and health. The overall effect is to drive us away from inner harmony: Alcohol creates the desire for more alcohol, and so we become addicted. This escalation occurs because the bodymind no longer thinks it has to produce that which it most needs, and more and more of the substance is required from the outside. The bodymind, blocked by ama, forgets that what it really needs is available on the *inside.* In a sense, it forgets its own worth; it forgets it has the most well-stocked pharmacy of all, right there in the brain, and that its internally produced drugs are 100 percent pure. Here is where we look to overcome addiction, in our own brain chemistry.

How does the brain supply us with what we desire? A synthetic drug molecule either reproduces the activities of an internally made molecule, or it blocks its effects. Dr. Candace Pert and her colleagues at Johns Hopkins University were the pioneer mindbody scientists who, in the early seventies, identified the opiate receptor, a molecule on the surface of a cell that is receptive to opiates, either synthetic or internally produced. These receptors allow us to both feel good and control pain. Women in labor, for example, have the ability to access the midbrain area, which is filled with opiate receptors and receptors for neuropeptides. This discovery of the opiate receptor led to speculation about why we would be born with receptors for morphine-based opiates: If your body has built-in opiate receptors, why doesn't it just produce its own opiates? The answer is that it does. This is the biochemical reason why we can overcome drug and alcohol dependency by returning the bodymind to its own natural program.

Ideally, we could all be making our own pleasure-producing drugs continually, whether endorphins or other opiates, in just the right dosages for our individual needs.

When our bodies are functioning well, we feel the joyful effects of inner psychological and physiological harmony and the "high" of perfect health, manufacturing our perfect sense of soothing endorphins, and there's no further need to seek outside supplies. But if we start to rely on outside opiates, our brains get a different signal, and to try to maintain homeostasis, starts to produce *fewer* inner opiates.

Sometimes we do need to take outside substances to normalize our physiology, especially if we suffer from pain, particularly long-term or chronic pain. Yet as a society we are more fearful of causing addiction than of causing pain. This fear often prevents adequate medical treatment for patients in pain. But this kind of need does not generally cause addiction. People in pain take drugs because they want to feel normal, not because they want to get high. They don't want to escape their lives, they want to enter into them more fully. As a result, they don't become addicted as quickly. Psychologist Ronald Melzack, a leading pain expert, reports, "Patients who take morphine for pain do not develop the rapid physical tolerance to the drug that is often the sign of addiction. . . . [They] do not need sharply rising doses for relief." He identifies a major difference in the effect of morphine on the addict who craves its mood-altering properties and the "psychologically healthy patient" who takes it to relieve pain.[4] Our psychological health is of course as essential as our physical response in the elimination of addiction. However, the deeper desires of the bodymind to be healthy interpret the drug differently from the body or mind separately. The Ayur-Vedic approach to addiction seeks a resolution that is both deep and integrative.

### AYUR-VEDA AND CHEMICAL SELF-SUFFICIENCY

Like its other approaches, the Maharishi Ayur-Veda approach to addiction is a combination of physical, mental, and emotional interventions, each having as its goal access to the inner healing field. Each intervention is understood to directly accentuate the self-referral awareness of body and mind, to help us return to a normal state of balance.

Ayur-Vedic intervention to overcome addiction involves restoring the bodymind's natural ability to enliven feelings of happiness within. All pleasurable experience can produce pleasurable chem-

**173**

icals in a healthy body. This happens only when we eliminate the blocks to feeling happiness. We know, for example, that the pleasurable feelings of enjoying music create natural opiates. In this same way, all our physiological abilities can bring us real pleasure, as we relearn how to enjoy our own chemistry.

Postaddictive functioning is first enlivened through self-knowledge. We start to remember what the body is like when it feels good and recognizes automatically what it needs to create that good feeling on its own, using its natural desires to awaken its pharmacological resources. As one young woman recovering from a drug addiction so aptly put it, "You can get high on the experience of self-knowledge."

Negative addictive behavior whether to drugs, food, or alcohol (or even to people) is easy to eliminate if we have regular contact with our own resource of self-nurturing happiness and establish chemical self-sufficiency. Research on the effects of Transcendental Meditation, the primary approach of Maharishi Ayur-Veda to addiction, indicates that when the powerful process of self-created bliss is allowed to occur, uninhibited by the intake of any outer substance interfering in the process, the use of the addictive substance spontaneously decreases.

In a 1993 statistical analysis of nineteen studies on the effects of TM on substance abuse, the rates of reduction of alcohol, cigarette, and illicit drug use were significantly larger than for standard treatment programs in the field. These included drug counseling, self-esteem programs, and educational programs. Moreover, the results from TM were generally sustained over time.[5]

What follows are a few simple guidelines to help our bodymind remember its own resource of biochemical happiness.

1. Learn and practice Transcendental Meditation. A large number of research studies indicate that TM really does reestablish a natural state of health and bliss.[6]

2. Detoxify the bodymind by following the ama-reducing program and consulting a physician, if necessary.

3. Keep to a daily Ayur-Vedic routine of proper eating, rest, and appropriate exercise (see chapter 4).

4. Refer to the *behavioral rasayanas* regularly (see chapter 8).

## The Ayur-Vedic Ama-Reducing, Ojas-Increasing Eating Program

Since the most common cause of ama is improper digestion, the following guidelines for reducing ama and promoting ojas focus primarily on dietary factors, including *what, how,* and *when* it is best to eat.

### Food Selection

1. As a rule, "nature knows best." Food should be unprocessed and free of pesticides and additives. Avoid frozen and canned foods where possible.
2. Favor warm, cooked foods. Avoid cold or iced foods and beverages. (Cold foods and drinks automatically decrease digestive power, because our digestive enzymes function at body temperature. Lowering the temperature in the stomach lowers the rate and efficiency of digestion.)
3. Eat mostly grains, vegetables, and fruits. Minimize meat, fish, and fowl.
4. Include *freshly* squeezed fruit and vegetable juices in your daily diet.
5. Avoid excessive amounts of refined sugar, caffeine, alcohol, and chocolate. (You knew that . . .)
6. Eat a balanced diet that includes all six tastes (see chapter 4).

### Liquids

1. Plain hot water with your meal is best. Room temperature water is acceptable, but your drinks should never be cold or iced.
2. Drink milk with cereal, breads, or other sweet-tasting items, but not with a full meal or with fish, chicken, or meat.
3. Non-iced juices are also appropriate to drink with the meal.

**175**

### *Ayur-Vedic Food Preparation Tips*

1. Prepare food as close as possible to the time when you'll actually eat it.

2. Prepare food from scratch as often as you can to ensure freshness and purity of ingredients. Ideally, avoid old or left-over food.

3. Try to cook in a pleasant environment, when you are in a happy or contented mood. Cooking tastes best and nourishes best when we put our loving attention into it.

### *Ayur-Vedic Eating Habit Tips*

1. Eat when you are hungry. Try not to delay or skip a meal because you are "too busy."

2. Try not to eat when you're *not* hungry. If you feel an urge to eat when your stomach's full, have a cup of plain hot water. This will usually clear sensations of "false hunger" by directly clearing out the ama that prompted it.

3. Eat to about two-thirds of your stomach's capacity. This is approximately equal to the amount of food that fits into your two cupped hands. (Bigger hands, bigger body, more food . . .)

4. Always sit down to eat.

5. Eat in a pleasant, settled environment.

6. Have your attention on what you're eating—really savor and enjoy it.

7. It's much, much better not to read, work, watch TV, or drive while eating.

8. Sit and relax for at least five minutes after the meal before returning to your other activities.

### *Timing*

1. Have your main meal at lunchtime and a lighter meal in the evening. Digestion (Pitta) is strongest at noontime, and food will be utilized most efficiently at that time. Studies have shown that most people can eat a certain number of calories early in the day and not gain weight, whereas if they eat the

same number of calories in the evening, they put on weight. Also, you will sleep better.

2. Eat your meals at about the same time each day, if possible.

3. Eat your midday meal between noon and 1:00 P.M., if possible.

4. Eat your evening meal by 6:00 or 7:00 P.M., if possible. If you must eat later, be sure to eat extra lightly. Monitor how well you sleep and how you feel the next morning as a gauge to how well you digested the meal and whether you need to further modify your evening mealtime.

### *The Four Main Ways to Eliminate Ama*

Even if you can only do the following four simple things, you can make a dramatic difference in your health.

1. Sip plain hot water frequently throughout the day. This helps the body digest and eliminate ama and metabolic wastes, so that your internal balance can be restored and maintained. You can add lemon to the water if you like.

2. Eat a full, warm, cooked meal at lunchtime, with all the six tastes described in chapter 4.

3. Take *at least* twenty minutes to eat, and sit for a few minutes at the end of the meal.

4. Eat a light, early dinner and have only liquids after 8:00 P.M.

Now that we have explored some perspectives on bodymind illness and bodymind health, let's look at the vision Ayur-Veda brings to understanding and healing our emotional lives.

# Chapter 7

RESPONSIVENESS

## Feeling and Healing in
## Our Emotional Bodymind

*The little space within the heart
Is as great as this vast universe.*

Chandogya Upanishad

Not only is there a "thinking body" inside us, there is also an emotional body; our emotions tell our bodies how to respond, creating a passionate, angry, exhilarated, or fearful physiology at different times. When we blush or throw something across the room or tremble in the night upon hearing a surprising noise, our hearts are as much involved with our responses as our minds. Within the Maharishi Ayur-Vedic model, it's more accurate to say that we have *thinking* hearts and *feeling* minds, as they are inseparable within the deeper field of consciousness.

Objectively, we know we have an emotional body that conducts our physiological responses. Consider the following:

- The feeling of joy, defined as mental resilience and vigor by researchers, was the second strongest predictor of survival time among women with recurrent breast cancer, following "length of disease-free intervals."
- The two highest risk factors for a first heart attack in men under fifty are not the ones taught in medical school—

overweight, smoking, diabetes, family history, or high cholesterol—but a lack of job satisfaction and a low level of general happiness.

• Herpes infections recur more frequently in people who are depressed.

• Bereavement causes a drop in the number of T-cells, an indication of the diminished capacity of the immune system to respond, which subsequently normalizes as the grief lessens over time.

• Some terminally ill people, especially women,[1] are able to "postpone" imminent death until after an event they cherish and long to see, such as a family wedding or the birth of a grandchild, or even until a meaningful holiday has passed.[2]

• In one study, flu was found to be most common among the employees whose morale was lowest.

The real question is, of course, whether these situations would occur without the underlying integration of body, mind, and emotions. It seems unlikely. We can then ask the next question: If the chemicals of desire can postpone death, can the self-made chemicals of happiness increase our good health and decrease our chances for illness?

### Health and Happiness

Nearly three decades ago, in their pioneering study of how emotional conflict could influence the onset and course of rheumatoid arthritis in women, Stanford University researchers George Solomon and Rudolph Moos compared two groups of women with a genetic predisposition for this kind of arthritis. They found that women who remained free of disease "were emotionally healthy . . . not depressed . . . and not alienated." Said Solomon in a recent interview, "We felt that emotional health protected them from rheumatoid arthritis."[3] Solomon's work was regarded with cynicism by many of his colleagues at the time; today he is renowned as a pioneer and a founder of the field of psychoneuroimmunology, or PNI.

Recently, researchers at Georgetown University discovered that mental stress can significantly alter the way a heart pumps and fills with blood. The results demonstrate that mental stress can be as damaging as physical stress. The researchers concluded that silent thought can affect the hemodynamics of the heart.

We now know that neuropeptides (information molecules) and the cellular structures to which they attach throughout the body are the physiological correlates of every emotion we have. This is why watching a funny film can lower our stress hormone levels and even open up our creative thinking processes. Laughter also has been found to increase respiratory activity, produce endorphins, reduce depression, and help us live longer. "Happy cells" can and do keep us free of disease.

Loving feelings are indeed healing. This is what PNI research is demonstrating. For example, the survival rate of male patients hospitalized for heart attacks is most highly correlated with the perception that their wives love them and only secondarily with medical factors. The *feeling* of being loved creates an internal life-supporting milieu, a collective emotional desire among all the cells which is so potent that it proves to be the determining force for the bodymind to organize itself in favor of continuing life in the face of death.

Your neuropeptides circulating throughout your bodymind ultimately help to determine which experience—pain or bliss—finally registers in your consciousness. There is now evidence that we experience bliss *before* our body produces serotonin, a neurotransmitter associated with relaxed states of our physiology.[4] Our experience of the world is literally being filtered by these internal messengers, by the collective psychophysiological hum of all the ongoing conversations between the cells, conversations that might sound something like: "Are we enjoying this concert or are we bored?" "Does this needle only hurt us or is it also beneficial?" "Does our spouse love us? Yes, indeed!"

These internal conversations within the bodymind actually may be more important than the nature of the stimulus itself, explaining why there is such a wide individual variation in pain threshold and why such feats as walking barefoot on burning coals without feeling pain are possible.

## How Emotions Hurt or Heal:
## The Desire-Fulfillment Cycle

In Ayur-Vedic practice, it is understood that it takes very little to change your physiology via your mind or your attitude. Just a small notion, "Oh, I think I'll be loving now," can cause the bodymind to completely regroup. One gentle tug on one leg of the table and the entire structure moves. When you can reset your whole physiology simply by a thought or a feeling, you are practicing first-class Ayur-Veda.

How does this emotional bodymind response come about? When we are functioning in a healthy way, things flow smoothly, the bodymind is well coordinated and well integrated. In these circumstances, our emotions are self-healing by nature. So when we tap into our own self-referral chemistry of love, however it may be triggered, we release neuropeptides and their pleasure-making properties into our blood. We experience a sense of well-being which we feel as love, happiness, or our deepest moments of creativity, defined by University of Chicago psychologist Mihaly Csikszentmihalyi as "flow" or "involved enchantment."

The ongoing experience of this heightened level of health is the result of an integrated "feeling-bodymind." Dr. Candace Pert and her colleagues have identified the role of the neuropeptides, the chemical substances released by the brain cells, as the "communication specialists" or "messengers" that link the mind, body, and emotions. Dr. Pert's early research, undertaken in collaboration with her colleague Dr. Solomon Snyder, identified how the opiates, our internally produced, pain-relieving chemicals, attach to neuropeptide receptors located throughout the body and in the brain, primarily in the thalamus, which organizes pain impulses, and also in the limbic system, which activates emotions in the brain. According to Dr. Pert, the receptors for the neuropeptides are the keys to the biochemistry of emotion.

This biochemical system is quite elegant: A very small number of types of neuropeptides—sixty or so—are thought to account for all the varying physiological manifestations of emotion. In the field of PNI, these are important keys to the healing processes of the bodymind, helping us understand why some patients with certain attitudes and emotional states can heal or hurt themselves. It also helps us comprehend how our emotional biochemistry translates precisely into a body receptive to and changed by any emotion— joy, grief, skepticism, anger, or any other.

Maharishi Ayur-Veda integrates this bioemotional process into its treatment programs, recognizing that emotion has a purpose beyond the experience of random feelings called up by a variety of outside circumstances. The inner purpose of emotion is to stir the body to fulfill the wishes of the heart and the desires of the mind.

Suppose you have a desire to be very wealthy. If it's only an intellectual thought, because you think you ought to be wealthy, you won't have the accompanying energy impetus of emotion to carry out your daily activities to fulfill this desire. You have to deeply and one-pointedly desire this in your life.

But even if you achieve this goal, you may find that it hasn't brought you a sense of ultimate satisfaction. You may then feel another desire stirring inside, for a materially good life for those nearest and dearest to you. And then you may desire for your community to become economically self-sufficient or begin to feel a passion to help change the economic disparities in the world to a more equitable situation. And despite what others may think, you know these are not merely lofty goals, empty of feeling. They are strongly felt personal desires, coming from within, conducting the physiology of your bodymind toward an ever deepening level of fulfillment.

From the Ayur-Vedic perspective, the ultimate goal of any desire is to move our personal evolution in a progressive and integrative direction, toward more satisfaction and more happiness. In this context, emotion is like the engine that moves and motivates the bodymind toward a given end. It energizes our commitments and enables us to carry out the activities we embark on with the exuberance of love and joy.

But there is also an opposite effect of the cycle of "desire-action-achievement-fulfillment," leading to a new desire. Just as a delicate impulse of desire changes our emotional biochemistry, *not* fulfilling the desire also changes us. Thwarted desires have a biochemistry, too. Lack of fulfillment can create emotional ama and eventually perhaps illness. Blocked desires can turn into psychophysiological blocks.

The emotional stress or ama from unfulfilled desires is associated in Maharishi Ayur-Veda with physiological restrictions that have come from the accumulation of emotionally stressful events in our lives, creating three kinds of hurt: doubt, disappointment, and rejection. Every instance of hurt can settle into our bodies as a deposit of stress, which can make us physically uncomfortable.

Any kind of doubt can lead to hesitation, lack of confidence, and a fearful heart. Doubt also creates an emotional disintegration, which can cause conflicted behavior if we receive opposing messages from mind, emotions, or body. For example, if you look at a piece of chocolate cake, your intellect may say, "Ah, yes, five hundred calories, this is not good," whereas your heart may say, "Oh, yes, I remember the chocolate cakes my mother used to bake for me for my birthday with such love and joy. What a nourishing item, this cake." And your body may respond to the chocolate cake with "Yes, this smells good, it will taste good, this will make me feel good, I want it." Or your body may say, "The cake looks great but I'm not hungry." And the pull of these very different messages causes an uncomfortable doubt, no matter what decision you make. The goal is to integrate all aspects of the bodymind so there are no conflicting messages creating doubt. Unless we do, we can become confused and have difficulty making decisions. Just adding the ingredient of harmony through a more life-encompassing desire offers bodymind integration and resolves any doubt with a deeper kind of joy.

Disappointment can occur if our experiences fail to meet our expectations or hopes. The solution is always to find the bigger picture, to remember the underlying wholeness. We can recognize that the smaller the picture, the more we are experiencing pragya aparadh, permitting our intellects to mistake the tiny part for the whole. We need to trust in the workings of nature; to recognize, for example, that a year from now, not getting a certain job might turn out to be the very best thing that could have happened. We have to remember that nature actually wants our happiness and bliss certainly as much, if not more, than we do. Even rejection can be resolved by this kind of surrender to nature's guidance. When we think of the hurt of a rejection, most of us reflect back on a relationship that involved our being turned away. But rejection is as much our refusal to accept or receive love as it is being rebuffed.

The less we reject love, the less we are rejected in love. When we reject others, we also damage our own hearts. And it can even be as subtle as not seeing the greatness, the wholeness, in yourself or others.

Modern medicine is just beginning to seriously examine the strong link between emotions and physiology and how it affects our behavior and health.

## Emotional Expression and Health

PNI researchers remind us that, as a form of prevention, it is very important to allow our physiology to express its emotional truth. If we are feeling happy or angry or sad or whatever, "bottling up" our natural responses appears to make us ill. In one study of physicians conducted at the Johns Hopkins University School of Medicine, the group characterized as "acting out and emotionally expressive" had the least incidence of cancer, whereas the group characterized as "loners," who were thought to have suppressed their emotions, were sixteen times more likely to develop cancer.[5] (One could argue, however, that the factors that made them unexpressive when they were young, perhaps certain stressful events, were more related to causing the cancer.) Recently, PNI pioneer George Solomon demonstrated that assertiveness is a factor in disease resistance and that being nice to the point of self-neglect can compromise the functioning of the immune system.[6]

A "cancer personality profile" has been established by several groups of research psychologists. One team at the University of California at San Francisco describes a "Type C" personality as one who is unable or unwilling to express anger or other negative feelings. Type C people tend to worry more about the effects of their illness on others than on themselves. Similar research has been carried out at the University of Pittsburgh, as well as in England and Germany. The Type C personality may be the typically "nice person" who even apologizes when she or he is sick, and this and other Type C traits are often praised in women in particular. But when we are sick, the emotional expressiveness of negative as well as positive feelings is called for. The more immediate bodymind purpose is to mobilize our inner resources to decrease tumor size and increase immune system response. And expressiveness does seem to help.

Studies have shown that, in women with breast cancer, those with a fighting, "this is unacceptable" personality outlive those with a stoic, "carry on as usual" personality. We can actively reorganize the bodymind to remind the cancerous cells and tumors to return to the collective good, to the healing response within. Mere acceptance gives permission to the cancer, whereas fighting back—not simply with anger at the cancer but with a powerful desire for life—helps open the way for normal functioning. Once a woman realizes that she has considerable power to influence her condition by her ability to organize her desires within consciousness, her Type C personality can change to a fighting spirit.

While there is some debate over the validity of this cancer personality profile, from an Ayur-Vedic viewpoint, it does not go far enough. Yes, there is benefit for a person "fighting" cancer instead of merely accepting it. But a deeper bodymind perspective enables us to see what attitudes are genuinely and deeply healing, not merely anxiety-driven combativeness.

A woman artist who has been healing herself with Ayur-Vedic techniques put it this way: "I don't 'fight' my illness. That's a kind of old imagery that doesn't work well for me. I believe I heal myself best by *allowing,* by taking it as it comes, by going *with* life, rather than opposing it. I don't even oppose my own illness. It's not that I want to be sick; it's that I don't feel afraid of it or overwhelmed by it anymore. I don't let it absorb me. What I do is *surround* my illness with my good health. I feel I am the artist of my own healing. And as a result, I'm feeling well."

But positive thinking alone doesn't get us well. The thinking has to represent the true expression of every emotion and cell in our body flowing together. There was a patient who always seemed just "too positive" about having cancer. When her physician gently confronted her on this, she broke down in tears and admitted she was petrified of having a negative thought. Her crying over her situation was probably healthier for her than any "false" positive thought because she was obviously very sad and frightened, two emotions that do not integrate well with positive thinking. By straining to hold back the tears, she was further separating her mind, emotions, and body. In fact, researchers have found that emotional crying (as opposed to cutting up an onion) is a good way to release toxins.[7] Since women are culturally "permitted" to cry more than men, we might as well take advantage of it. Many of us do, sometimes going to the movies or reading novels, just to "have a good cry."

The bottom line seems to be that there are some real health benefits when we fully feel and express our emotions. However, we also need to be aware that continually expressing anger in chronic antagonism has *not* been associated with a lower incidence of heart disease. Just the opposite.

Psychologist Paul Costa at the National Institute on Aging says, "The key factor in the development of heart disease is whether a person feels angry all the time," not whether the anger is suppressed or expressed. When, instead of letting go, our bodies literally hold on to the stressful emotions at a deep level, we can create further damage and imbalance. These become toxic emotions that we want not to express so much as to eliminate, such as inappropriate anger, anxiety, and depression.

## Ayur-Veda and the Physiology of Anger, Anxiety, and Depression

Dr. Redford Williams, director of the Behavioral Medicine Research Center at Duke University, noted that "hostility, particularly the anger that is fired by our cynical beliefs about the motives of others, sets in motion the chain of biological events that leads on to disease and death."[8] Researchers have found that while occasional anger may be fine and even healthy in a normally functioning individual, the same anger in an already overly hostile person is injurious. It's not the aggression but its interaction with the underlying distrust that causes problems.

A constant vigil of mistrust is found to raise not only blood pressure but also testosterone levels, which speed up plaque formation in the arteries. There is evidence that because women have far less testosterone than men, they have far less toxic anger and therefore live longer. "Like salt for people with high blood pressure, anger is poison to the hostile person," reports Williams.

Maharishi Ayur-Veda reminds us that hostility comes from

**186**

somewhere—a lack of fulfillment of desire—and that anger is thus not itself the primary cause of the subsequent illness. Anger, in Vedic terms, occurs when desire is blocked: "When the flow of a particular desire is obstructed by another flow, energy is produced at the point of collision, and this flares up as anger, which confuses and destroys the harmony and smooth flow of the desire." As a result, "the very purpose of life, which is the expansion of happiness, is marred; the very purpose of creation is thwarted."[9]

Anger is mainly understood as a Pitta imbalance, associated not with the hard-driving Type A purposefulness and achievement orientation, but with a subset of Type A behavior that includes chronic aggression, hostility, and cynicism. These components can cause disease of the heart muscle and related illness by fostering disturbances in metabolism, especially in the level of "bad" cholesterol and plaques in the coronary arteries. According to psychologist Costa, "It's the cold-blooded variety of hostility that puts you at risk for heart disease, not the hot-blooded kind." Forgiveness of both ourselves and of others helps decrease the physiological damage of unrelenting anger.

In terms of the doshas, anger should be recognized as a signal from our physiology that there is (usually) a Pitta imbalance that deserves to be addressed. Ayur-Vedic treatment for anger focuses on bringing Pitta back into balance.

While imbalanced Pitta is generally the harbinger of anger, imbalanced Vata is the grande dame of anxiety. Whereas fear is commonly thought to be associated with something specific, anxiety is understood to be often "free-floating" or nonspecific. We know how debilitating anxiety can be, a feeling of fear flying in the face of rationality. Anxiety often comes when we feel we have to take responsibility for, or carry the burden of, a problem or a situation all by ourselves. Or it can be caused by a work and/or family overload leading to a feeling of fragmentation and disorganization.

But recall that anxiety also has a specific origin. It is strongly associated with imbalanced Vata dosha, with its accompanying restlessness, inability to focus, and airy, dissociative qualities. In people with Vata dosha dominant, emotional ama very often takes the form of fear and anxiety. It occurs when we lack stability in our lives, when we do not have the feeling of being "at home," of "being seated in the self." We may feel disconnected to any established

source of love. We can overcome these feelings of anxiety by reducing Vata through appropriate Ayur-Vedic regimes. In addition,
by tuning in to our own inner support systems, as well as by learning to receive fully from others and from nature itself, we can learn
to take it as it comes, instead of trying to control an outcome and
thus worrying endlessly about it.

Phobias are also understood as Vata disturbances, albeit extreme ones, which can cause high anxiety and panic attacks. Many
neuroscientists now believe that there is a biochemical explanation
for a panic attack thought to be initiated by a single fear triggering
an extensive chemical reaction and causing a flood of frightening
images, feelings, and scenarios. We can begin to deal with phobias
by first reducing the conditions in the bodymind that support un-
warranted fear through balancing Vata dosha and then participating
in a gradual step-by-step program to break the grip of the triggering
fear and subsequent panic.

Depending on our constitutional type, the season, and other
factors, Vata, Pitta or Kapha imbalances can cause depression. If
the Vata imbalance is more dominant in the depressive symptoms,
we may experience insomnia and/or weight loss and may feel
anxious and "empty" inside, resulting from an unsettled nervous
system. If Pitta imbalance has created the depression, anger, frustration, and resentment will be the more dominant features. If it results from a Kapha disturbance—manifested in the "I can't get out
of bed" syndrome—the depression will take on the sluggishness,
lethargy, excessive sleep need, and immobilized feelings associated
with Kapha imbalances. Just as the overly jumpy physiology of imbalanced Vata, which we call anxiety, may shun food, creating a
further Vata imbalance, the overeating often associated with couch
potato–style depression can create a further Kapha imbalance. The
emotional ama here is blocking our biological intelligence, and
thus we can be inappropriately guided to seek comfort and
warmth in food. What we really need to reverse the lethargy of
Kapha-type depression is a Kapha-reducing eating regime, more exercise, and more social interaction, so we can get rid of the ama,
become lighter, less congested, and more mobile physically, mentally, and emotionally.

In general, the onset of depression can usually be traced back
to some combination of overly intense activity, disrupted routines,

lack of rest, and emotional stress. Any treatment for depression must also attend to a central question: "What do I need to be happy? What is standing in the way of my personal fulfillment?" Even a genetic tendency toward depression can be eventually overcome by keeping the bodymind in balance on a daily basis. We can benefit from following the Ayur-Vedic routines to realign biological rhythms and rebalance the doshas according to which symptoms are more predominant.

All these psychological situations have specific physical symptoms associated with them. And although they are usually identified as separate and distinct from physiological situations in modern medicine, Ayur-Veda identifies them as highly individualized doshic imbalances and treats them accordingly.

## Restructuring Our Emotional Patterns

Maharishi Ayur-Veda helps us clarify another consideration for understanding the physiology of emotional healing. Our emotions don't just come out of the blue or even out of the blues. Just as there are emotional causes for physiological events, there is also a physiology of emotion that acts as a *predeterminant* of the emotions and feelings themselves.

Take the example of trust, an absolutely vital component of good health. Despite its value, it can be elusive. Some of us actually have a built-in bodymind tendency toward mistrust. Our bodies simply don't produce enough neuropeptides to help us feel comfortable around others. The reasons for this bodymind setup will naturally vary, depending on life experiences. There are those of us, for example, who have grown up with overly critical and/or abusive parents and have biochemically internalized our self-protection needs into a general distrust. So the tendencies created early in our lives may be set in our brain responses, and we are inappropriately blocked in our openness and trust of others, the very basis for the intimacy that we really need. Fortunately, Ayur-Veda can help us deal effectively with this situation, by enabling us to "reset" our brain responses. Let's see how this resetting process occurs.

Generally speaking, our emotions, like our thoughts, are organized in patterns that have been literally grooved into the brain. If deposits of stress or ama block our functioning, we become caught in habit patterns that are not life-supporting. Our nervous system returns time and again to the familiar, and we lose the flexibility associated with creativity and developmental growth. Ultimately this loss inhibits the fulfillment of our desires and detracts from the emotional satisfaction we require to bring about good health.

Caught in old patterns, we respond physiologically in an overly self-protective way to a new situation. The offer of a loving friendship is turned down by habit, despite what our hearts might long for. Our creative and loving impulses are overshadowed or, as the eminent psychologist Abraham Maslow put it, "drowned," by habit. We may have a thousand apple trees but still pick apples off the one tree that doesn't produce very healthy apples. Stuck in this habitual response, we eat the same apples over and over, whether they make us sick or not, because we don't have a way to move on to the next tree. So how *do* we learn to move on?

The tenets of Maharishi Ayur-Veda suggest that *because habitual patterns are fixed at the level of the nervous system, they must be dissolved at the very least at that level.* In other words, to overcome emotional ama, to free our hearts from being closed and distrustful, we need to alter the associated neural and biochemical patterns: For this we need something deeper than thinking or talking about our problems on the level of the problems themselves, something beyond psychotherapy or analysis. *We need a full psychophysical shift into a healthier bodymind.*

Maharishi Ayur-Veda offers the technique of Transcendental Meditation to enable us to let our minds go beyond their usual intellectual thinking modes. By dissolving stress in our nervous system, we erase the old programs, the useless bodymind patterns, and free our minds and hearts for the kinds of loving and unifying life experiences we most desire. The TM program provides a way to spontaneously cultivate a nervous system that supports all healthy emotional, mental, and physical possibilities, as it dissolves deep stress and ama that may hold us back. With a regular daily TM program, one's bodymind is easily moved from producing an overpatterned, restrictive mental and emotional response system to creating a fluid mode of responsiveness rooted in an ability to contact the nurturing unified field of consciousness within.

An elevated point of view, a positive belief system, can dynamically change our DNA, nervous system, and immune cells, giving us maximum opportunity to alter the course of disease. We can accomplish this only by changing our bodymind, by eradicating ama and stress where it was originally deposited, through a mental technique such as TM. Or we can first eliminate ama from our body and thereby create an eventual shift in our thinking and emotional responsiveness. Maharishi Ayur-Veda has brought out a number of different approaches by which we can create this bodymind change and thereby create more integrated health patterns. All the approaches are highly compatible and move in concert toward the same goal: a permanent state of total health. Some approaches are physical, including oil massages, eating regimes, and some yoga exercise stretching routines; others are more on the level of mind, such as TM. One approach offers a kind of medicine for bettering relationships called "behavioral rasayanas." This program (described in detail in chapter 8) can help to overcome anger, hostility, and distrust to free us from the grip of stress and clear out mental and emotional ama, enabling our entire physiology to be more fully open to the nurturance we desire.

## Dhatu Transformation and the Emotions

We've been looking at the effects of emotions on our physiology and behavior, but our emotions are also interdependently connected with our bodymind at an even deeper level, via our tissues, specifically in association with the entire cycle of digestion.

In the last chapter we discussed how all the levels of digestion come into play in our bodymind through the transformations of the dhatus. The dhatus give us a picture of how our physiology supports love and how love supports our physiology, and how the two are simultaneously structured to bring this ultimate nourishment directly into our physical, mental, and emotional lives.

"*I love you.*" Few other words produce such good medicine.

The Ayur-Vedic sages understood how love produces subtle transformations in your psychophysiology just as the digestion of food does. In this sense, the act of loving is an act of self-nourishment, the digestion of another kind of nourishment to enhance your emotional and spiritual growth. The idea of digesting love may seem unfamiliar, but remember that everything you experience through the senses, the mind, and the emotions affects you physiologically. As we've noted, watching a movie about Mother Teresa can benefit your physiology. The bodymind ingests and digests everything, whether in the air you physically inhale, the landscape you visually take in on the way to work, the social and emotional behavior of the people you care for and respond to, the love that you express and receive in all aspects of your life.

Vedic wisdom teaches, "All love is love of Self." Even if we are pining for the other, or fully immersed in devotional feelings for the other, what is really occurring is that we are awakening to our own inner self. We are transforming inside, growing in self-awareness and expansion of the heart. We nourish ourselves in order to grow and evolve within. It is a self-referral process of growth within our consciousness. However it may appear, union with another is really a union with one's innermost self as well, providing a vehicle to this more essential nourishment.

In this way, all the love one feels even as it extends outward to others is still love of self. Thus, even "unrequited" or one-sided love can have the same transformative effect as reciprocal love, if we understand that what is essential to our development is our *capacity to love*. It's not the object of love but its subject, the loving person, which expands. One important sign of good health is that the feeling of love is always requited within the self. Let's see how this self-referral process takes place throughout the bodymind.

### From a Full Stomach to a Full Heart

We can understand the development of our emotional health in terms of the Ayur-Vedic principles of transformation of the dhatus. While the function of the dhatu agnis, or each dhatu's "fire," is to transform experience into bodily nourishment, on a deeper level, the dhatus structure transformations of consciousness. We can envision how the seven-stage transformation process of digesting food can also represent the digesting of emotion. Indeed, the first dhatu, rasa, is also defined as "emotion" in the Ayur-Vedic texts. The first taste of food is thus transformed into chyle and blood plasma, but also nourishes the first awakening of feeling, the first satisfaction of a desire, resulting in bliss. Therefore, it is said, the first bite should be sweet.

Any imbalance in the rasa dhatu can be involved in both the emotions and the physical symptoms of eating disorders. If the rasa dhatu is out of balance and ama is created here, we can become lethargic, malnourished, underweight, and depressed. We may literally lose our appetite, our taste for food, and perhaps our appetite for other aspects of life. Whether we eat or not, we don't feel nourished. This imbalance can affect the transformation to the second dhatu, rakta. In some situations, there could be too much "heat" in the blood. As a result, along with the accompanying physical conditions, lack of the first sweet taste of love (rasa) can turn into anger in rakta: We could become emotionally "hot-blooded," ill-tempered and jealous; ego and possessiveness may come into a relationship either with the inner self or with another. To be healthy, we can let go and allow nature to help us take things more lightly, with less attachment, to lose more of the ego in order to gain more of the self.

The third dhatu agni, associated with mamsa, converts the product of rakta into the body's muscle. If the first two dhatu agnis have done their job well, we will develop strength and fortitude, both in body and in relationships. If we are digesting physical and emotional nourishment properly, we will feel solid and stable, as well as deeply protected and loved. But if the two preceding dhatus are weakened, the muscle fiber will not develop its strength and vibrancy. Emotionally, we won't feel secure in relationships, either with ourselves, others, or the world; a lack of "muscle," and a feeling of disempowerment could result and leave us feeling defenseless.

When nourishment is next transformed via the fourth dhatu agni, associated with medha, muscle is converted into fat. If the preceding dhatus are healthy, then our bodies easily transform muscle into fat and emotional strength and security into committed relationships with our deepest self and with others. If, however, the tissues are not well nourished to this point, the bodymind will send signals that we need more food, creating an overproduction in medha or fat tissue. This medha level can represent the sharing of love between couples or between parent and child. But it also can represent our deepest connection with self; in our society, overweight may reflect the result of lack of fulfillment in our most essential relationships and our lack of access to the self-nurturing field within.

The fifth dhatu agni, which is related to ashti, transforms fat into bone. It is associated with integrity, whereby the supportive mechanisms of emotional stability and loving allow us to stand tall, to have "backbone"; to be an upright, vital, personal and social force. With a weakened ashti, we can end up feeling a lack of real presence or depth in relationships. Even a committed love relationship doesn't make us feel strong when we don't feel supported inside.

The sixth dhatuagni is associated with majja and converts food and love into the central nervous system and also supplies our bone marrow. We may have had a relationship or an inner experience in which we have the feeling, "It touches me to the marrow," a feeling of being deeply known, loved, and nurtured. This is where, when majja is strong, the bone structure can be filled with life-supporting nourishment, with fullness, with self-fulfillment, where love is nurtured in the self from the deepest source.

When this occurs, majja can be successfully transformed into the seventh tissue, shukra, which is expressed as ova or sperm. The shukra tissue is extremely potent, the end product of the entire process. It is the delicate final blossoming of all the dhatus. It can create its own reproduction (a child) and it can create ojas. Ojas, as we've seen, is the subtlest physical essence of our bodies, expressed not only as a final substance but found between all the dhatus, supporting each of the levels of transformation. It is both the product of digestion in the bodymind and also the fulfillment of self-referral love, which is self-sufficient, needing nothing from outside itself to feel whole. Ojas integrates our bodyminds, emotions, and spirituality.

## The Integrating Results of Self-Nurturance

It's clear that from the Ayur-Vedic point of view, having an emotionally balanced life starts within our consciousness and gets expressed in our metabolism; if our digestion and elimination processes are dysfunctional, so too will our emotions be off-balance. The responses of our emotions and physiology are interdependent events; neither process "comes first." With this approach, Ayur-Veda addresses the problem of why many otherwise intelligent women participate in negative addictive love relationships. When our physiological balance is off, we may crave a certain kind of relationship that can create further imbalance and further addiction in the same way that nervous people become addicted to caffeine, to the very quality that is causing the problem. Women "who love too much" and make "foolish choices" in partners may be doing so because their physiological body type is off-balance. By becoming balanced physically, a woman can spontaneously choose healthier relationships that promote rather than negate her emotional needs and growth.

While a great deal of attention is paid to the emotional basis for good physical health—"Love yourself and you will be healthy"—from an Ayur-Vedic perspective, psychiatric and psychotherapeutic interventions that neglect nutritional and other physiological issues are as negligent as surgeons who disregard the emotional effects of surgery. To correct this situation, a number of clinicians are incorporating physical treatment modalities, such as nutritional, sleep, and meditation techniques, into their therapy practices. Every therapist knows that clients are often dealing with physical symptomatology along with mental and emotional issues. Ayur-Veda enables the field of psychotherapy to reassess mental, emotional, and addiction problems by addressing their equally significant physiological basis.

### Trust and Distrust, Health and Separation

Not surprisingly, having a heart that trusts others has been found to be medically sound. Its opposite, distrust, creates illness and emotional ama. It also seems that the many physiological and emotional consequences of a lack of basic emotional nourishment can cause great harm to health, especially when they occur in infants and children. Unless one has internalized the feeling of "mother is at home," a feeling that one is safe and secure, being and feeling alone can induce highly stressful long-term physiological reactions.

At the Primate Lab at the University of Wisconsin, researchers isolated six-month-old monkeys from their mothers and other caregivers for only twenty-four hours. As a result, white blood cell regulation was disrupted for at least a month after the babies were reunited with their mothers. Dr. Christopher Coe, chairman of the lab, noted, "When prolonged, this response can have a mutagenic effect on surrounding cells that might increase susceptibility to disease. . . ."[10]

Because infants and the elderly may be most at risk, fostering emotional stability in our young children and in the elderly by minimizing loneliness is a health measure that could avert the onset of serious illness. Certain research also has linked separation stress to such varied diseases as asthma, arthritis, and leukemia. Coe suspects that "divorce, hospitalization, or the death of a parent might cause immune suppression" as well.

Other research suggests that, all other factors being equal, there is a perceived lack of closeness with parents in individuals, both men and women, who have developed cancer. The researchers concluded that the quality of human relationships may be an important component in the development of cancer.[11] This was corroborated in another study at the Johns Hopkins University School of Medicine: A significant increase in cancer (including lung cancer in nonsmokers) was found among subjects who indicated through projective tests that their interpersonal relationships were less than satisfactory.

A trusting heart is one of the secrets to enjoying the best of health, allowing us to withstand life's ups and downs without feeling deeply shaken emotionally by every difficult event. Such trust is generally established when we are children. A secure child learns to ride the waves, having internalized a sense of being loved no matter what. But many of us are not so lucky as to have had such a sense of security internally established when we were children.

Maharishi Ayur-Veda can provide us with the means to learn to trust, even when we have been deprived of such stabilizing influences early on. It gives us a way to experience an inner self that never changes, without having to revisit the stress of the past. This happens because when we transcend to deeper aspects of the self, we meet up with nature's emotional support system, that eternal mother within, Mother Divine herself. Whatever name we give her, she is never far away; she appears within our own hearts. Once we become reacquainted with this most intimate source of nurturance inside, we find her everywhere, in the hearts of our friends and even in the eyes of strangers. We become fearless; not out of foolishness but out of genuine freedom.

A complete state of trust can come only from being connected to the deepest, most stable sense of inner selfhood. From a psychological view, lack of trust stems from the fear of losing a relationship that we feel we depend on. But we know that relationships always change, even in the best of circumstances: A spouse or parent dies, we get a divorce, the children grow up and leave home. So despite some psychological arguments to the contrary, a relationship is not the best basis on which to establish a permanent sense of security.

To find real emotional security, we have to develop our inner lives to the fullest, not in a narrow, self-indulgent way, but in the sense of developing faith in the sustaining value of our own experiences Emotional stability occurs as a quality of our consciousness, within which we can experience the unshakable unity of life. From this inner awareness, we can love fully, like a trusting, openhearted child who knows that her mother is watching over her, even if she cannot see her. Here is where we find the reservoir of absolute trust. And here our bodymind finds its most constant support, secure in the knowledge that we can go into and even out of relationships if we have to, without feeling emotionally, mentally, and physically demolished. Once we are living in absolute trust, we feel far more intimately connected to others, not because we are necessarily "good" at relationships, but because we can give fully of ourselves, unafraid, holding nothing back, moving effortlessly beyond the boundaries of self-isolation and loneliness. We can give love, and perhaps even more important, we can surrender at last, and allow love in. By welcoming love in, and not pushing it away, we permit the essential lubricant of aching bones and inflamed joints to soothe away our pain, a most wonderful kind of bodymind medicine.

In the next chapter, we're going to look at relationships from the point of view of our health and consider why some relationships are healthier for us than others and why love is the sweetest medicine of all.

# Chapter 8

LOVE

## The Physiology of Personal Relationships

*A loving heart, a heart full of love,*
*Is the precious essence of human life.*
*Love is the supreme blessing of life;*
*Love as love is universal.*
*Personal love is concentrated universal love.*

Maharishi Mahesh Yogi[1]

All relationships flow from consciousness. Realizing that our emotions move physically through our bodyminds, we can recognize that our loving relationships with others as well as ourselves create a powerful and direct physical influence on health or illness. In Maharishi Ayur-Veda, there are relationship guidelines that remind us that the purpose of relationships is to produce the bliss of vibrant health *simultaneously* within ourselves and within others. You can tell if it's a healthy, healing, and evolutionary relationship if it is nourishing. This happens when you experience a wave of love or touch the heart of another deeply and sweetly: A wave of bliss is created where the mind and body meet, rinsing away the effects of old stress there. We can draw to us a powerful healing influence through choosing, where possible, interactions that heal by creating wholeness. In this context, mutuality of interests, desires, depth, and loyalty produce holistic growth and create the essence of a healthy relationship.

## Women as the Scientists of Interpersonal Relationships

A long history of care-taking relationships permeates the responses and interactions of modern women. Through centuries of devotional service to others, whether as wives, mothers, nurses, or teachers, women's heart orientation has been well developed. Even today, we are still primarily guided in our behavior by the learnings of the heart: Researchers have found that even the most successful career women, when asked what brings them the most happiness, place their relationships ahead of their work achievements.

This heart orientation obviously does not preclude intellectual, social, or creative development; it suggests rather that there is another force at work here. In her ground-breaking research on women's moral development, decision making, and relationship styles, Dr. Carol Gilligan of Harvard University identified women as scientists of interpersonal relationships who base their decisions on the effects they will have on others.[2] It is a personal system of caring, responsibility, and dependency, as in dependability. (Gilligan found that little girls consider "dependency" a positive word, as in "you can depend on someone.") She concluded that women's moral decisions are based on relative judgments structured in the ability to empathize, affiliate, and identify with others; our intentions and actions are based more on feelings relative to circumstances than on a predetermined intellectual principle of right and wrong. This caring nature of women runs even deeper than our culture, suggests Gillian, because the culture itself has not particularly upheld or respected these perceived "female" values. But that situation is changing. These female values are now becoming far more highly prized in our society. They have even become associated with good health. For example, researchers at the University of Nebraska School of Medicine reported that elderly individuals, both men and women, who had at least one good woman friend they could confide in had better immune function and lower levels of cholesterol and uric acid in their blood—i.e., less stress effects—than those without a female confidante.

Given our psychophysiology and our history, it's no surprise that women often seek a profound level of fulfillment within relationships. Studies have demonstrated that women of all ages have greater ability and desire than men to discern emotions and feelings. This naturally gives men and women a different set of expectations in relationships. For women, relationships are understood to be, if not *the* essential vehicle for growth, at least among the top two or three such vehicles. So we look to our relationships as fundamental for bringing happiness into our lives.

To this end, much of our time may seem to be spent "working" on our relationships, to establish lines of communication and improve feelings between our spouses, parents, children, coworkers, and friends. These are certainly worthy and necessary social, and even spiritual, goals. But how do we go about accomplishing this?

Many women are familiar, through experiences of individual and group psychotherapies, with the ongoing and widespread psychological, process-oriented approach to love and relationships, which is essentially based on personality and developmental theory. But most of what we currently recognize as "therapeutic" in our culture tends to ignore the *physiological* structures of relationship. Indeed, we spend a great deal of time and energy analyzing compatibility in our relationships, focusing on interpersonal communications, mutual perception, social identities, and so forth, but in all our discussions, almost nothing is said about *physiological compatibility* which is based on consciousness. Yet this may be a far more essential consideration for getting along with someone. As one physicist has observed, "The quality of a relationship depends upon the 'ground state' of the persons involved in it. . . . Two people who are in the same state will have a more harmonious intimate relationship than two people who are in different states."[3]

Ayur-Veda offers a system of understanding relationships that can be seen in the light of balance and health. The expression "healthy relationships" takes on a more integral meaning when we start to recognize the choices we are spontaneously making, and have made, from the Ayur-Vedic perspective. Of course, most matters of the heart are generally beyond the intellect—"The heart has its reasons that reason knoweth not"—and with that understanding, we can take a lighthearted look at doshas and relationships.

## The Unifying Nature of Relationships

Although the process may not be an entirely conscious one, we are always seeking balance. Since the doshas are found in all of nature, the ways to balance our own are infinitely available to us. Hearing the birds on a spring day in Iowa, looking up at the sky on a starry night in Vermont, or smelling the fragrant eucalyptus trees in Northern California—this is our dosha-balancing medicine.

You may feel a great desire to be at the ocean or on a mountain or in the woods, often depending on which dosha is predominant. Your decisions about where to live or where to go on vacation and when may well be physiologically based. This can cause conflicts for families taking a vacation together. A Vata-type family member may sincerely need a time of sun and ocean, warmth and quiet during a dry, cold, Vata-imbalancing winter; a Pitta may require a week in the cool mountain air during a hot, humid summer; a Kapha type may find herself longing for the excitement of wind-surfing or the lung-clearing, drying experiences at a desert resort. We also balance our doshas by being around certain people. For example, the recent integration of child-care services within elder-care facilities has been of great benefit both to the children needing adult love and the adults needing the children's warmth and affection. Perhaps we could say that the Vata of the older person is balanced by the Kapha of infancy and childhood.

Ayur-Veda reminds us that our personal relationships, although we may treat them as a special category in our lives, are part of nature and therefore subject to nature's laws as well. Just as you metabolize the ocean breeze, you metabolize your relationships; that is, you take in the psychophysiological being, the consciousness of others. If we regard others as separate and different from ourselves, we have more difficulty digesting them. Racism and other forms of people-hating actually create far more ill health for those who experience the hatred than for those they hate, just as those who surrender in love benefit from the healing that such devotion creates far more than the beloved.

Quantum physics offers us an interesting perspective on relationships within the unified field. What is known as the Einstein-

Podolsky-Rosen Paradox, or the "EPR phenomenon," suggests that "once two particles have been near each other, they continue to instantaneously affect each other no matter how widely they may be separated."[4] They can be separated by time as well as space, yet still maintain that intimate connection. A corollary of this is the concept of "action at a distance," according to which one bodymind influences another as if the two were never really separated at all. If this holds true for people as well as protons, twenty-five years or three thousand miles means nothing. If you have ever attended a reunion, you know what this feels like; the connections don't really disappear, even if everything else has changed.

Once we have interacted, we become part of each other's physiology. And because we are together on this earth at the same time or feel Bach's music in our hearts five hundred years after he composed it, the entire phenomenon of bodymind interaction still permeates our genes and our behavior. We have always been and will always be in each other's worlds on a very basic level; there is really no division between selves, between "I and Thou," between where I end and you begin. When this happens in a group of people, we enter into pure connectedness and allow ourselves to venture beyond fear and separateness into the experience of the recognition that we are all expressions of the unified field. Of course, we are still separate and individual and very much our own persons, but our essential connectedness enables us to enjoy the expansion of a greater and deeper territory for interpersonal relationships and social responsibility.

In this light, when we want to consider our specific personal relationships in Ayur-Vedic terms, it's important to keep in mind that in the eyes of Mother Nature we are always "in love" and can never really be out of love, because we are all joined within the unified field where the differences disappear. And if we want to work on a particular relationship, it makes good sense to first work within ourselves, to reawaken the source of love within our hearts by accessing this unifying resource of love and bringing it to the friendship table. Without it, our sense of being separate can never really be resolved; with it, our sense of being united can never really disappear. This is the highest goal of all relationships, to cultivate the experience of unity with and within each person we love.

Now let's look more closely at constitutional compatibility within relationships.

## Doshas and Relationships

On the one hand, like doshas attract. It's the comfort and joy of the familiar. Vatas adore each other's high, light energy and those endless phone conversations where fourteen topics are left dangling as a fifteenth starts; Pittas relish the keenness of purpose and achievement orientation they share, and their mutual intensity in any activity; Kaphas take pleasure in their mutually experienced, secure, graceful pace of life. And it's nice to have dinner with someone who eats as slowly and speaks as evenly as you.

A more intuitive, simpler relationship can occur when we understand why our friends are the way they are, using as a basis of understanding the responses of our *own* physiology. For example, a Vata naturally recognizes why her Vata friend just started another new project; a Kapha realizes why her Kapha son prefers to save his money rather than take a vacation. And a Pitta fully understands why her Pitta spouse did not enjoy losing that Sunday afternoon tennis game. There can be a delightful, easy "frictionless" flow between likenesses.

On the other hand, like doshas can be uncomfortable together. Two Vatas often can go nowhere together fast—all air, no substance, dust in the wind. And two Kapha types can go nowhere slowly; their mutual lack of mobility and disinterest in change could make for a very noncommunicative, undynamic pairing. Two Pittas can subtly and not so subtly compete and continually annoy each other with their own need to be "right." So while there may be lifelong comfort in similarity, there also could be a tendency for two individuals with the same constitution to create further imbalance in the predominant dosha, since like increases like.

We can and do more easily balance our doshas through our opposites. It can often be difficult to be with a slow Kapha if you are a fast Vata, but it also helps you experience balance. And these multiple combinations add interest and dynamism within our various relationships. For example, if your dominant dosha is Vata and your employee's is Pitta, what might happen? Sometimes you will find a benefit in this fire and air combination; the excitement and intensity can be very productive. Vata can benefit from Pitta's goal orientation and focusing power and accomplish a great deal more, while Pitta can enjoy the expansiveness and vision of Vata's creativity. At other times it's literally an explosive combination; Vata's air can fuel Pitta's fire too well, turning the relationship to ashes. And lacking much Kapha, long-term stability might be somewhat tenuous.

Or if your dominant dosha is Pitta and your sister's is Kapha, there can be a marvelous feeling of "temperature" balancing; Kapha feels warmed up and alive, and fiery Pitta feels the soothing cool Kapha on her fevered brow. But watery Kapha also can extinguish Pitta's flame and Pitta can overheat Kapha. The combination can "boil" the relationship down to nothing. And without much lighthearted Vata, these two can get ponderous and pontifical.

In the Vata and Kapha combination, Vata can feel very happy, even mesmerized by the gracious, stabilizing, earthy influence of her Kapha neighbor, while Kapha may fully enjoy Vata's ability to lighten, brighten, and energize the relationship. On the other hand, Kapha may find herself digging into a more fixed position, unable and unwilling to move with Vata's mutability and impulsivity, while Vata can begin to find Kapha's initially charming stability more a quality of stubbornness that slows down or inhibits Vata's free-wheeling-ness. Without fire, the Vata and Kapha relationship can be a bit disconnected, distant, and cool.

Since most of us have more than a single dosha dominant, the dual-dosha combinations in romantic, working, or friendship relationships are perhaps more typical. A Vata-Pitta individual, for example, meeting up with a Pitta-Kapha person, brings Vata dosha to the table and is offered Kapha in return. And in this way, all three doshas are available in the relationship. Their mutual Pitta fire is a great meeting place, while the Vata and Kapha balance each other. Similarly, a Vata-Kapha interacting with a Pitta-Kapha will enjoy the mutual stabilizing and leisurely quality of being together, while the other doshas are in balance as well. And a Vata-Kapha with a Vata-Pitta will share the airy exuberance of Vata, and yet have enough forcefulness and silent settledness between them to last more than a Vata hour.

It appears that relationships that are long-lasting have both some opposition and some similarity. For many if not all long-term couples, the doshas are in some deep sense shared. The two may start to look alike. This is not surprising; their lives are intimately intertwined and so is their physiology. This kind of true union is often very beautiful when it occurs and very devastating when it ends, not just emotionally but physically.

*Joe and Beth were married for fifty-five years. They had six children and eight grandchildren and were always each other's nearest and dearest. Beth's Vata-Kapha constitution complemented Joe's Pitta-Kapha. Their mutual Kapha traits let them establish a very habitual life that pleased them both enormously. When Joe died in his early seventies, the huge loss that Beth experienced was not only emotional but also required an entire realignment of her bodymind, which took several months of her feeling very out of control. Grieving his loss, she felt alternately "spacey" (imbalanced Vata) and dull (imbalanced Kapha). She lost her appetite; her gastrointestinal system was entirely out of whack, alternating between diarrhea and constipation.*

*She started on a Kapha- and Vata-balancing program, which increased the "fire" in all aspects of her life. She started to eat more Pitta-increasing kinds of foods. She also found herself enlivening Pitta in other areas. She began to take some courses. And she started doing all the focusing tasks that her husband always had done. She was put into a far more active financial role, which she enjoyed, and then started her own investment management program, learning on her own with a financial computer service. Her success at finances brought her into a more balanced frame of mind; her organizing skills and clarity developed quickly.*

*Beth also felt physically better, not just mentally and financially, once her doshas were more in balance. Her digestion returned to normal. Her acceptance of her emotional loss obviously took much longer, but with improved overall health, eventually she was able to overcome the physiological longing, sadness, and heavy heart. The sense of loss, although present, was much lighter and less disruptive to her bodymind functioning.*

## Object-Referral and Self-Referral Relationships

Why do relationships have such different qualities, such different effects on us? Some seem to foster very good feelings, others seem to only make us feel bad. Often we have great difficulty, despite our best intentions, distinguishing the good relationships from the not-so-good ones in advance, or even when we are in the middle of them.

Maharishi Ayur-Veda makes it clear that relationships are opportunities for the growth of the self, ways to ultimately create health within the bodymind by awakening our inner awareness. But sometimes, in our desire to love and have that beautifully expansive feeling, we forget that all love is directed toward the self. We mistake the object of love for the subject of love. We experience desire coming from a feeling of something lacking. We may believe, for example, that a change in a particular relationship would make us feel more whole; if only that other person behaved in a different way, it would make us fulfilled. The less we are caught in this feeling of lack, the more likely we are to have healthy relationships. In this light, there are two essential kinds of relationships: object-referral and self-referral relationships.

### OBJECT-REFERRAL RELATIONSHIPS

You are "in love." You may be exhausted or sick but you don't care. You may have isolated yourself from your usual sources of support and love, your friends and family. Your work, generally a source of pleasure for you, holds no interest and your attention is very divided. You are "in love." You experience the feeling of what is called "losing yourself" in the relationship.

When you are operating from an "object-referral" state of awareness, you believe that something outside yourself is going to make you happy: It could be a new car, a certain award, or a particular person. When you lose yourself in a relationship, you have lost the knowledge of the self in its wholeness, and you find yourself identifying with the objects of experience.

The feeling of being overshadowed by or even "addicted" to another person, as opposed to feeling the fullness of unconditional love, is really an indication of an imbalance in the doshas. You may find yourself seeking object-referral experiences that heighten already overstimulated emotions, causing further imbalance. When you are able to balance your doshas physiologically, these love addictions disappear. Your feelings of deprivation and sadness, which seem to accompany all obsessive longings, are alleviated by the addition of physiological nurturance. You may still be attracted to certain people, but without the addictive quality of life-or-death attachment.

Once you are more in balance physiologically, you are freer to choose what you really want in relationships.

### SELF-REFERRAL RELATIONSHIPS

You are constitutionally in balance, bodymind and emotions. You feel as though you are humming along with good fortune on your side. You don't need to paint this state of consciousness, or write about it, or even express it intimately to another person. It just *is,* in its own glorious, unbounded way. You have a sense of deep self-sufficiency and don't feel you need anything from outside yourself to experience this happiness. You interact with that infinite resource within, in a self-referral way. You feel healthy, dynamic, productive, and yet rested. You enjoy the silence inside. It is not an isolated feeling, or a too proud or too scared feeling. You feel very open to others; you perceive them at their most beautiful and most cherishable.

Your awareness is dominated by the unifying aspects of life, not the distinctions, although you can make them. You recognize that others are not separate from you, but a part of you. You feel free to choose to be with someone and free to choose not to. When you meet someone, you may feel deeply interested but not needy. Your interest is based not on imbalance but on equality. You may be joyfully attracted but not overwhelmed or out of control. This state of balance does not deny love; just the opposite, it can give and receive love fully and unconditionally.

In this self-referral state, you can enjoy a heart that is full of love and full of life. According to the well-known Vedic text, the Bhagavad-Gita, "When love is full, life is full like the ocean, it is full like a silent ocean for it ceases to flow in any direction, it just is, it is free from desire."[5] And this status of the fullness of love is a wonderful goal; just by *being,* you are living the fullness of your life.

This is the goal of Ayur-Veda, providing far more than medicine for the body, offering the ultimate nourishment for the heart. To accomplish this, it provides us with special prescriptions, medicine for *behavior* that can actually help create deep integrative health within each of us.

## Prescriptions for the Heart:
## The Behavioral Rasayanas

A *rasayana* (ruh-sah-yuh-nuh) is an herbal or mineral preparation taken through the body to rejuvenate our physiology, balance the doshas, and support our longevity. Behavioral rasayanas do the same for the personality. They are some of the most beneficial Ayur-Vedic prescriptions, the Ayur-Vedic "herbs for the heart." They may sound simple and very familiar, because they are really not new, yet their simplicity doesn't detract from their truth. They remind us of what we have always known but may have forgotten during the morning rush hour.

Each of these "prescriptions" deepens the experience of the real self, serving to heal mind, body, and heart simultaneously, by producing the biochemicals that create ojas and the experience of bliss. If followed and lived continuously, they are said to promote a state of completely invincible health, "twenty-four-hour-a-day" bliss, where your heart feels happy for no other reason than the experience of its own natural state, not dependent on a promotion, winning the lottery, or a perfect relationship.

As you look down the list of behavioral rasayanas, try not to think of them as something *outside* yourself to be introduced, but as something *within* you, ready to be reawakened. You may feel deep familiarity with them, because you are already living many of them and are enjoying their healthy effects in your daily life. You will notice they are actual qualities of self—not advice on how to *behave,* but reminders on how to *be,* in order to maintain good health. You can't do them; you just have to be them.

*1. Speak truthfully but sweetly.* Maintaining a good connection with your own inner resource of integrity is the key to smooth and harmonious relationships. Use a daily technique such as TM to make firm this connection, and then be sure you are settled within before you speak. Being truthful frees us from any worry and fear arising from deception and complication, which can lead to illness. Being truthful is a health-producing process, but only when we speak the "sweet truth," which does not cause unnecessary pain to another.

*2. Speak well of others.* Speaking well of others allows for refinement in thinking and feeling. It is a beautiful opportunity for eliminating fear and anger, thereby healing your own heart. It enables you to enjoy your positive feelings fully, while remaining neutral toward your less happy ones. Complaints don't improve anything or anyone. It helps to remember that what you put your attention on grows stronger in your life.

*3. Be free of anger.* Avoid getting caught in a world of redress or revenge. Of all the psychophysiological correlates of behavior, hostility has been found to be the most toxic and most damaging to one's own body, whether we direct the hostility toward someone else or toward ourselves. Postpone any discussion when your bodymind feels agitated, angry, or otherwise unsettled. If you can't put off an uncomfortable exchange, try not to mind the emotions of the other person. Just listen and respond to the *content*.

No matter how different we are from one another, one thing is the same in all of us—the unity of our being that lies in the depths of our hearts.

*4. Abstain from immoderate behavior.* Balance is the key not only to health but also to healthy behavior. We can feel most deeply and love most fully while maintaining emotional balance through moderation. When we are calm, even, and contented, the most positive aspects of our friendships will be most sweetly nourished.

*5. Be nonviolent and calm.* Ahimsa (uh-hihn-suh) is the experience and expression of nonviolence or harmlessness. Keep a quiet attitude of friendliness, compassion, and receptivity. Eighty percent of what you "say" is communicated to the other person nonverbally. Nonviolence should permeate our thoughts, speech, and, of course, our actions. A demeaning remark can do harm and put a crimp in the heart, actually inflicting some physiological as well as emotional damage, both within oneself and within the other person: "Words can be scalpels. They can generate thoughts, feelings and beliefs in our brain which can be communicated to the cells in our body and even to the chemicals within cells."[5]

Speak and behave in a way that produces ojas and keeps it flowing, in order to communicate healthiness, not illness, as much as possible.

*6. Maintain cleanliness of yourself and your environment.* Attend to creating ojas in your bodymind and beauty and harmony in your environment with equal diligence. Ingesting and digesting the orderliness of each, of the inner and outer environment, will mutually enhance the healing, enlightening value of the other. This applies to your thoughts as well, as they structure your inner and outer home. A sound mind *is* a sound body.

*7. Be charitable.* Give your time, your attention, your money, your energy where and when they are needed. Yet remember always to treat yourself charitably as well, taking the time you need to replenish. Don't allow your light to become extinguished. If you give light to others from a lit candle, your light is not diminished; rather, more light becomes available to you as well.

*8. Be respectful to teachers and elders.* Respect includes an open heart and the ability to listen sincerely, so that the deepest exchange can occur, beyond the social or informational exchange of words alone. Listen to your teachers from your heart as best you can. Learning from a mentor or teacher gives the invaluable advantage of verifying your own experiences of knowledge. Someone who has been there before you can point out the signposts along the way. The long-lasting traditions of our elders, whether within our immediate family or culture or from other cultures and other centuries, have real value and allow us to go more deeply into knowledge and experience, providing the essential foundation on which creativity thrives.

*9. Be loving and compassionate.* When you are "calm" and "passionate" at the same time, you can deeply feel for others without losing yourself in their needs. The calm power of love is limitless. It produces maximum good with minimum energy. The more deeply settled within you are, the more you can feel for the struggles of others, while at the same time being capable of dynamic, responsible, life-augmenting actions.

*10. Keep a regular routine.* A regular routine allows you to focus well, and not get scattered. It provides rest, energy, coherence, and a settled mind and heart and enables you to bring the value of your expanded consciousness to any activity. It will provide you with the best conditions under which you can be the person you most want to be, the person nature most wants you to be.

*11. Culture a simple state of awareness and simple, guileless behavior.* Practicing TM twice a day easily develops that most desirable bodymind integration, a simple state of awareness, from which we spontaneously behave in accord with the magnificent guidance of nature's laws. By trying to manipulate events and other people for our own ends, we produce illness in body and mind, especially if we are trying to swim against the tides. Innocence is the key to getting nature on your side, giving you maximum support, fullness, and success without any superficial distractions and unnecessary machinations complicating the most direct path.

*12. Keep the company of the wise.* The incandescent light of consciousness is compelling. Being around individuals whose physiology is balanced helps you restructure your own. A wise person can thus bring you to your own wisdom. Whenever possible, choose to be around the people who uplift you, those who bring you up, not put you down, who bring out the best in you.

*13. Maintain a positive outlook.* Whenever you recognize that you have a choice, choose the positive over the negative, and happiness over unhappiness. In order to attain the best in life, you will do well to direct your spirits to absolute gladness, bringing hope and the least possible discouragement to others.

*14. Be self-controlled and follow the precepts of your religious beliefs.* To be self-controlled means to be one-pointed on the highest path, settling for nothing less than your full development, doing what you know intuitively is right for you. Finding such a path, a religious teaching that attracts you, will provide you with the opportunity to enliven your devotional nature, to develop higher states of consciousness, and to help cultivate a feeling of surrender to your best self. Allowing nature to express herself through us is the greatest blessing of all.

*15. Devote yourself to the knowledge and development of*

*higher states of consciousness.* Learning to fully develop and use the full capabilities of your bodymind is nature's way of optimizing, of evolving, through you. The desire to enjoy higher states of consciousness is the most natural desire of all. The knowledge of higher states of awareness is the most satisfying knowledge, the most personal, the most intimate, the most healing—producing life-supporting influences in your entire physiology, beyond the development of your mind alone. Such knowledge is the greatest purifier of all, a perfect way to keep healthy, enriching every aspect of daily life with ever greater depth of experience and unity.

## Three Healing Principles

Along with the behavioral rasayanas, there are three principles that can help us to heal ourselves through love, upholding the deepening stability of our emotional and mental health: transcending, self-nurturance, and integrity.

### LOSING THE EGO AND GAINING THE SELF: THE PRINCIPLE OF TRANSCENDING

Women seem to cherish above all the experiences of the deeper values of life that transcend the separateness of individual ego and allow us to feel united with others. This depth of interior life, often in concert with the interior life of another, keeps us feeling full and happy. It is the process, not the goal, the present moment of openness and not the potential future, which seems to bring us the greatest joy. For example, in a study of men and women artists, researchers found that when other factors were equal—money earned from art, critical acclaim, gallery representation—the one thing that distinguished men artists from women artists was their orientation to the future. Whereas the men were consciously taking steps to ensure their future reputation, the women were not preparing for the future of their art and, perhaps most significant, *had no desire to do so.* Similarly, when compared with their male counterparts, women doctors were found to be less interested in gaining (future) status and recognition in their field than in the (present) process of caring for their patients.

These studies give us some indication that women may have developed a greater ability to be less attached to the fruits of their actions, more liberated from the boundaries of ego without losing any of the accomplishment that might accompany such ego attachment. We seem to have learned the secret of letting go because we have had to let go. As Virginia Woolf wrote, "Often nothing tangible remains of a woman's day. The food that has been cooked is eaten; the children that have been nursed have gone out into the world." This is the lesson of nonattachment, of surrender. This is a natural state that comes about innocently. And it's an important illness prevention measure as well.

For both males and females, there is a close link between how fully you experience the expansive values of life and how fully healthy you are. Every time we divide life up into objects and things and pieces of time and partial views, we cut ourselves up as well. And every time we let go and allow in a feeling of trust and expansion and surrender, we enliven the wholeness value and we build a stronger bodymind.

The Ayur-Vedic prescription is that we put our attention on what we want to happen and then we let go and allow nature to organize the outcome. To capture a wave you sink back into the ocean.

This principle supports our emotional and physical health in all aspects of life, even as we progress toward our various goals. Being able to accept the processes of life and to exercise a loving, nonjudgmental attitude toward them enables us to let go and enjoy the present. By holding too tightly to what we think we want to achieve, we may miss other more significant opportunities to grow and may also create a lot of internal distress. By freeing ourselves from the desire to "win," we can focus on the process of achievement, on the steps to the goal, not merely on the goal itself. We learn to favor the "being" aspect of life over the "doing" aspect. We can benefit from culturing the ability to lose the ego and gain the self.

Quilting is an example of the cooperative style of creation that grew out of the deeper, interconnective feelings of the women who created quilts. There is a certain egoless maturity in allowing the group effect to take precedence over one's individual contribution. Research has corroborated this assessment of interconnective orientation; even highly individualistic, high-achieving women have also been found to be collectively oriented and concerned about the greater good.

This "self-in-relation-to others" modality is thought to be a function of a higher level of development. It allows for maximum enjoyment along the way and, not coincidentally, maximum success—without creating dis-ease—as we rise to the top. It also presents the opportunity to create the integrity of a win-win situation, where competence, not competition, is the key. Competition at the expense of good health is generally stressful and unnatural. It prohibits the benefits of all-around winning, of loving and nurturing ourselves and others simultaneously. It often leaves us feeling defeated even when we have "won," and it never satisfies in the way that mutual benefit does. This same principle applies to all our relationships, at work, with our families, and with our friends.

### HEALING THE SELF: THE PRINCIPLE OF SELF-NURTURANCE

The most important relationship any woman has must be with herself. How she treats herself, in sickness, in health, for better, for worse, can be the only basis on which she becomes capable of loving and cherishing others, of creating genuine health. If a woman starts to lose touch with the self-nurturing resource within, she often loses the ability to nurture others. None of us, no matter how well-intended, can offer real sustenance from an empty cup. The cup must be full and even running over, so we don't feel drained or feel a loss in nurturing.

If a woman gives to her family to the point of exhaustion or to her husband to the point of resentment, because she does not feel his emotional support in return; or if she is so busy and so tired that she no longer has time or energy to give to herself, she will be risking ill health. She will be highly susceptible to the common syndromes of burnout, depression, and chronic fatigue, which so many women today are experiencing. The inability to self-nurture is very likely an underlying cause for a variety of health problems associated with a lack of loving, especially for "women who do too much" and end up feeling too little.

Losing connection with a source of love inside may start as a

feeling of loneliness even in the midst of a great whirlwind of social and professional activity. We may term it a lack of self-love or
self-esteem, but it is essentially the result of being out of touch
with our own nature. We know that real nurturance, whether one
is in a happy relationship or not, comes from deep within ourselves. We can access the reservoir of creativity, love, and intelligence that guides all nature, and certainly each of us, if we can just
remember to keep in touch with it. We can then give easily from
a full heart instead of struggling to do so from an emptied vessel.
With self-nurturance, our needs and expectations of receiving all
our missing love from others can subside, and we can enjoy a more
powerful self-sufficiency within our relationships.

### THE INTEGRATION OF SELF: THE PRINCIPLE OF INTEGRITY

Many women today suffer needlessly from the fear of success, pop-
ularly called the "imposter syndrome." This fear is most easily overcome with the recognition that the person we want to be is the
same as the person we are. If we constantly separate aspects of the
self from the feeling of wholeness within, if we think about how
we should look and how we should behave and how we should
achieve some goal as separate endeavors, our self-image and selfhood become separate as well. And because the innermost self is
the only place where our integrity is fully realized, anything less *is*
is a kind of imposter.

To go beyond a fragmented sense of partial self, we need a
deeper understanding of what and who we really are. What
women fear is not success but the loss of a richer, more satisfying
level of fulfillment that comes not from external success but
from inner congruity, from the knowledge that what you want to
be and what you are *already* are joined within. This level of self-
acceptance is the belief that Mother Nature is guiding us and we
need only listen to her sweet whisper of abiding encouragement.

It seems we can only enjoy our successes and not mind our fail-
ures when we know how little they have to do with who we really
are inside. Then waves of achievement and their opposites move
by us, leaving us undisturbed, full, and unbounded. No job opportunity, no relationship, no financial windfall, can ever offer more

than the satisfaction of simply knowing, "I am being fully myself."

Enjoying this deep personal integrity is no doubt the healthiest way we can live. To struggle against our natural inclination even to follow a seemingly "right" behavioral code would in the process create more ama than ojas, more stress than bliss. To stay healthy requires not compromising our integrity, although we can certainly compromise our attachment to anything outside the self, to any particular person or activity. In the strength of the integration of self, we can be infinitely flexible. With a bedrock of inner integrity, we are free to enjoy "the lightness of being," unencumbered by tricks, falsehoods, and manipulation.

Dr. Brihaspati Dev Triguna, considered the premier Ayur-Vedic physician in the world, has offered some very powerful descriptions from the texts of Charaka for making life "fully enlightened and blissful." There are four types of life *(ayu)* described in Ayur-Veda: *hita-ayu* (hih-tuh-ah-yooh), *ahita-ayu* (ah-hih-tuh-ah-yooh), *sukha-ayu* (soo-khuh-ah-yooh), and *duhkha-ayu* (dooh-khuh-ah-yooh). Hita-ayu is what you do for the good and benefit of the life of others, for the happiness of society. Ahita-ayu is the opposite of this, that which is disadvantageous to others and for society. Sukha-ayu is for the good of the individual physiology, to keep it healthy and blissful. Duhkha-ayu is its opposite—any type of life that is not good for the individual physiology. Choosing hita-ayu and sukha-ayu and avoiding their opposites gives us what we need to "keep ourselves pure, working for others, and doing good for the future."

As women, we have another way to promote effortless health and happiness. We have the advantage of a uniquely female biological cycle whose purpose is to keep us maximally healthy.

# Chapter 9

❀

# PURIFICATION

## The Monthly Cycle as Our Health Advantage

*Truly there is in this world
nothing so purifying
as knowledge.*

Bhagavad-Gita

Dr. Balaraj Maharshi, one of India's most highly esteemed Ayur-Vedic authorities, noted that in his nearly fifty years of medical experience, he has never seen anything like the number of gynecological disorders common in the West. Western medicine, it seems, has had little to offer women in the way of menstrual cycle knowledge and care. In fact, until the 1940s, and even into the next several decades, discussion of the topic was pretty much taboo. Instead of educating women about the healthy effects of menstruation and menopause, women were offered such unwelcoming concepts as "the curse," "being unwell," and the dreaded "change." Fortunately, these negative constructs of female physiological functioning have not been part of most world cultures. Ayur-Veda especially views the menstrual cycle in a most positive and evolutionary way.

217

## Our Beneficial Menstrual Cycle

One of the most powerful aspects of a woman's physiology is a self-healing mechanism for keeping the bodymind prepared for wholeness, a purpose beyond reproduction. Menstruation is a uniquely female physiological function, intimate to the health and even happiness of women during their childbearing years. Yet few of us actually appreciate and realize the benefits of this cycle for promoting our good health and long life in general. We more typically see it as a nuisance at best, and so we fail to recognize its health-giving purpose.

The most obvious function of menstruation is allowing the body to slough off the inner lining (endometrium) of the uterus to prepare for another reproductive cycle. The shedding of the endometrial lining—the menstrual flow—is like a lawn that's been mowed, so the top layer is removed. As a lawn is stimulated to growth by various amounts of sun and rain, the endometrial lining is affected by amounts of hormones during the month, involving a cyclic interplay between the pituitary gland and the ovaries. The menstrual cycle will thus change in length, in the amount of flow, and so forth, as hormonal levels change.

Ayur-Veda offers us new understanding and appreciation of the role that menstruation plays in keeping us healthy. It does not revile menstruation as a kind of ritual disorder; rather it honors its purifying value. It clarifies how the cycle provides a phenomenal cleanup system, a perfect renewal opportunity. A number of research studies support this understanding, that menstrual cycles keep women healthy, providing significant long-term benefits. But we need to examine how this process works, so we may fully enjoy its results and reduce any discomfort along the way. Ayur-Veda also suggests precise ways to identify and treat various menstrual disorders that may develop.

Once we understand the menstrual cycle as a purifying mechanism for keeping the bodymind prepared for wholeness, we recognize its purpose beyond reproduction as a regular opportunity for eliminating the accumulation of ama or waste products that have the potential to give rise to illness.

## A Syndrome of Symptoms

For many healthy women, the menstrual cycle is a normal, easy, monthly elimination; for others, it is a time of intense pain, emotional upset, and debility. Some women waver between a little discomfort and a great deal of discomfort from month to month or from year to year. What accounts for this wide range of menstrual experiences? Modern medicine offers no clear answers as to why such variable dysfunction occurs.

Activated by the monthly hormone cycle, a syndrome of symptoms known as premenstrual syndrome (PMS) was defined back in 1931. By now over 150 symptoms in nearly every organ system have been attributed to PMS, although many of the attributed disorders, such as binge eating, volatile emotions, and so forth, have never been adequately researched or significantly associated with the menstrual period itself. PMS theories abound, both biological and psychological: Researchers have investigated theories postulating hormonal or biochemical causes, such as progesterone deficiency, estrogen excess, vitamin B6 deficiency, vitamin A deficiency, elevated prolactin, excess aldosterone, decreased serotonin uptake, endorphin deficiency, prostaglandin excess or deficiency, and allergic response to food, hormones, or environmental agents. Psychologists have looked at the concept of stress as either a cause or an effect of PMS, expectation of symptoms as cause, and neuroticism and inner conflicts of various types. None of these theories has proved definitive, and the specific cause(s) of PMS remain a mystery. As a result, treatments based on them have limited success.

Although most doctors today recognize that stress, lack of exercise, poor diet, and other life-style factors all play a role in creating menstrual difficulties, there is little agreement on how to provide relief for PMS, other than through the use of medications that may have negative side effects and whose effectiveness in alleviating all symptoms remains unproven or even disproven. Neither the Pill, progesterone supplements, vitamins nor tranquilizers have been able to take care of the whole job. The most promising of these treatments, progesterone supplements, was recently found, at least by one group of researchers, to be no more effective than a placebo.[1] Nearly all treatments appear to work to a certain extent, yet none any better than a placebo, which seems to work exceptionally well in 40 to 95 percent of the cases studied.

Perhaps the most plausible model of PMS offered thus far is the "state model" theory of researchers Rubinow and Schmidt,[2] who suggest that PMS is due not to an excess or deficiency of any one biochemical or hormone, but is rather a disorder characterized by a "menstrual-cycle-linked transition into a particular experiential state," an emotional state usually marked by irritability. But why this happens is still unknown. How a woman's bodymind transits into this experiential and physiological state is the missing link to understanding and treating PMS.

This is exactly the element that Ayur-Veda supplies.

As we've seen, the Ayur-Vedic theory and practice of medicine is based on the understanding of the connection of our individual bodymind to an underlying field of intelligence. Any disconnection at this junction can create a host of symptoms of imbalance throughout our minds and bodies. From this perspective, PMS is basically a bodymind disturbance, an overall imbalance, manifesting from a variety of imbalances within the doshas.

PMS is difficult for modern medicine to deal with because the wide variety of symptoms means that there is no one universally effective treatment, no one vitamin, hormone, or drug that solves the entire problem at the biochemical level. In Ayur-Vedic terms, because each symptom is an expression of an imbalance that has its source at a deeper level of the mind-body system, treating all symptoms at once occurs only at that deeper level. This may be why PMS seems to respond so well to placebos, because the placebo response takes place at the junction point where mind and body meet. A particular thought that something will work, a mental state of expectation, gets conveyed at that precise junction and expresses itself in the body, bolstering immunity, hormonal balance, and central nervous system stability.

Ayur-Veda proposes that PMS and other menstrual cycle problems happen if and when we experience any or all of three interdependent conditions: (1) Our biological rhythms are off, (2) one or more of the doshas is out of balance, or (3) there has been a build-up of ama or excess metabolic by-products during the month.

We will explore each of these causal conditions and see how each can be treated to take care of particular menstrual cycle symptoms.

## The Relationship Between the Menstrual and Other Biological Cycles

Most of us are aware that our changing moods and outlook can be very much affected by the menstrual cycle, reminding us in both subtle and dramatic ways of how completely interconnected our bodies, minds, and emotions are. But we can experience another level of interdependence—our connection with nature itself, not only in a poetic way but also in a biological sense. When you take a look at nature, you see that the cycles, whether the winter cycle of hibernation, the lunar cycle of tides, or the twenty-four-hour circadian cycle of rest and activity, all have some kind of renewal component that promotes growth in the particular system they govern.

Human biological rhythms too are cycles of rest and activity within your physiology. They are present at every level—from your DNA to your hormones to your cells to the more complex levels of your biological functioning, from breathing in and out to psychophysiological behavior patterns such as sleeping, eating, and menstruation. Within the menstrual cycle, the rhythms of hormonal activity are highly significant. In fact, the time of month chosen for breast cancer surgery (in premenopausal women) has been found to influence the survival outcome dramatically. In a 1992 study of surgical treatment between 1975 and 1985, published in the *The Lancet,* researchers found that of 250 women, those treated from Day 3 to Day 12 of the cycle (higher estrogen output)—counting the first day of flow as Day 1—had a 54 percent rate of survival, whereas those treated in the first two days or from Day 13 to the end of the cycle (lower estrogen output) had an 84 percent survival rate.

We can recognize that these natural cycles don't just happen over and over purposelessly; they are highly well-organized and well-timed events, meant to renew and revitalize and even transform. Bio-logical thus conveys a sense of the "logic" of biology.

There is a reason why things happen. Indeed, nature hasn't given women 450 or so monthly menstrual periods over approximately forty years time just so we can discard the fertilizable eggs not used for reproduction. Nature is far more efficient than that. The shedding of the endometrial lining is in and of itself purposeful: It is health-producing. Our personal hormonal cycles are not independent events either; they are extremely intimate to the functioning of our bodymind and pull us into close association with all natural cycles. Many of us have noticed, for example, and research also is indicating, that our menstrual periods occur far more frequently during the times of the full moon. Moreover, it is well known that women who are close friends or who are living in groups start to have their menstrual periods simultaneously, in tune not only with the environment, but with each other.

If we recognize that our biological rhythms are the rhythms of nature, then we readily understand the need for a balance of rest and activity within our monthly menstrual cycle. And we can further understand why anything that throws off our biological rhythm can create menstrual problems. Since each cycle operates in phase with every other cycle, if we are off-rhythm in our sleep cycle owing, say, to jet lag, this can easily throw off our menstrual cycle. Changing shifts at work from day to night and back again can also adversely affect a woman's cycle.

The presence of PMS generally indicates that our monthly rhythm of menstruation and hormone production is not properly aligned. By rebalancing the *daily* rhythm of our lives through a good routine, the *monthly* rhythm of the menstrual cycle can become stabilized, fully alleviating PMS symptoms for some of us. Others of us, however, may need another kind of balancing, beyond our biological cycles. Ayur-Veda takes us into some very interesting new territory in considering a second cause of menstrual problems, imbalance in one or more of the doshas.

### The Doshas as a Key to Solving Menstrual Problems

Just as they conduct and carry out all other physiological functions, the three doshas are each intimately involved in the menstrual cycle. Vata is responsible for the downward flow, Kapha for the

**222**

mucus, fluids, and tissues, and Pitta for blood, hormones, and cleansing. Imbalance in any of the three doshas can result in a disruption in the normal menstrual process, which will eventually be experienced as a symptom. The type of symptom usually indicates which of the doshas is responsible. Researchers are presently discovering that PMS occurs in symptom clusters, with certain types of symptoms tending to occur together more often than others. These clusters clearly parallel the grouping of PMS symptoms by doshic imbalance.

In a 1990 preliminary study, Dr. Nick Argyl and his colleagues[3] surveyed women between seventeen and forty-five who met the criteria for having PMS, and grouped the participants into four symptom clusters that paralleled those delineated by other PMS researchers.[4] One group's symptoms were associated with Vata imbalances, another with Kapha imbalances, and a third with Pitta imbalances. Half of those in each group had participated in a variety of Ayur-Vedic programs, including TM, dosha-specific eating programs, herbal supplements or rasayanas (see chapter 12), Panchakarma (also chapter 12), drinking hot water, monthly internal cleansing, daily oil massage, and keeping a regular bedtime. Specific bodymind types were found to have responded best to specific interventions. As Ayur-Vedic theory predicts, those with Vata dosha predominant noticed most benefits from rest, TM, and regular bedtime; Pitta types found the purification of a monthly internal cleansing most helpful; and Kapha types responded best to the ama-reducing eating regimes and the herbal supplements.

Ayur-Veda categorizes PMS and other menstrual symptoms with reference to the underlying imbalance(s) in Vata, Pitta, or Kapha and treats them not as single illnesses but according to the dosha(s) that are out of balance. If Vata is out of balance, we might experience symptoms such as anxiety, insomnia, feeling "spaced-out," constipation, and cramps. If mainly Pitta is out of balance, we'll notice symptoms such as irritability, diarrhea, heavy flow, and increased hunger. If a Kapha imbalance predominates, we generally experience water retention, bloating, swollen breasts, and perhaps lethargy. If two or three or all three doshas are out of balance, any of these symptoms can arise. Correcting any imbalance in the doshas helps eliminate PMS symptoms.

Here is a summary of symptoms categorized by dosha.

## PMS AND MENSTRUAL SYMPTOMS BY DOSHA

### VATA TYPE

*Premenstrual*

Nervous tension
Mood swings
Anxiety, depression
Insomnia
Forgetfulness
Constipation
Abdominal bloating
Fatigue

*Menstrual*

Pain, cramps, backache
Extended length of period
Light amount of flow
Dark, clotted flow
Irregular periods
Spotting

*Common diagnoses:* Endometriosis, dysmenorrhea

### PITTA TYPE

*Premenstrual*

Irritability, anger
Increased appetite
Sugar craving
Headache (especially
 migraine)
Excessive body heat or
 sweating
Diarrhea or increased
 bowel movements
Skin rashes, acne

*Menstrual*

Excessive bleeding
Increased frequency of
 periods
Headache

*Common diagnoses:* Menorrhagia, endometrial hyperplasia,
dysfunctional uterine bleeding

KAPHA TYPE (AND AMA-RELATED)

*Premenstrual*

Weight gain
Fluid retention
Breast enlargement
Lethargy
Vaginal yeast infections
Slow digestion

*Menstrual*

Stiffness in back, joints
Pale, mucuslike menstrual
 flow
Clots

*Common diagnoses:* Fluid retention, fibrocystic breast disease, ovarian cysts, uterine fibroids, vaginitis (yeast type)

You may notice that you have symptoms in two or even three categories. This can happen when an imbalanced Vata affects the other two doshas. Most likely your imbalance started with Vata dosha. So correct Vata imbalances first and then choose the dosha category or categories that include a majority of your symptoms or the symptoms that you find most troublesome, referring back to the food and rest recommendations in chapter 4 along with the guidelines at the end of this chapter. You can also determine your current dosha imbalance through learning self-pulse assessment (see chapter 12) or by consulting an Ayur-Vedic physician.

It's necessary to remember that all the Maharishi Ayur-Veda programs work together as a whole system to structure balance. They work best if you follow all the recommendations, not just one or two, so you can gain all the benefits.

One important note: The categorization of symptoms here according to the doshas is, of course, not a substitute for proper medical evaluation and diagnosis. The degree to which a dosha imbalance can manifest spans the range from mild functional symptoms to malignancy. While mild menstrual pain, backache, or cramps are fairly common and are due generally to an imbalance in Vata dosha, more severe or incapacitating pain should always be evaluated by a physician, as it may indicate that a more serious condition has developed. But regardless of the degree of imbalance developed, whether a minor complaint or a serious illness, following the guidelines for correcting the doshic imbalance (at the end of the chapter) will help bring about better bodymind conditions for healing in conjunction with modern medicine.

As an overall guideline, pain is always less "Ayur-Vedically correct" than straining to adhere to any healing routines while suffering. We do not suggest that any woman should endure severe pain and certainly encourage taking a pain reliever for menstrual cramps. However, it is important not to substitute this symptomatic treatment for correcting the causative imbalance. We can do both simultaneously, and many women who do so find that their need for medication decreases and eventually they may need none at all.

### Identifying the Menstrual Subdosha

In the Ayur-Vedic system, each of the doshas is divided into five component functions of *subdoshas,* which represent the function of each dosha in various areas of the bodymind. Vata is the subtlest, most pervasive dosha, and "leads" the other doshas. Therefore, understanding the functions of the specific subdivisions of Vata and how to keep them in balance is important for most preventive health-care measures. One of Vata's subdoshas, *Apana* (uh-pahn–uh) Vata, specifically governs the menstrual cycle and plays a significant role in women's health.

Apana means "downward moving." Apana Vata functions in the lower abdominal and pelvic regions and is responsible for the downward flow through the intestines, the urinary tract, and the reproductive tract. If Apana Vata gets disrupted, the menstrual flow can be irregular, clotty, painful, start-and-stop, or disrupted in some other way. As we'll see, almost every menstrual problem involves an imbalance in Apana Vata.

### Ama and Menstrual Discomfort

Ayur-Veda identifies ama as another cause of menstrual problems. Menstruation is an opportunity for ama cleansing; if our elimination has been off during the month, or if we've taken in a lot of toxins because of improper diet, poor digestion, or some environmental pollutants, an extra heavy buildup of wastes occurs. Many symptoms of PMS are due to this accumulation of ama and its effects on the doshas and dhatus.

If your diet, your sleep and rest, and your exercise are balanced during the month, you'll notice far fewer PMS symptoms than if you've been eating poorly, going to bed late, and not exercising much. Menstrual cramps, nausea, diarrhea, and/or heavy flow are all more likely to occur during your period if your body requires increased cleansing in order to eliminate more ama. If your symptoms are mostly ama-related, you may also notice that you feel great after your period; the effects may even last two or three weeks, but if you continue with a poor diet and little exercise, too much ama begins to build up prior to your next period, and PMS symptoms can flare up again.

If you are more careful during the entire month, lessening your consumption of caffeine,[5] alcohol, and junk foods (foods high in sugar, salt, and additives), you'll find a significant decrease in PMS symptoms, with fewer cramps and discomfort.

## Ayur-Vedic Perspectives on Endometriosis and Dysmenorrhea

As the result of ama, a much bigger job than ordinary may need to be accomplished during the cleansing week of the cycle (possibly including incomplete menstrual elimination from the previous month). The intensity of the cleansing often exacerbates the menstrual difficulties and can cause a whole range of psychophysiological symptoms, such as those associated with endometriosis or dysmenorrhea.

According to one modern medical theory, endometriosis occurs when sloughed bits of the uterine lining, instead of moving down through the vagina and out of the body during the period, move upward and adhere to the pelvic or abdominal organs. This usually results in severe pain during the period, as these bits of tissue, stimulated by monthly hormones, begin to bleed inside the abdomen and set up an inflammatory reaction. At its worst, this can result in infertility, owing to scarring of the ovaries or Fallopian tubes, or severe pain in the abdomen. Most cases can be successfully treated with laser surgery, followed by hormonal therapy. But endometriosis may be able to be avoided through preventive Ayur-

Vedic routines. Modern medicine has no explanation for what causes pieces of uterine lining to move and adhere to the organs, and therefore provides no advice on how to prevent it. In Ayur-Vedic terms, endometriosis is a problem of imbalanced Apana Vata, a reversal in downward flow; women with this condition are frequently constipated, a related symptom also due to imbalanced Apana Vata (see next section).

Dysmenorrhea, which means "painful periods," generally affects women under age twenty-five. It is experienced as severe cramps resulting from uterine spasms that temporarily deprive the uterine muscle of oxygen, a kind of "charley-horse" of the uterus, perhaps triggered by the release of prostaglandins. The pain can be blocked by over-the-counter pain relievers such as ibuprofen. This may help the symptoms temporarily, but it is important for women with severe menstrual pain not to ignore this not-so-subtle signal that something's wrong.

*Renee, a thirty-four-year-old Los Angeles management consultant, had suffered from dysmenorrhea and PMS symptoms. For twenty-two years, ever since she started menstruating at age twelve, she had had almost no relief from a dual condition that she experienced fifteen days out of every month or one-half of her teenage and adult life.*

*The PMS symptoms started about ten days before each period, when she would be so bloated that she could not wear her usual clothes; she would be spotting enough to have to wear a tampon or pad. Always extremely tense and irritable, Renee would feel a big drop in self-esteem and be on "a giant emotional roller coaster." When her period arrived, the menstrual cramps were so severe that she was bedridden two or three days each month. She missed school and work. Her relationships, including her marriage, and her sexuality were negatively affected by the monthly ordeal.*

*Renee found no relief from the usual menstrual-relief drugs such as aspirin or Midol, nor from stronger pain medication such as Motrin. She eventually tried birth control pills, which improved the cramps and pain somewhat, but caused an increase in PMS symptoms. She finally had to resort to taking narcotic pain relievers, which she took for many years.*

# PURIFICATION

*When Renee first came to a Maharishi Ayur-Vedic health center for an evaluation, she was identified as having a Pitta constitution with a severe Vata dosha imbalance. To achieve balance, she was asked to avoid Vata-aggravating foods such as raw vegetables and cold foods and drinks; to take special herbs to balance Vata; to cut back on her excessive exercise routine; and to rest at home for the first two days of her period.*

*Over the following six months, her symptoms were reduced by 50 percent. She experienced cramps for only several hours on two days instead of enduring five days of constant pain and she was able to stop taking the narcotics. She then started receiving regular seasonal Panchakarma treatments, which resulted in the total elimination of the PMS symptoms and the need for all drugs except for an occasional aspirin tablet on the first day of her period. Having experienced almost an entire lifetime of menstrual disorders, three years later Renee describes her "new" physiology as "unbelievable—I'm walking on cloud nine."*

## The Subdoshas of Vata: Once Apana Time . . .

The Ayur-Vedic texts describe the five subdoshas of Vata as divisions of the one "life breath" that upholds all living systems. This life energy is identified as a fundamental law of nature, the motivating and evolutionary force of creation. It creates, sustains, and evolves within our bodymind. It is essential for good health—it is after all the breath of life; without it, there is no life. And as Vata governs all movement and flow in the mind and body, its five subdivisions are also recognized as *types of flow,* which Ayur-Veda refers to as five types of "breaths."

First subdosha: *Prana* (prah-nuh)—the forward breath
Second subdosha: *Udana* (oo-dah-nuh)—the ascending breath
Third subdosha: *Samana* (suh-mah-nuh)—the assimilating breath
Fourth subdosha: *Apana* (uh-pah-nuh)—the downward breath
Fifth subdosha: *Vyana* (vyah-nuh)—the diffusing breath

Each of the subdoshas is concentrated in various parts of the bodymind.

1. Prana is located in the head, heart, and lungs. Its functions: To sustain all mental, emotional, and sensory experience and to maintain normal breathing and heart activity.

2. Udana is located in the ears, nose, throat, and chest. Its functions: Speech, breathing, coughing, hiccoughs, and sneezing.

3. Samana is located in the stomach and duodenum. Its functions: Peristalsis, digestion, assimilation, separation of nutrients from wastes.

4. Apana is located in the pelvic area, intestines, and reproductive organs. Its functions: Elimination (via bowels, bladder), menstruation, sexual functioning, labor, and delivery. Apana also plays an important role in the settling down of mental activity.

5. Vyana is located throughout the bodymind. Its functions: Circulation, nervous system activity, and sense of touch.

Although the proper functioning of all five subdoshas of Vata is important for good health, none is as critical as the balanced functioning of the first, Prana, and the fourth, Apana. Prana is said to maintain life and health through awakening our innate impulse toward greater happiness, progress, and fulfillment, while Apana is said to maintain that progress by moving wastes, impurities, or other obstacles out of the way. Apana is also the primary cite of potential imbalance. According to Ayur-Veda, *the most common initial pathway of disease in both women and men is via an imbalance in Apana Vata subdosha.*

In essence, the "forward" and "upward" movement associated with Prana and responsible for energizing the nervous system must be properly balanced by the "downward" action of Apana, associated with the removal of wastes and impurities and the menstrual flow from the body. When these two subdoshas or breaths—Prana and Apana—are balanced, all the functions of Vata are more likely to be in balance and the body as a whole to be healthy. When their balance is upset, not only do the other functions of Vata become disturbed, Pitta dosha and Kapha dosha often become imbalanced as well.

**230**

Here's what happens: When Apana Vata gets out of balance, instead of flowing *downward,* it moves *upward,* ultimately interfering with the function of the other subdoshas.

This mechanism of Apana Vata moving upward is one of the most common subdosha imbalances. Whether it results from too many late nights followed by rushed mornings, intense mental or emotional stress, and/or poor eating habits, when Apana Vata becomes imbalanced and travels upward, a number of symptoms can arise. We could notice a disturbance in the lower abdomen, such as a tendency toward constipation, irritable bowel, or we might experience menstrual discomfort. If the imbalance continues, then Apana moves farther upward and causes imbalances in the other Vata subdoshas in the bodymind.

When this happens, a wide variety of symptoms can occur that follow a specific pattern. This pattern results from the interaction of Apana Vata with the other subdoshas, as it pushes its way upward from the lower abdomen. The natural reaction of your body is always to maintain balance, so the affected subdosha tries to "push" Apana back to its natural place, with varying degrees of success, and can lead to an uncomfortable feeling of pressure, tension, or constriction in the area involved.

For example, if Apana Vata moves upward past the stomach, it begins to exert pressure on the chest. It may then affect the functions of the heart and circulatory system, the domain of Vyana Vata, leading to palpitations or, in more severe cases, to high blood pressure.

Other symptoms such as sinus congestion, hay fever, and light-headedness can occur if Apana Vata moves farther upward into the area of Udana Vata, which includes the ear, nose, throat, and sinus passages. If Udana Vata pushes down in an attempt to maintain its homeostatic status quo, tension and tightness in the neck commonly result.

Finally, if Apana Vata has overridden all attempts by the other subdoshas to prevent its inappropriate course upward, it reaches the head, the domain of Prana Vata, resulting in symptoms such as worry, anxiety, insomnia, headache, or head pressure.

It is apparent that Apana Vata, when it becomes severely imbalanced, can cause a number of problems. What follows is the case of one woman who developed an imbalance of Apana Vata which also caused an imbalance in Samana Vata, as Vata moved up. This resulted in serious menstrual and digestive problems.

*Rebecca D. came to a Maharishi Ayur-Veda health center at age thirty-two. For the preceding fourteen years she had been dealing with a severe condition first diagnosed as a constriction of the muscle controlling the valve between the stomach and small intestine. Her ability to eat was limited by her constant nausea. Her menstrual periods stopped for eight years. She had a number of bouts with mononucleosis and ended up having the wound-up, rubberband-tight stomach muscle surgically removed when she was twenty-four.*

*The condition came about, Rebecca believes, as the result of her feelings surrounding the sudden death of her father when she was eighteen. "I felt such deep sadness and loss, particularly because I never got to say good-bye to him." She was on her own very quickly, holding back her very real emotions in order to be "grown up."*

*The surgery had only minimal effect; she still felt nauseated a lot. Her periods started up again and became regular but were accompanied by chills and vomiting. At age thirty she underwent further tests but no abnormality was found that could account for her continued symptoms. The distress would grip her so forcefully that she would constantly blow up at those closest to her, including her husband. She started psychotherapy, where a great many anger issues came up. She felt somewhat better emotionally, but her body continued to "explode" in bouts of diarrhea and vomiting.*

*After seeing several chiropractors, Rebecca went for a Maharishi Ayur-Vedic evaluation. She was prescribed four courses of Panchakarma treatments over a year's time. In addition, she was advised to prepare for her periods with internal cleansing and was given certain Ayur-Vedic herbs to reset her physiology. She started an eating program to balance Apana Vata. She learned to take her food cravings seriously, as indicative of specific imbalances. She learned TM, which she believes gave her a deeper way to be self-loving and interact with others to draw more love and support to herself.*

# PURIFICATION

*Five years later she says, "I finally feel truly nourished inside and all the symptoms have virtually disappeared, except for some mild cramping during my period. My eating has improved. I've gained the weight I wanted to. There is no more nausea. And I am finally feeling ready to consider having a child, something I only dreamed of years ago but never thought my health would allow."*

Now let's look at another woman's experience with an imbalance in Apana Vata that centered around a hysterectomy.

### APANA VATA IMBALANCE BEFORE AND AFTER HYSTERECTOMY

*Alice F., a fifty-eight-year-old physicist from Chicago, had been suffering for five years from a myriad of seemingly unrelated complaints that doctors had finally concluded must be "psychosomatic." By the time Alice went for Ayur-Vedic treatment, she had had multiple workups and had undergone several years of psychotherapy, which she said "helped me understand myself better, but did not help how I feel— nothing has helped that."*

*Alice's most troublesome symptom was a constant pressure and pain in her jaw and at the back of her head which occasionally involved her entire head. The pressure was associated with mental fuzziness and a lack of coherent thinking. In addition, she experienced frequent emotional ups and downs that she had never experienced before in her life. This loss of inner stability was quite demoralizing to her.*

*The onset of Alice's symptoms five years before coincided with a hysterectomy for fibroid tumors of the uterus, associated with heavy bleeding. She felt she never completely recovered her previous level of vitality following the surgery. She developed a series of symptoms that her doctors were unable to explain other than to say that the numerous tests showed nothing serious; hopefully, her symptoms would go away. These included irregular bowel movements and flatulence, which were diagnosed as irritable bowel syndrome, along with pressure in her head, which had been only temporarily relieved by pain medications, chiropractic treatment, or acupuncture.*

*When Alice sought out a Maharishi Ayur-Vedic evaluation, examination of her pulse revealed an imbalance in Udana Vata, with an underlying disturbance in Apana Vata in the lower abdominal region. The connections were clear. The imbalance had begun in Apana Vata, probably long before her hysterectomy, as evidenced by the long-term growth and presence of the fibroid tumor. Vata dosha usually becomes disturbed at least temporarily by surgery, and when the surgery involves the abdomen or pelvis, Apana functions in particular are disrupted. Alice experienced the gaseous distention and temporary bowel dysfunctions commonly experienced after abdominal surgery.*

*Her Ayur-Vedic treatment was directed toward balancing Apana Vata first and subsequently treating Udana Vata. After a month of at-home treatment, which included daily oil self-massage, herbal supplements to balance Apana and Udana, and dietary modification to reduce ama, Alice reported an almost complete reduction in head pressure—"It's virtually gone"—and a growing sense of control over her health. She was very relieved. "It's comforting to finally know what has been happening to my health and why, and to have such a simple and precise way of treating the problems. I'm beginning to feel like myself again."*

Alice's experiences before and after hysterectomy are unfortunately not unique. What is questionable is the use of hysterectomy as a treatment for a benign condition. From an Ayur-Vedic point of view, the Apana Vata disturbance should be treated first to see if the symptoms subside before a hysterectomy would be considered an appropriate intervention.

A recent book by Winnifred Cutler, Ph.D., *Hysterectomy: Before and After,* includes information collected from a review of over 3,500 recent studies. She concludes that every aspect of a woman's health may be affected by hysterectomy, including her personality, her outlook on life, her moods, her sex life, and her rate of aging. Cutler is among a growing number of Western researchers, physicians, and medical workers who are seriously rethinking this all-too-common procedure. She counsels, "There is an understandable panic when [a woman] is bleeding unexpectedly. However, if she can muster the patience to have a thorough diagnostic process, she has a good chance of finding a healthful resolution to her problem that does not include hysterectomy." We would simply add that the diagnostic process might do well to include an Ayur-Vedic evaluation to identify and address the underlying causes.

## Ayur-Vedic Treatment of Apana Vata Imbalance

To prevent and treat all of these menstrual cycle disorders, deep rest and the avoidance of excessive mental and physical activity during menstruation are recommended. Often very active women try to push aside the symptoms and pretend nothing is wrong. These are the very women who will benefit most by taking their conditions seriously and dealing with them directly and effectively. The habit of taking pain relievers such as ibuprofen or aspirin and then blithely barreling ahead as though nothing were happening physiologically is a short-term convenience that can cause real problems later on, as ama continues to accumulate month by month and Apana gets more out of balance. Many effects of what is called aging, including arthritis, are due to this dual condition of ama and imbalanced Vata, which you can reduce or prevent through proper attention to a Vata eating program and adequate ama elimination earlier in life—and by taking a real rest during the first few days of each menstrual period.

Some Western women already have figured it out for themselves. As writer Judy Grahn has said, "Now . . . I eat quite differently—and I love my period. . . . I try to spend time by myself because I feel pleasantly introverted and a little spaced-out (or in)." Grahn goes on to report that other women "are attempting to find this personal seclusion as well. Often this state [during menstruation] includes strong feelings of renewed purposefulness in life, self-respect, and good will and gentleness toward other human beings."[6]

The Ayur-Vedic key is to maintain the proper function of Apana Vata, which is actively moving wastes, impurities, and the menstrual blood downward and out of your body. If Apana is disturbed and moves upward at this time, your period will not provide as much opportunity for purification. The general idea is to go with the body's natural impulse to stay quiet and not be so active. Downward and inward, not outward and upward, is more or less the bodymind dictum during your period.

Here are some simple guidelines for enjoying, not simply enduring, menstruation, *whether or not* you are experiencing any symptoms.

### The Ayur-Vedic Prescription for Menstruation

#### 1. TAKE TIME OUT FOR REST

In general, Ayur-Veda recommends resting during the heavy days of flow (the first two to three days for most women). But resting doesn't necessarily mean lying in bed, unless cramps or other symptoms are incapacitating. Rest can be anything that enables you to adopt a slower pace to minimize any stress or fatigue.

In general it is not advisable to sleep during the day because this promotes sluggishness, poor circulation, and a tendency for blockage in the shrotas, the channels in the body through which ojas flows. This is especially important for Kapha types, or if you have a Kapha imbalance. However, a brief rest lying down is fine.

If you can, plan to take those days off each month for light, enjoyable activities around the house, such as reading, organizing, etc. If you must work outside or in your home, plan a lighter schedule and try to avoid staying late at work or school. When at home, eat a light supper, minimize evening activities, and go to bed early. One woman who followed these rest guidelines for a year commented, "I used to feel like a traitor to women by resting, by not working, and by not running around oblivious to my physiology throughout my period. But now that I've experienced how it benefits my health and relationships, I've come to feel I'd be a traitor to myself if I didn't rest."

If you are a mother, plan shopping trips, appointments, entertaining, and so forth around those two or three days as best you can; try to take some extra rest time for yourself in the afternoon and retire early, if at all possible. If your responsibilities do not permit you to rest adequately during your period, try to rest during the weekend before or after and pay extra attention to other measures for Vata pacification (see chapter 4). And do the best thing for Vata that you can: Don't worry about it!

As a mother of four has found, "It's a relief to know I'm not only justified but 'wise'—as opposed to feeling irresponsible—when I tell my family not to expect me to cook or go with the kids on a long hike, and that I'll be taking it easy instead. I've learned not to strain to accomplish what I can't do easily at that time."

### 2. KEEP YOUR EXERCISE EASY

A walk each day for about fifteen to thirty minutes during a period is ideal for most of us. If you are in the habit of exercising, whether running or participating in an aerobics or dance class, it would be better to reduce your exercise workout during your period to no more than a brisk walk. This smooth, steady, lighter activity is more conducive to normalizing menstrual flow and maintaining balance in Vata dosha. No one doubts your ability to get your pulse rate up to 160 while you're menstruating, it's just physiologically inappropriate. You can, however, use your exercise program to *prepare* for your period. Women commonly experience fewer cramps and have an easier period when they have been exercising regularly throughout the month. Consistent, moderate exercise is one of the best preventive measures for menstrual health in general, especially when you follow a program that considers your bodymind type as well as your level of conditioning (see chapter 4).

### 3. LET YOURSELF TURN INWARD IF POSSIBLE

This is a time for rejuvenation, the best time to attend to your own needs and happiness. To keep Vata settled, it's better to avoid lengthy conversations or matters that involve a lot of mental work. If you can take extra rest, allow your awareness to be more inward and pay attention to your body. Try to do the things that you enjoy during your period. Don't save up all the chores just because you know you're going to take a little time off. In general, say the Ayur-Vedic texts, positive emotions at this time help culture more refined feelings throughout the month.

If you are more inward, one woman noted, "The period itself is smoother—there's less discomfort and irritability, and I have a lighter flow, so I don't need painkillers to make it through. It also leads to a much greater sense of mental well-being, because I'm not straining to focus and be active when my mind and body want to be more quiet and settled. This sense of well-being carries through the rest of the month."

### 4. ENJOY A VATA-PACIFYING EATING REGIME

Your diet should be full of light, warm, Vata-pacifying foods that are easy to digest, because your digestive fires are weaker during your period. Avoid carbonated beverages, which aggravate Vata. The second focus during your period, after keeping Vata balanced, is to minimize ama production. The most important points are to eat a little less than usual, especially in the evening, to avoid cold drinks and cold foods, and to avoid ama producers such as cheese, yogurt, red meat, chocolate, and fried foods.

### 5. HANDLE CRAVINGS COMFORTABLY

Many women experience cravings for sweets or for salty foods before or during their periods. This craving time is not at all unusual; it represents your bodymind's desire to pacify Vata or Pitta. It also can be the result of ama that is blocking proper delivery of nutrition to your digestive tissues. As a rule, you will usually do less damage by satisfying the salt craving first; you may then notice that the sugar craving disappears. Salt cravings can be more fully satisfied for a longer time by having a cooked dish seasoned with salt than by eating chips or other quick-fix snacks.

If you still want sugar, fresh whipped cream with honey can be a surprisingly satisfying substitute for ice cream, without the latter's digestive fire-extinguishing effect. Warm milk with honey is an excellent choice as well; add the honey after the boiled milk has cooled down.

### 6. BATHING AND OILING

Bathing in cold water tends to reduce flow, while bathing in hot water tends to increase it. While baths can be relaxing and soothing to Vata, for most women a shower is ideal on days of heavy flow to minimize any interference with the natural pace of the menstrual flow. Vata can also become aggravated if there's a lot of massaging, especially around the head area, so it's advisable to keep shampooing to a minimum and postpone having a facial or other head or face treatments during the first few days.

Gently massaging your head with warm sesame oil on the fourth or fifth day of the cycle, leaving it on for several hours or even overnight (keeping a towel on your pillow) and then shampooing it out has a wonderfully soothing effect on Vata.

The daily abhyanga or oil massage described in chapter 12 needs to be modified during your period. Leave out any vigorous massage—or you may want to skip abhyanga altogether.

### 7. SEXUAL ACTIVITY

The classic Ayur-Vedic texts say that menstruation is not a good time for sexual activity. This recommendation is not based either on the desirability of a woman at this time or on a woman's desires; it is based on a sound principle for health. Sexual activity tends to disrupt the smooth flow of Apana Vata during your menstrual flow and can thus promote the development of Vata imbalances.

### 8. HYGIENE

Tampons are not as healthy as they are convenient. Even though concerns have abated about Toxic Shock Syndrome (TSS), tampons in general impede the free passage and clearance of the menstrual blood. Use external absorbent pads if possible. If you find it too inconvenient or impractical to forgo tampons entirely, at least use external pads at night and whenever you are just taking it easy around the house.

## The Ayur-Vedic Prescription for Premenstrual and Menstrual Problems

Some pain during the monthly period is common, especially when we are active and focused. Menstrual pain, backache, or cramps are the result of imbalanced Vata. So are the severe pain of dysmenor-rhea and the attachment of uterine tissue to the abdominal organs that occurs in endometriosis, although these are far less common symptoms. Incapacitating menstrual pain should always be evaluated by a physician.

You can also reduce the symptoms of PMS by following the advice given under the menstruation section above, in addition to the following:

1. Vata pacification through diet and rest is a general principle. If you habitually have menstrual problems, this may indicate that your Vata dosha is out of balance. You may really need to rest more during your period.

2. Drinking plain pure hot water frequently, as often as every thirty to sixty minutes, during your period will help regulate the flow and reduce menstrual cramping by promoting the normal downward movement of Apana Vata. Drink just a few sips up to a cup, according to your thirst at the moment.

3. A regular eating and rest routine *throughout the month* is very helpful. Remember that harmony in your daily rhythms can help balance your monthly rhythms. The imbalance of Apana Vata often happens when you haven't stayed on a regular eating, exercising, and rest routine.

4. Daily oil massage, *abhyanga,* is also highly recommended throughout the month. (See chapter 12 for instructions.) Focus the massage on your abdomen; massage it gently with sesame oil, using a clockwise circular motion, for a few minutes every day. Follow with a warm tub bath.

5. Heat and oil are great Vata-pacifiers. During your period, gently massage the abdomen and low back, if it is hurting, with warm sesame oil and then apply a hot water bottle to the abdomen and/or low back. This often helps to alleviate the pain enough to

sleep at night or to feel reasonably comfortable during the day.

6. A liquid diet (juices, dhals, soups, or blended solid foods made from vegetables, grains, etc.) is also very beneficial on the first day of the period when your agni is naturally slowed down. Liquids are digested more easily. This procedure helps prevent and eliminate ama, reduces bloating, and helps promote a normal flow without cramps or pain. You might also want to avoid eggs or anything fermented such as vinegar, ketchup, or soy sauce, as well as very spicy or very sour foods.

7. Take two tablespoons of pure aloe vera juice after lunch and dinner every day of the month until one week before your period. Resume after completion of the menstrual flow.

### INTERNAL CLEANSING INSTRUCTIONS

You can also help alleviate menstrual problems by the following monthly internal cleansing program. This Maharishi Ayur-Vedic program is suitable for women in overall good health who have no serious gastro-intestinal diseases. Its purpose is to clear your digestive tract of toxins and other ama-producing substances. (This program can also be beneficial for menopausal symptoms, which we discuss in chapter 11.)

Perform the cleansing once a month for three months in midcycle, at ovulation, i.e., between the fourteenth to twentieth day of your cycle, counting from the first day of the last period.

On a day when you can remain at home (or at night if you prefer), take a warm bath or shower, then take four teaspoons of castor oil mixed well with one-fourth cup of fruit juice (other than grape), for palatability. Lemon or orange work best. This will usually result in three to four bowel movements over the next four to six hours. If you've had no bowel movements after the first three hours, take an additional two teaspoons castor oil. Do not eat until the majority of the laxative action has ceased, although small amounts of warm water or juice are all right if you feel the need.

Your diet for the remainder of the day should consist of warm, cooked food that is not too oily, preferably liquid or semisolid, such as soups, lentils or dahl, or cooked cereal. Avoid any cold drinks or foods, and have a restful, easy day.

* * *

If these measures are not helping, you may want to consider a consultation with a Maharishi Ayur-Vedic physician. He or she may be able to prescribe specific herbs for Apana and other imbalances and may suggest some Panchakarma treatments (see chapter 12).

Now that we've explored this very vital aspect of women's health care, let's look at the reproductive aspect of the menstrual cycle. In the following chapter, we'll see how Maharishi Ayur-Veda can help support you through pregnancy, childbirth, and being a new mother, and can expand your conception of motherhood.

# *Chapter 10*

### ❁

# NURTURANCE

## Pregnancy, Childbirth, and Other Conceptions of Motherhood

*We should know that the purpose of creation is the expansion of happiness.*[1]

Maharishi Mahesh Yogi

Ayur-Veda defines human life span in terms of a sequence of the three doshas. The Kapha cycle starts at birth and lasts to around "thirty-something." It creates the psychophysical and social structure through which we experience rapid physiological growth and change, as well as mental development. During the Pitta cycle, which governs the middle years, from about thirty to seventy, we put our development to use. This is the most active and interactive cycle—the "metabolic" time of life, a time of focus, when we experience the processes of transformation and learn to make things happen, whether we are raising a family and/or making other contributions to society in dynamic activity. The Vata cycle of life can start as early as age fifty-five or as late as age seventy, depending on one's personal psychophysiology, and can last a very long time thereafter. The Vata cycle is associated with expansion, related to its elemental qualities of wind *(vayu)* and space *(akasha)*. It is a time when intuition and other aspects of inner development can blossom, when we can grow to higher levels of awareness, and can contribute the depth of our wisdom, our counsel, our healing powers, to ever larger communities.

Within each of these doshic cycles are biological and psychological opportunities for experiences having to do specifically with being a woman, including pregnancy, childbirth, and motherhood. For some women, the experience of being a mother may not require raising one's own children. We can express this aspect of our nature in relationship with any child, with friends, partners, spouses, parents, students, within a community, with the environment, with the world. We can be pregnant with thought; we can give birth to songs, books, scientific discoveries, paintings, inventions, and, ultimately, through the full expression of creativity, a woman can give birth to her Self.

"I believe," wrote the poet Adrienne Rich, "that a . . . reinterpretation of the concept of motherhood is required which would tell us, among many other things, more about the physical capacity for gestation and nourishment of infants and how it relates to psychological gestation and nurture as an intellectual and creative force."[2]

## The Journey Home: Considerations for the Meaning of Motherhood

"Women, as nurturers, use power to empower others," writes psychologist Jean Baker Miller. There are those who believe that the contributions of a mother to society are not really significant—that their influence is only "indirect," through the achievements of their children. But what mothers learn to do is exactly what the great mentors and teachers do—they develop the skill and art of eliciting the potential in others, of helping them to express their best qualities. And no one would argue about Socrates' contribution to Plato or Annie Sullivan's to Helen Keller or about their true accomplishments in their own right.

The only common factor that influential women and men have identified as the basis for their life achievement is the positive influence of their mothers. This influence seems to coincide with the predominance of first-born children among the eminences of history; they are said to have received the most maternal attention. A Roper Poll of American men and women also reported that both sexes considered their mothers to be the most important influence in their lives, before fathers, spouses, or friends.

From the Vedic perspective, "mother" means not only a family mother but also the nurturing creator who represents inner life, the true home of humanity. Being the mother at the center of "the home" in this sense does not mean waxing the floors and organizing the lunches. Rather, "home" is understood as the silent basis for the inner progress of life. In the most developed cultures, home has meant this inner self, and the "journey home," like Ulysses' journey home to Penelope, means returning to the essential self, to the healing silence of one's inner nature.

Women, whether as societal or spiritual mothers, become the essential guides in this journey. Simply by virtue of being a woman, one is a mother to all creation. The development of the inner nature of women—subtle intellect, a loving heart, and intuitive refinement—are the preparation for the primary role of woman as creator.

In the Vedic tradition, all love is said to be "by, for, and of" the Self. Therefore, when we love another fully, we love ourselves fully. Motherhood in this sense is the creative and nurturing principle of life that expresses in its highest form the quality of unconditional love. And the mother or "motherer," with her own children or with others, guides best through her attention, allowing growth to blossom as nature desires, providing deep loving nourishment with even the quietest look. To handle the multiple roles of motherhood well requires deep personal integrity, a life so well integrated that it can adjust to every little change: Like an artist finely tuned to nature's laws, motherhood brings the highest levels of development when a woman can keep this balance fully maintained.

When Ayur-Veda was first developed as a system of medicine, there were a number of great men and women seers who cognized the universal laws that structure the natural world. These Vedic cognitions are thought to contain the seed form of all the various levels of life's expression—they are the DNA of the universe, codified as sound and the vibrations of thought. Among the enlightened women seers was a woman named Vak (vahk), whose name means "speech." Vak cognized what she called "the expanse of my own unbounded nature." She saw all creation as emanating from herself—as her child—and realized:

*The universe is but my own expression....*
*One who eats does so through me;*

*One who sees, breathes or hears*
*Does so through me.*[3]

Hers was an exemplary vision of the creative function of motherhood. By finding "each of the glories of life to be an aspect of my own Self," she found herself in all of creation.

## The Motherhood Envelope: Mother as Healer

The mother's attention is the child's best medicine from the moment of conception. The physiological ties between mother and child create the strongest bonds of intimacy we know. This connection gives mothers an extended "bodymind influence" over their children. So the real understanding of the physiology of motherhood goes far beyond breast-feeding and hormonal changes. Research psychologists have identified no biological force greater than the desire of a mother to protect her child from harm. The mother's awareness envelops the child within the protection of her own consciousness, as an agent of Mother Nature. This protection—a kind of "motherhood envelope"—contains a profound health-giving and healing component from consciousness alone.

We know that healing occurs only through nature. If our consciousness is awake and we are connected to the laws of nature directly, our intentions and desires have a direct line of command to the functioning of our bodies. We read about the mother who single-handedly lifts a 2,000-pound car off her six-year-old son and saves his life. Later she tries to recall what happened. She remembers tapping into a source of super endurance within, a flood of strength that allowed her to perform a seemingly impossible feat. It came from her body's response to a message from her brain, producing instant activity in the pituitary gland to manufacture the strength-producing hormones required to enable the muscles, joints, and bones to act on her single powerful thought "I must rescue my child." Researchers such as geneticist James Roberts at Columbia University have found that the body normally uses only about 1 percent of its endurance capacity but that under demanding environmental conditions, latent dormant cells in the pituitary gland will increase their hormone production a hundredfold. It seems that when every molecule in your body says, "YES, I want only this to happen," when there is no mixed, confusing message, when doubt does not cloud your mind, then your body can respond fully: Every cell, nerve, muscle, and bone can act in accord with your desire.

Children quickly learn the value of their mother's healing power of love and attention. Two-year-old Elliot, when he has hurt himself, runs to his mother for a kiss. If she doesn't kiss him exactly where it hurts, he holds his arm up and points to where she must deliver the kiss. She has taught him to come to her when he is hurt; he has figured out on his own how to have her healing awareness fixed just at the right place.

If, when they are small, children have a consistent sense of their mothers being there when needed, as they grow older they learn to take in lasting love and can "remember" the feeling. This leads to the security of knowing that Mother loves you even when she's in the other room. Or at an office. As they grow, they feel safe away from their mothers as they realize that the feeling of "mother" is really a feeling inside. They learn to love themselves not on the basis of something from outside but from the inside, from their own reservoir of security, self-acceptance, and self-love. This inner security and happiness offers the basis for a lifetime of freedom from fears and stress.

To establish this health-giving feeling of security, Ayur-Veda encourages a mother and father to spend as much time with the baby as possible, especially during the first two years of the baby's life. True, in our society, where a majority of mothers as well as fathers need to work, most have few choices about whether or not to leave young children. So we do our best and try to keep rested, well nourished, and openhearted when we are with our children. The feeling of being fully loved will be transmitted to the child, even if we can't spend as much time as we might like.

Whereas we may not have a choice about being a working parent, most of us do have the choice of having a baby under the best circumstances we can. In this regard, Ayur-Veda offers some interesting guidelines.

## What to Conceptualize When You Are Conceiving: Natal Attraction

The Ingalik Indians of North America believed that babies choose their parents, looking down from the sky to pick the right couple. This is not a unique idea: The Ayur-Vedic texts also support this conception of conception, that the coming together of parents and infants is more than just happenstance. Parental preparation for a child takes on a deeper value in this context; after all, we want to be well worth choosing!

Ayur-Veda thus places great emphasis on pre-conception and on the ideal development of potential parents via a highly detailed and sophisticated prenatal preparation program. Ayur-Veda addresses four significant areas regarding conception and pregnancy:

> 1. The balance of the mother's reproductive system and overall physiological functioning, including her mental and emotional health
> 2. The strength of the ovum and the sperm (which is said to be better strengthened by a month of celibacy prior to conception)
> 3. The time in the menstrual cycle, and the mother's biological as well as chronological age
> 4. The mother's diet during pregnancy

According to the ancient Ayur-Vedic physician Charaka, a baby is made of four parts: one part from the mother, one from the father, one from the mother's "intake" during pregnancy (food, drink, the inhalation of air, perceptions, feelings, etc.), and one from a generalized aspect of nature or consciousness.

Of those things over which we have some control, nothing is more important than maintaining optimal maternal and paternal health to ensure the optimal health and happiness of the child. In this regard, the following preparatory techniques are recommended:

> 1. Pre-conception Panchakarma treatment (see chapter 12) for *both* parents is ideal, but especially for the woman.

2. Follow the daily routine in chapter 12, emphasizing the daily oil massage (abhyanga).

3. If you are a would-be parent, optimize your diet, emphasizing milk, ghee, almonds, fresh fruits and vegetables, whole grains, fresh juices, and plenty of water. Eliminate junk food, meat, alcohol, and caffeine.

In comparing these Ayur-Vedic pre-conception considerations to our Western outlook, it's interesting that we in the West are just now paying the slightest attention to preparation for conception, primarily because pre-conception care can improve the chances of preventing low birth weight and potential reproductive risks.[4] (Some studies report that older mothers, because of their added interest in proper pre-conception and prenatal care, are giving birth to healthier babies on average than their younger counterparts.) Ayur-Veda offers its own approach to prenatal care as well as to fertility concerns.

### Infertility

While some infertility is thought to be due to inadequate sperm count or motility, blocked Fallopian tubes, or hormonal imbalances, in approximately half the cases of infertility, defined as a couple's inability to conceive after one year of unprotected intercourse, no physiological explanation is ever found.

Many doctors believe that anxiety about the possibility of infertility alone is enough to impede the conception process. If the couple, particularly the woman, follows a program to reduce stress, pregnancy very often follows. Researchers have recently demonstrated that women who have had difficulty conceiving who are taught meditative techniques to reduce their stress and also participate in a supportive group environment increase their chances of becoming pregnant by about 35 percent within six months.[5]

The daily practice of the stress-reducing program of TM and other Ayur-Vedic approaches may help rectify most of the usual causes of infertility cited above, with or without concomitant modern medical treatment.

Often the problem of infertility is too subtle to be detected by medical testing and lies in the realm of early imbalances in the doshas or dhatus. In these cases, following the Ayur-Vedic measures for preparing for conception may be sufficient to result in a pregnancy. In addition, other more specific treatments can be prescribed on an individual basis following an Ayur-Vedic evaluation.

### Enjoying Pregnancy Ayur-Vedically

Whereas modern medicine recognizes the importance of the mother's diet from a nutritional standpoint, Ayur-Veda also considers the effects of specific foods for balancing a woman's entire physiology during pregnancy to minimize stress and discomfort. Her food cravings—which in our culture are often considered more amusing than important—can serve as a useful guide to balance doshas through recommended foods. Ayur-Veda also considers a woman's food cravings during pregnancy to be related to the desires of the child as well.

Maharishi Ayur-Veda gives specific dietary guidelines to combat morning sickness, fluid retention, constipation, dryness, hemorrhoids, and other pregnancy-related sources of discomfort. Here are a few:

#### How to Eat When You Are Pregnant

1. Follow the general guidelines of the Vata-pacifying diet plan (see chapter 4). This does *not* mean only eating foods listed under "favor" and never having foods listed as "avoid." Sweet tastes are considered the best during pregnancy. This includes all breads, grains, rice, sweet fruits, and common sweeteners such as raw sugar or honey. Large amounts of refined sugar are not recommended. Avoid hot, spicy foods, too many raw green leafy vegetables, and dried beans and lentils. In general, a well-balanced diet with adequate protein and plenty of fresh fruits and vegetables is best.

2. Enjoy warm, cooked, fresh foods. Avoid leftovers as much as possible. In general, avoid foods with artificial flavors, preservatives, and other chemical additives.

3. Milk (warmed) and ghee are considered two of the most

beneficial foods to include in your diet at this time. Hot cereals such as cream of rice or cream of wheat are also good.

4. Honor specific food cravings (in moderation), especially from the fourth month on.[6]

5. If you are experiencing nausea, try the following:

a) Roast cardamom seeds, powder them, and eat a pinch as needed throughout the day.

b) Drink a little plain hot water (which has been boiled for ten minutes) every fifteen to thirty minutes. Add one-eighth teaspoon powdered or freshly grated ginger, if desired.

c) In the mornings, on an empty stomach, have a cup of room-temperature water with lemon and honey.

d) While napping or if you awaken in the early morning, try to sleep in a semireclining position rather than flat.

### EMOTIONAL NOURISHMENT DURING PREGNANCY

Ayur-Veda suggests paying as much attention to your emotions as your physiology during pregnancy. Your thoughts and feelings, as well as your food, will all have an effect on the baby. This is the time to be particularly attentive to the movies you watch, the books you read, the friends you associate with, and so on. An expectant mother can benefit especially from a "mother" network and peer-group support from other mothers-to-be, experienced mothers who can serve as mentors, and life-supporting people in general. For many women, traditional support within the extended family has reemerged as peer support. The value of some kind of positive social support in preventing premature births was recently demonstrated in a study which found that "women who experience conflict within their immediate support system and are unable to resolve those conflicts are at greater risk for premature births."[7]

### Nine Bodymind Considerations for Pregnancy

1. The most important principle to remember is that your happiness during this time is probably the most vital nourishment you can give the baby.

2. Your mate needs to give you lots of attention and affection during this time, staying home in the evenings as much as possible, and keeping you happy and fulfilled in your desires.

3. A daily walk of about thirty minutes is the ideal exercise for now, although swimming is fine, too. Try to avoid running, lifting, or straining, and any sharp movements. It is also good to minimize sexual activity.

4. Daily oil massage is especially beneficial during pregnancy (see chapter 12). In the eighth and ninth months, spend extra time massaging the nipples to help prepare for nursing. Apply oil to your abdomen gently and lightly throughout the pregnancy.

5. Sleeping during the day is not recommended, as it can create imbalances.

6. Have your attention on uplifting subjects and events. Avoid books, TV shows, and movies with frightening or violent themes. Be with loving friends and relatives as much as possible.

7. During the eighth month, in accord with Ayur-Veda, you should rest at home as much as possible, as this is the time when the subtle nutrient ojas is passed between mother and baby.

8. If you are practicing the Transcendental Meditation technique, have your meditation checked (by a qualified TM teacher), as there are special recommendations for pregnancy.

9. Continue regular care with an obstetrician you like and follow his or her advice regarding your pregnancy.

One final note: Many mothers report feeling very good during their pregnancy. Beyond hormonal changes, which can make us feel quite awful in the first few months (as our bodies are purifying) and quite wonderful in the remaining months, according to Ayur-Veda there is also the good effect the child can be having on the mother. Specifically, the child's influence can balance the mother's doshas, and many women are aware of feeling well balanced and settled inside later in the pregnancy.

## Optimizing Blessed Events:
## Ayur-Vedic Guidelines for Childbirth

In classic Ayur-Vedic childbirth practices, as well as in many other traditions, women giving birth are helped through the process by the presence and support of other women, by a collective female consciousness. Belly-dancing, for example, originated in Middle Eastern childbirth traditions. The natural birthing movements were facilitated by the imitative movements of other women present giving powerful nonverbal support. This is not a minor contribution.

In a study to determine the effects of a supportive companion during the birth process,[8] one group of first-time mothers underwent labor alone except for infrequent checks by hospital staff, while another group received continual support from an untrained woman companion. The companion was unknown to each mother but provided hand-holding, backrubs, and friendly conversation. The results were dramatic: While 75 percent of the mothers birthing alone had complications, only 12 percent of the mothers with companions did, and of the mothers who were alone but had an uncomplicated birth, the labor time was more than twice as long as for the supported mothers. The observed interactions of both groups following the birth indicated that the supported mothers were more talkative, friendly, and open with their newborn babies, and touched them more than those mothers without labor support.

### Ayur-Vedic Suggestions for Labor

1. Have a trusted, loving, knowing labor companion, if at all possible.

2. Walk to enhance the progress of labor.

3. Deep breathing can help maintain Vata in balance.

4. Utilize Maharishi Gandharva-Veda music therapy to facilitate relaxation (see chapter 12).

5. Apply sesame oil to waist, sides, back, and thighs.

6. To aid dilation, apply gentle outside pressure to a point one-half inch up from the tip of the coccyx.

## Ayur-Vedic Postpartum Care of Mother and Infant

### POSTPARTUM CARE OF INFANT

1. To initiate respiration, instead of spanking, sprinkle the newborn's face with water—cool in summer, warm in winter.

2. Dry off the newborn and rub a small quantity of slightly warm sesame oil on the head. Cover the fontanelles (soft spot on skull) with gauze saturated in sesame oil.

3. Before the first bath, massage the newborn with sesame oil, then wrap (swaddle) in silk or soft cotton after the bath.

### POSTPARTUM CARE OF THE MOTHER

Following delivery of the placenta, the mother can be gently covered with sesame oil and bathed. Ghee and sesame oil can be applied to her abdomen and then wrapped loosely with a long cloth strip. This binding prevents accumulation of Vata in the now empty abdominal space. The first nourishment after delivery should be liquid, either warm milk or herbal tea. A new mother's digestive power is generally weak, so warm liquid foods such as soups are best. Follow the Vata diet guidelines for the first six weeks.

Until the baby is sucking well, a new mother needs to massage her breasts daily to prevent blocked milk ducts. Whether breastfeeding or not, respect and respond to the baby's natural hunger, but leave adequate time between nursings for the previous feeding to be digested.

## The Maharishi Ayur-Veda Mother-Baby Program

Although there are a number of prenatal programs for women, there are almost no postnatal care programs available for new mothers outside of exercises designed to get your figure back. Pregnancy and delivery significantly alter a woman's constitutional balance, physically, mentally, and emotionally. Postpartum depression is real, but its treatment is not well understood in Western culture. After giving birth, most mothers feel very overwrought and/or fatigued. They need maximum rest and revitalization. This is provided by the Maharishi Ayur-Veda Mother-Baby Program, one of the most powerful of the Maharishi Ayur-Vedic programs available. One second-time mother observed, "After my first baby, it took me five months before the mood swings, roughness, and fatigue went away. With my second baby, I participated in the Mother-Baby program and started to feel good immediately. Now, six months later, it feels like someone has rebuilt my body, and it's true, they have. And the baby is also very settled and seems very healthy."

From the Ayur-Vedic perspective, a new mother's recovery depends on restoring her natural psychophysiological balance. Ayur-Veda attributes many Vata-related disorders such as constipation and gas, as well as postpartum depression, to improper care of the mother after delivery.

*At thirty-five, Margaret K. experienced a virtually problem-free pregnancy and delivery of her second child. But twenty-four hours later, a doctor discovered a prolapsed uterus and told her that she would probably have to undergo a full hysterectomy, and the sooner the better. Instead of having the recommended operation, Margaret started the Maharishi Ayur-Veda Mother-Baby Program, which she had arranged to do before the birth, consisting of a Vata-pacifying diet, cooked fresh daily by friends and family; a quiet, full-attention breast-feeding program for the baby; and daily warm oil massages for both mother and baby.*

*With this extra attention and help, Margaret was able to stay quite rested for six weeks and remain mostly off her feet. She did some Ayur-Vedic stretching exercises on a daily basis and put her attention on self-healing. She remembers reminding herself, "I have the resources inside to keep it together. It's my uterus, and I want to have it as long as possible."*

*The day after the program ended, she went to see the same doctor, who told her, in a surprised tone, that her uterus was back in a healthy position, and that she no longer needed the operation. Two years later, Margaret con-*

*tinues a Vata-reducing eating program, regular Panchakarma treatments twice a year, and plays a vigorous weekly game of tennis without fear of prolapse.*

If possible, try to organize ahead of time to participate in the at-home "Mother-Baby Program" made available through the Maharishi Ayur-Veda Health Centers. The program is simple: Three to five days after delivery (or ten days following a cesarean birth), a technician comes to your home; she administers a warm herbalized oil massage (abhyanga) and tucks you into a freshly made bed with hot-water bottles, where you rest until a hot bath is ready for you. One or both of you also massages the baby (see below). The treatments can be enjoyed daily or a few days a week, for from one to six weeks. Clara Berno, who established the Maharishi Ayur-Veda Mother-Baby Program, says, "This program gives mothers a chance to come out of the postpartum period with even more energy and better health than ever before. You can change postpartum blues into postpartum bliss."

Whether or not you can avail yourself of the complete Mother-Baby Program, here are some Mother-Baby Program suggestions for postpartum care.

### SUGGESTIONS TO AID POSTPARTUM DIGESTION

1. For reducing gas and constipation
   - Put one teaspoon whole fennel seeds in two quarts of water. Boil for five to ten minutes. Drink warm throughout the day.
2. For promoting healthy breast milk
   - Snack on almonds (blanched are best) and coconut.
   - Have one to two cups daily of boiled milk with a pinch of saffron, one-eighth teaspoon cardamom, one-eighth teaspoon ginger, and add brown sugar to taste. Also add one-half teaspoon ghee (clarified butter) if desired.
3. Foods to favor
   - Milk, rice, warm rice pudding with milk and sugar
   - Pumpkin, sunflower, and sesame seeds
   - Summer squash, asparagus, and coconut

4. It is also very helpful to follow a Vata-pacifying eating program (see chapter 4).

(see chapter 4)

### SUGGESTIONS FOR REST

Maharishi Ayur-Veda strongly recommends that mothers get as much rest as possible after delivery. This may mean readjusting priorities in a major way, eliciting the support of family members and friends to help with work around the house, grocery shopping, etc. A new mother should lie down and rest or nap when her baby naps, at least once a day, to try to complete the rest she is missing at night because of the baby's feeding schedule, crying times, etc.

A real shift from a high-activity life to a slower pace may be required. For Pitta types, this may mean moving away from a tendency to make the most of every minute to get "things done." For Vata types, it may mean ceasing to try to do several things at once. (Kaphas don't usually have to slow down; on the contrary, they may need to gear up for a higher level of activity and the disruption of routine that a new baby can bring.)

The purpose of a postpartum "slow-down" is a commitment to getting enough rest for the multiple purpose of staying healthy, producing adequate, nutritious breast milk, and being physically prepared to really enjoy the tender, blissful experience of a new baby with minimal fatigue and anxiety. To this end, Maharishi Ayur-Veda recommends that mothers attempt to take time for their own oil massage, even five minutes in the morning before their bath or shower, and that they take a five- to ten-minute bath afterward.

You'll notice that we have been focusing on the mother's postpartum care, as the mother's ability to remain stable, alert, and loving is the most important care she can provide the baby. Now let's look at the baby's care.

### THE AYUR-VEDIC BABY MASSAGE PROGRAM[9]

Abhyanga is equally important for the newborn, because it increases circulation and improves respiration, giving more oxygen to each cell. This results in improved digestion, healthy muscle tone, better development of sleep patterns, and resistance to disease. We know that circulation isn't developed fully until after the first few months. A daily baby massage can warm up and make flexible the infant's feet and hands. But it can also do far more.

Research conducted by psychologist Tiffany Field at the University of Miami School of Medicine provides convincing evidence for the benefits of infant massage, apart from its obvious help in promoting intimacy and bonding between babies and parents. In one of Dr. Field's landmark experiments, a group of premature babies were massaged fifteen minutes three times a day for ten days while a similar group were not. The massaged infants gained 47 percent more weight than the control group, although they did not eat more, and were observed to be more alert. Even eight months later, long after the massages had stopped, those infants who had been massaged still weighed more, and their mental and motor skills were more highly developed and mature.[10]

The Maharishi Ayur-Vedic Baby Massage Program can generally begin as soon as the umbilical cord falls off, usually within the first week of delivery. In the meantime, daily sponge baths help to keep the baby fresh. The total massage usually takes about twenty-five to thirty minutes; the massage itself takes only about five or ten minutes maximum, but with the setup time and bath time, allow about fifteen minutes more.

INSTRUCTIONS FOR BABY MASSAGE

You'll need:
- Three large towels
- A baby bathtub full of warm water
- Two pillows covered with plastic
- A clean diaper
- A baby washcloth
- Warm sesame oil in a plastic flip-top bottle

The bathroom is an ideal place to give the abhyanga. If you don't have a baby bathtub, you can use a large sink, or put a sponge cushion in your bathtub. Be sure that the room is kept warm and try to avoid drafts, which may make the baby uncomfortable.

Remove your shoes, all sharp jewelry, and your watch, and check your nails to see if they need trimming. Spread a sheet or large towel on the floor near the bathtub. Place your materials nearby so you can easily reach them. Put a pillow on the sheet so it's more comfortable. Run water in the bathtub, a bit warmer than normal, since it will cool down during the time of the abhyanga. Sit comfortably on the pillow with your back supported against the bathtub or wall and your legs spread out in front of you. Your legs can be bare or protected with a towel.

The first position is with your baby on her back with her head toward your stomach, or if you prefer, you can begin with her head toward your feet, so you can look at each other. She's easy to handle when she's lying on your lap. As you do the massage, speak gently and sweetly to your baby and tell her what's going on; let her know what you're doing as you progress. It's a nice opportunity to express how much you love her and how good she is.

Begin with the baby's head. Apply a small amount of warm oil to your hands, rub them together, and apply the oil in a gentle circular motion to the top, sides, and back of her head. Be very gentle over the soft spots, or fontanelles. Having her head massaged is very soothing and calming to a baby. Then massage her ears, avoiding the inside of the ear. Then her face: Move your hand gently back and forth on the forehead, use your forefingers over the sinus area, and make gentle circles with your palms on the temples and cheeks, making sure not to get any oil in the baby's eyes. Now use your forefinger across the upper lip and chin. If there is any skin irritation such as a rash or pimples, it's best to not use any oil on that area until it is clear. Sweep gently up her neck, if you can easily get to it, and be careful of the windpipe.

Re-oil your hands as needed, though it's not necessary to use a lot of oil. Your baby's skin will absorb some oil, but it should not be greasy. Just use enough oil so your touch is smooth with no friction. However, be very careful also to keep the slippery (!) baby well protected. Sweep up the chest and out the arms to the tips of the fingers. Repeat this three times. You'll notice that your baby will begin to look very relaxed. The baby massage helps to release stress and tension and even the muscular tightness that has accumulated from being in the fetal position for nine months.

Massage each arm. Use a circular motion on the shoulders, and a straight back-and-forth movement on the upper arm. Do each motion three times on each. Use a circular motion on the elbow, a back-and-forth motion on the forearm, and a circular motion on the wrist; make circles with your thumbs inside the palm of the baby's hand and on the back of the hand. *Gently* pull each finger.

Massage her abdomen slowly and carefully from left to right in a clockwise motion. This is helpful for digestion and elimination and helps to move along any gas bubbles she may have. If your baby becomes fussy, just continue easily. She may be uncomfortable because of gas. Most babies really enjoy this experience, even with a few moments of discomfort.

Next, massage the legs. Begin by sweeping your hands down both legs at the same time from upper thigh all the way to the toes three times. Use a circular motion with your thumbs on the inner thighs, which are the most constricted from diapers; this helps her circulation. Massage each leg using a circular motion on her hip, knee, and ankle. Move straight back and forth with your palm on her thigh and calf.

Next, do her feet. It's good to give special attention to the feet and massage each part gently and thoroughly. Massage some circles around the ankles, back and forth on the Achilles tendon, on the top of the foot, and at least ten times on the sole of her foot with the palm of your hand. Massaging the sole of the foot is said to have a beneficial effect on the whole body. Then gently pull each toe.

Now carefully turn the baby onto her abdomen. You can place your baby face-down lengthwise with her head toward your feet if that's comfortable. In this position be sure your baby has an area for breathing and that a towel or sheet is not in the way. Or you can place her across your lap and hold her with one hand under her chest if needed. Gently massage up and down her back utilizing your full hand. If you spend six to eight minutes on the entire baby massage, spend about three of those minutes massaging her back; this is a most important area for relaxation, even for a baby.

After the abhyanga, gently cleanse the baby. Be sure to use a very gentle soap because baby skin is very tender. It's fine to shampoo her hair, but Ayur-Veda usually recommends doing this only about once a week, to avoid drying the scalp. Dry the baby with a soft towel, especially her head.

If you want, you can massage your baby twice a day. Fathers often enjoy giving the second massage, which can be done in the evening and can become part of the night-time routine. Many fathers have found that this is one of the nicest ways to interact with their newborn babies. The procedure is so soothing that the baby usually settles down easily before sleep. At night, use only a very small amount of oil so that there's no need for a bath.

Note: If the baby has a fever or some congestion in her nose or chest, skip the massage for a few days until she returns to normal.

### BABY EXERCISE

After the baby's massage is a good time to do some exercises that can help a baby's flexibility, digestion, and neuromuscular integration.

Repeat the following exercises three times each:

1. While he is on his back, hold his feet and gently and slowly bend his legs from knees to tummy. This is very helpful for digestion and can be done at other times during the day. It's better if your baby doesn't have diapers on so there's no binding.

2. Gently bend the baby's legs straight up from the hips by holding the feet with one hand, keeping your other hand over the knees to help keep his legs straight. This is helpful for flexibility in the hips and also for digestion.

3. Extend his legs and cross one over the other.

4. Straighten the opposite arm and leg and then cross them over the tummy. Then repeat with the other arm and leg.

5. Spread his arms all the way out and cross them over the chest.

### TEN FURTHER SUGGESTIONS FOR THE FIRST SIX WEEKS

You are probably familiar with almost all the points that follow but just keep in mind:

1. A newborn baby's nervous system is very delicate and tender during the first few weeks. For this reason, Ayur-Veda recommends keeping the baby indoors for the first six weeks.

If you do take the baby outside, do so when the weather is mild and don't stay out too long. What seems to be normal activity for you may be uncomfortable for the baby.

For this same reason, as well as for the well-being of the new mother, it is better to limit visits during the first few weeks—perhaps immediate family only or really close friends.

2. After being in the womb for so many months, simply being out in the world is quite a contrast for newborns. They prefer a more quiet environment and dimmer lights. You may have noticed that new babies are easily startled by loud noises or bright lights. It's an excellent idea to limit intense sensory stimuli of all sorts during the first few weeks. Even the smell of perfume may be too strong for a newborn.

3. Avoid exposing the baby to cold winds or drafts.

4. To prevent damage to spinal-cord nerves, always securely support the baby's neck and head, until the baby can hold her or his head up without wobbling.

5. It is better not to rely on a pacifier to soothe a crying baby, because although the crying may temporarily abate, it usually means the baby needs more attention.

6. If colic develops, place drops of fennel tea on the baby's tongue. Apply extra sesame oil to the front fontanelle in the evening.

7. Never frighten an infant or young child even in "fun," as it is injurious to his or her mental state. Nor should a small infant be tossed in the air in play as this aggravates Vata and can produce fear and anxiety.

8. Spend as much time with the new infant as you possibly can. And more.

### Ayur-Vedic Feeding During the First Year of Life

Breast-feeding is recommended for the first six months to a year, especially because breast milk in a woman who is free of toxicity has a uniquely high content of ojas. Traditionally, a baby can be weaned starting at seven or eight months, around the time when she or he starts to develop teeth. According to Ayur-Veda, weaning is a gradual, natural process that ideally should be completed before eighteen months of age. The mother and baby can be viewed as a breast-feeding "couple": Either one can initiate the weaning process. Babies can give you signs that they are ready to be weaned when they are inattentive during feeding, when they nurse for only one or two minutes, or when they actually refuse to nurse. Mother-initiated weaning is best if it is a gradual process. The basic tenet for the weaning process is "Don't offer, don't refuse." You can devote extra time to nurturing the baby on other levels, through attention, play, music, and cuddling. As in every other aspect of Maharishi Ayur-Veda, it's important not to strain. The mother should consider it appropriate to nurse however long she feels it is comfortable for her and for the child. You can substitute a bottle or food or cup at the feeding that the baby seems to be least interested in. If you just stop the lightest feeding, the night-time or early-morning ritual can still continue.

The noontime meal is the best time to initiate the start of other foods, when the baby's digestive fire or agni is strongest. You can introduce one food at a time so as not to overtax the digestive system and cause ama; you can also detect any sensitivities to particular foods this way. (It's fine to continue to nurse during the time food is being tried.) First, introduce semi-liquids from grains such as rice or semolina—but it's better not to mix grains early on. After semi-liquids, start mushy solid foods such as strained fruits or vegetables. Introduce milk after a year. Milk is considered an acceptable food for older children, especially when warmed, which provides a calming effect. You may want to start with goat's milk because it is less Kapha-producing than cow's milk. The milk can be boiled first and served warm, making it more easily digestible and less mucus-producing.

Cheese and yogurt should be avoided, as they can increase mucus production, which can lead to earaches, colds, or fluid in the ears. Even though this is a Kapha time of life, however, we don't necessarily want to put our children on a long-term Kapha-pacifying diet. It's fine for children to have sweet treats from time to time, but limit highly concentrated sweets and avoid chocolate. All six tastes should be included for infants as well as for adults (see chapter 4). In general, an infant's diet should be more bland than an adult's diet, so avoid offering foods that are too salty, sour, or highly spiced.

The first preventative measure for constipation is to be aware of your child's defecation habits and to respond to any early variations by increasing the amount of ghee, fresh fruits, vegetables, and fluids in the diet. Try to avoid enemas, drugstore laxatives, and suppositories.

It's better not to insist that babies or young children eat foods they do not like. Unless they are ill, they usually have normal, balanced physiologies; their food preferences are innocent and they know instinctively what they need.

## Understanding Babies' "Temperaments": Prakriti Types

As we mentioned in chapter 3, every newborn can be identified by his or her "prakriti" or constitutional type. This is not unlike what infant development specialists such as psychologists Jerome Kagan at Harvard University and Nathan Fox at the University of Maryland call "temperament." But prakriti is a more inclusive concept than temperament in that it adds an essential physiological component. A baby will be naturally more Vata, more Pitta, or more Kapha structurally, mentally, and emotionally. The prakriti can be identified when the baby is about ten days old, allowing time for all the doshas to rebalance and recover from the birth experience.

Knowing the prakriti helps parents to understand the behavior of the baby from a broad yet personal perspective and helps them to separate the behaviors and qualities of their own physiology from the baby's. When mothers or fathers know, for example, that their baby has a Pitta nature, they will be more likely to respond appropriately to the baby's needs, rather than reacting to the baby's behavior on the basis of their *own* doshas or prakriti. Later on, knowing the prakriti or dosha predominance will aid in determining dosha-pacifying foods for various childhood illnesses.

Always remember that parents have the first priority. If you are happy and settled in yourself, your ability to nurture your children becomes far more effortless. The simple Ayur-Vedic wisdom is, If a parent is happy, then the child will be happy. Use common sense and take care of yourself.

\* \* \*

Let us now explore Ayur-Vedic perspectives on another aspect of a woman's life, the expansive Vata cycle, menopause, and what is called aging. What Maharishi Ayur-Veda proposes and what modern science is beginning to recognize is that our whole vision of time passing, understood as aging, is really a fallacy. It's not the number of years that determine age; it's our state of bodymind awareness while we're living that makes us old or young.

# Chapter 11

### ❀

# FULLNESS

## Menopause, Life Span, and the New Aging

*Ayur-Veda is for those who desire immortality.*

Charaka Samhita

*Let us go forward to dancing and laughter,*
*assuming a longer and a better life....*

Rig Veda

Within the next twenty years, the number of women reaching the age of menopause in the United States will be almost 40 million. Unfortunately, our society often turns this universal stage of life into an ailment-based process. We are asked to see it "as a medical event—even a disease process," writes Sadja Greenwood, M.D., in her pioneering book, *Menopause Naturally.*

In many cultures, especially non-Western, menopause is looked upon as a time of greater freedom and increased status for women, and little or no emphasis is placed on psychophysiological symptoms. And often, when a woman reaches menopause, she is admitted into a powerful society of women healers, her wisdom at this stage of life more highly regarded than ever before. Similarly, in her book *The Silent Passage,* author Gail Sheehy cites the work of anthropologist Martha Frent, who found that 80 percent of women of the Rajput caste in India had no symptoms of depression related to menopause, as they feel liberated from the restrictions of youth. In Japan, where the language has no phrase for "hot flashes," 65 percent of the women report an uneventful menopause. In China, too, there are few reported menopausal symptoms. These differences were presented at the Sixth International Congress of Menopause in Bangkok in 1990, confirming extensive cultural differences regarding menopause between Eastern and Western cultures, even though the average age for this transition was the same: about fifty-one years for nearly all women worldwide.

The essential difference appears to be in the perceived advantages. If menopause is interpreted as a greater freedom, fewer problems are associated with it. For example, African-American women are more likely to pass through menopause with no psychological problems, because the family structure is generally matriarchal, often run by a strong grandmother, and women are perceived as coming into their own as they become older. On the other hand, where the value of youth is emphasized over the value of age, menopause is often regarded as a start of a decline. That thought alone is enough to set off a whole chain of symptoms in the bodymind.

## The Natural Cycle of Menopause

Despite the shadow of "medical crisis" hanging over its arrival, menopause is not an abrupt event. It is a gradual process, part of a cycle that occurs over time, as our ovaries stop producing estrogen. Estrogen and progesterone production start decreasing as early as age thirty. Over approximately the next two decades, this decrease eventually leads to irregular cycles, shorter cycles, a reduction in the amount of the menstrual flow, and bleeding without ovulating. Menopause takes about five years to complete, beginning with irregular periods and ending with the cessation of periods between the ages of forty-two and sixty (although the possibility of conception generally continues for one or two years following the last period). About 10 percent of us go through menopause before age forty. The last episode of menstrual bleeding brought on by our cyclic secretion of ovarian hormones marks the actual beginning of menopause. Any bleeding that occurs a year following the cessation of the menstrual periods is considered cause for investigation.

Menopausal symptoms can appear but this is not always the case.

According to epidemiologist Sonja McKinlay at the New England Research Institute, who has been conducting a long-term study on women during menopause, most women experience a year or two of irregular periods, some fluctuation in body temperature, and perhaps a few sleepless nights. "They have a lot of apprehension as they approach menopause, and then they come through it and say, 'Oh, it's not such a big deal after all.'"[1] Similarly, psychologist Karen Matthews found that postmenopausal women did not have more depression and anxiety than premenopausal women of the same age.

Perhaps the most important feature of menopause is that it is experienced very differently by different women. Women who have healthier bodies in general experience a far easier menopause, although at least three-quarters of us do experience hot flushes or flashes, night sweats, and vaginal dryness, and most of us don't feel as clear and bright as usual, partly owing to insomnia and partly owing to a decrease in hormones.

Hot flashes are the most common discomfort of the menopause process, especially because they often happen at night and cause insomnia. On average, 20 percent of us will have hot flash experiences for less than a year, but for another 25 to 50 percent of us, they can occur for more than five years. It is worthwhile noting, however, that it is generally women whose bodies have grown accustomed to estrogen over twenty-five or thirty years who have hot flashes. Women who have their menopause in their teens or twenties due to surgery or genetic problems typically do not experience hot flashes. And women who experience a more rapid withdrawal of estrogen, perhaps following surgical removal of the ovaries in their thirties or forties, tend to experience more hot flashes than women going through menopause gradually. It therefore appears that even the hot flash is not due solely to a lack of estrogen, but also to the state of imbalance induced when the body loses a key hormone and has not yet adapted to that change. Our bodies, however, can and do adjust.

The issue for each of us is whether the adjustment comes easily or with difficulty. Some women may experience emotional changes at this time, such as anxiety, depression, and irritability, often associated with sleep disturbances caused by the hot flashes. We can also experience mood swings, short-term memory loss, migraine headaches, and a variety of other symptoms. On the plus side, fibroid tumors become smaller and symptoms of endometriosis decrease.

Modern medicine has discovered that some menopausal symptoms are controllable with specific life-style changes. It is well-known, for example, that a balanced diet, no smoking, decreased use of alcohol and caffeine, and regular low-impact aerobic exercise can minimize the difficulties associated with menopause. But some symptoms are not so manageable.

From an Ayur-Vedic perspective, premenstrual syndrome and menopausal symptoms are a reflection of the common underlying causes of both conditions: an imbalance in the doshas and the buildup of metabolic wastes that disturb tissue (dhatu) metabolism. With an understanding of these underlying causes of specific menopausal symptoms, we can take steps to speed up the body's adjustment phase, both lessening and cutting short the symptoms.

## Menopause and the Doshas

Let's consider how each of the doshas is involved in the physiological changes of menopause. First of all, since menopause marks a major transition in a woman's biological life as she moves from the time of life dominated by Pitta to that dominated by Vata, Vata tendencies will often start to increase around menopause, regardless of constitutional type.

Classic signs of this increase in Vata can include constipation; thinner, drier skin and drier mucous membranes; some thinning of the hair and bones; lighter, more interrupted sleep; and an increased tendency to worry. Rather than viewing these conditions as inevitable, Ayur-Veda proposes that they can be largely avoided by keeping Vata dosha in balance.

Imbalanced Pitta can also play a part in a symptomatic menopause. Because Pitta dosha regulates our hormonal balance, heat production, and metabolism, it is the dosha primarily involved in the phenomenon of hot flashes. During the years of menstruation, ama gets eliminated with the menstrual flow. When menopause occurs, excess Pitta can build up throughout the bodymind, especially if ama is present. The phenomenon is analogous to a heater turned up to "high" in a room with the doors closed. The heat has nowhere to go, so the room keeps getting hotter. The Ayur-Vedic solution to decreasing hot flashes lies in turning down the heater (balancing Pitta), and also opening the doors so the excessive heat can escape (clearing out ama).

As we've seen, Pitta dosha is also related to digestion and to the regulation of fat and hormone metabolism. The medha dhatu includes all hormonal activities—including of course estrogen—and, along with asthi, is particularly important during menopause. Estrogen aids in our metabolic processes, and if our metabolic processes are weak at menopause, the withdrawal of the supportive role of estrogen will reveal any blockage in fat tissues that may cause an elevation of cholesterol and an increase in cardiovascular disease.

As we saw in chapter 6, the tissues of the body are nourished in succession, with the nourishment of each tissue dependent on the proper metabolism of the previous tissue. Estrogen, along with all the other hormones, functions from the level of medha (fat) dhatu, which regulates fat and cholesterol metabolism. The activity of medha dhatu not only affects the processes of medha such as cholesterol metabolism but also the metabolism of the next successive dhatu, asthi (bone). At menopause, however, estrogen levels drop dramatically, and our metabolic processes lose that support. Ideally, since the drop in estrogen at menopause is natural, the body will adjust and no disease will develop. Increased cholesterol, heart disease, and osteoporosis will only occur if the body's metabolism has been affected by ama and imbalance over the years. In effect, the loss of estrogen may bring to light any underlying imbalance in metabolism.

If you have developed symptoms or complications at menopause, or feel you are at risk for them, you'll find Ayur-Vedic recommendations for menopause listed later in this chapter. These recommendations are individualized by each dosha.

You may also find that the doshas promote different emotional responses to hormonal changes during menopause. Vata imbalances can lead to erratic mood swings; Pitta imbalances to anger and irritability; and Kapha to lethargy. Imbalanced Vatas tend to be more fearful as they face uncertainty and change in their lives, but can become quickly accepting and expansive to new ways of being in the world. Some imbalanced Pittas may lament the loss of control associated with menopause; they then may fix their mental focus on menopause research, gathering information about studies and new approaches to deal with discomfort. Kaphas are less likely to notice any dramatic imbalances in their physiology and often go through this transition fairly easily. However, they need to keep active if they start to feel heavy or depressed.

Knowing your constitutional type, your doshic imbalances and ways to counteract them, and the differences between your symptoms and those of a friend with a different doshic profile can allay fears, offer symptom relief, and provide a more comprehensive level of knowledge, so your experience of menopause feels comfortable for you.

*Menopausal Symptoms Associated with Vata Dosha*

> Mood swings
> Dry skin or mucous membranes
> Constipation or irritable bowel
> Insomnia
> Worry
> Reduced libido

*Menopausal Symptoms Associated with Pitta Dosha*

> Hot flashes
> Irritability
> Heavy bleeding
> Skin problems

*Menopausal Symptoms Associated with Kapha Dosha
(or ama-related)*

Weight gain
Overweight
Fluid retention, edema
High cholesterol or triglycerides

## Bone Density, Calcium, and Exercise

Menopause does *not* have to induce a symptomatic "estrogen-deficient" state in our bodies. In fact, a woman's body continues to produce some estrogen after menopause, and for the majority of women, the amount is sufficient to prevent many of the symptoms and potential health problems that may be associated with menopause, including fractures resulting from osteoporosis, or decreased density of the bones. What helps to ensure the most favorable postmenopausal bone strength is good premenopause preparation through sufficient exercise and calcium, as well as through Ayur-Vedic regimes.

Recent research on osteoporosis has shown that it is not simply a disease of the postmenopausal woman, but represents a progressive imbalance in bone metabolism that begins in the early thirties for both women and men, resulting in progressive, gradual loss of bone mass over the years. Whether we develop debilitating osteoporosis depends on how much bone mass we lose yearly and also on how much we have built up. Calcium intake, exercise, and menstrual regularity all play a role in the strength of our bones.

These findings have led some specialists to refer to osteoporosis as a "pediatric disease," stressing how important it is for growing children, particularly young girls, to build up bone through adequate dietary calcium, regular exercise, avoiding excess protein in the diet, and by maintaining a regular menstrual cycle.

Calcium is important throughout our lives for the strength of our bones. Recent studies show that American children and adolescents need as much as 1200 to 1600 milligrams of calcium per day to properly nourish their bones. This is roughly equivalent to five cups of milk per day. Adult women need 800 milligrams per day;

after menopause the need increases again to about 1500 milligrams per day. (To calculate your intake, consider that an average diet, excluding dairy products, provides about 300 milligrams a day. Then add about 250 milligrams for each serving of a dairy product.) It is now known that calcium needs are higher in those people whose diet is relatively high in protein, such as those who eat meat on a daily basis, because calcium is lost in the urine when protein wastes are excreted. Calcium needs are considerably lower in women in other countries such as China, where a largely vegetarian diet is consumed. The higher rates of osteoporosis in the United States are now being attributed to a diet high in meat protein, and too low in certain vegetables and legumes which have a high content of calcium easily absorbed by the body.

A regular menstrual cycle is also important for building and maintaining bone strength throughout our reproductive years. A recent study by Jerilyn Prior, M.D., an endocrinologist at the University of British Columbia, found that more than half of all women ages thirty to fifty could be losing bone mass every year owing to subtle disturbances in their menstrual cycles. Women who missed ovulation one or more times had an average loss of 4 percent of their bone density over the year, whereas those women who had normal ovulation and cycles every month had no bone loss. (The runners among them showed increased bone density, highlighting the value of regular exercise, when the menstrual cycle is regular.)[2]

As the periods become irregular and cease at the time of menopause, estrogen is less available to help support bone metabolism. As a result, during the several years before and after menopause, bone mass typically drops off at an accelerated rate, and a woman can lose as much as one-fifth of her total bone mass. Neither calcium nor exercise have been shown to be very effective in preventing bone loss in this transition time, during which the body adjusts to a relative lack of estrogen. From the Ayur-Vedic point of view, if the doshas are balanced and the dhatus are free of ama, then the body's homeostatic mechanisms will more efficiently help our metabolism adjust. Bone loss eventually does slow down several years following menopause, after the body goes through this adjustment process. Some researchers have proposed that the extra weight women commonly gain during menopause reflects an attempt by the body to cope with the hormonal changes by increasing nonovarian sources of estrogen, such as fat, which assist the body in converting androstenedione (another hormone in the body) into estrogen.[3]

After menopause, regular exercise and adequate calcium remain essential and can reduce the rate of bone loss by 50 percent.

## Menopause and HRT

For women who are at risk for osteoporosis, taking estrogen can lead to bone mass increases of as much as 6 percent, also preventing the majority of the bone loss that occurs in the perimenopausal transition.[4] Considering the known and unknown risks of hormone replacement therapy (HRT), however, we do not recommend that every woman take hormones automatically. It should be a decision made in consultation with your doctor and based on a complete assessment of your health. If osteoporosis is the primary reason you are considering HRT, the evaluation can include an actual measurement of the bone density in your hip and spine, so you and your doctor will know precisely how dense your bones are and whether you are truly at significant risk for osteoporosis.

HRT is also prescribed to help women through the uncomfortable phase of their menopause.

The average length of time women usually choose to stay on HRT is about nine months. It is often given cyclically, to mimic the body's natural secretion of hormones. Estrogen is given the first twenty-five days of each month; progesterone is added from the fifteenth to the twenty-fifth day, and there is an expected flow between Day 25 and Day 30 of each month. (Unfortunately, this normal monthly bleeding can be difficult to distinguish from any bleeding that may indicate uterine cancer. If spotting occurs throughout the month, then further investigation is necessary.) HRT can be taken in pill form or absorbed through the skin from wearing a transparent patch. It is best taken in the smallest dose necessary to relieve symptoms; otherwise, nausea and breast tenderness may be experienced. These symptoms are usually more pronounced at the beginning of therapy, and tolerances do develop over time. Once you stop the treatment, your menopausal symptoms may return.

Let's consider some of the pros and cons of HRT. Since menopause is a natural phenomenon, our bodies can and do adjust to
the decrease in estrogen levels. However, modern medicine has
conceptualized menopause itself as a disease of estrogen deficiency, or "ovarian failure." In an approach analogous to the treatment of hypothyroidism with thyroid hormone, the current
standard medical approach to menopause involves giving women
hormones to replace hormones that the ovaries no longer produce.
The problem with this approach has been that many women never
develop negative health consequences from menopause, but are
still being treated as if for a disease with HRT.

In the recent past, HRT use was poorly understood, and estrogen alone was prescribed without progesterone (another important
hormone in the reproductive cycle). This imbalanced hormonal
state resulted in serious side effects, some of which are now prevented by giving both hormones together. While this combination
approach is far safer than giving estrogen alone, there is a growing
body of evidence suggesting that women on HRT nevertheless remain at some increased risk for potential health problems. These
include a form of PMS, migraines, fibroid tumors, elevated blood
pressure, symptoms of fibrocystic breasts, gallbladder disease, and
increased risk for breast and uterine cancer. Furthermore, HRT is
generally not recommended for women with diabetes, kidney or
liver disease, uterine or breast cancer histories, a history of deep-
vein thrombosis, a suspected pregnancy, or undiagnosed vaginal
bleeding.

On the positive side, HRT does offer some very important
health benefits. Besides eliminating incapacitating hot flashes in 90
percent of the cases and reversing the thinning of vaginal tissues,
HRT, as we noted, is highly successful in the prevention of osteoporosis for those who are at risk for this condition.

Studies have shown that perhaps the most significant health
impact of HRT is decreased mortality from acute and chronic arte-
riosclerotic diseases,[5] reducing the risk of heart disease in particular. This is important because after the age of sixty-five, women are
more likely than men to develop high blood pressure and have
twice as many fatal heart attacks.[6]

Fortunately, we will know a great deal more by the year 2002.
That is when the massive NIH-sponsored study, the Women's

Health Initiative, will conclude. The study is evaluating the effects of hormone replacement therapy, diet (especially calcium and fat), and other factors on the incidence of major diseases in 150,000 women between the ages of fifty and seventy-nine, including heart attacks, stroke, breast cancer, colon cancer, and osteoporosis.

All in all, HRT may be very appropriate for some women and not for others. For some, the benefits of postmenopausal hormonal replacement outweigh the risks, especially since rates of death from endometrial cancer are far less than from heart disease. But let's not forget that if lack of estrogen were the primary cause of heart disease, every postmenopausal woman would develop some form of this disease, and this is obviously not the case. Because the current research data shows some very positive benefits, we do not dismiss HRT by any means. Each of us needs to make her own decision on the basis of individual specific risk factors for the various diseases for which HRT has shown benefit, including heart disease and osteoporosis.

At the same time, any woman can make numerous changes in her daily life that can dramatically reduce her risk of heart disease, are good for her in other ways as well, and do not involve taking an outside drug.[7] Taking estrogen does temporarily reduce cholesterol and the risk of heart disease, but treatments such as diet, exercise, and meditation also reduce risk factors for heart disease and osteoporosis without side effects, by promoting the body's healing mechanisms.

### Free Radicals, HRT, and Ayur-Veda

From an Ayur-Vedic point of view, it is not estrogen loss that causes women to age and get ill after menopause. The use of estrogen merely sheds light on what is really going on in your body, which appears when the added protection of estrogen is missing. For example, as we saw in chapter 5, free radicals (unstable oxygen and other molecules) are normally produced by our bodies to fight bacteria and remove toxins, but they are also produced from radiation and other toxic elements in our environment. They break down our body tissues and lead to degenerative changes we associate with aging, such as wrinkles and stiffness in our joints. Researchers are now also recognizing that the clogging of the arteries as we get older is not only due to an excess of total cholesterol in the blood, or even to an excess of LDL, the so-called "bad cholesterol," but to *oxidized* LDL. It is LDL cholesterol which is attacked by free radicals and transforms into an unstable, oxidated form which damages artery walls and leads to arteriosclerosis, heart disease, and strokes. It is unfortunate that oxidized fats such as LDL are more readily created from polyunsaturated oils which are found in the margarine we've been encouraged to eat to *prevent* heart disease, than from saturated fats (such as butter and ghee) or monounsaturated fats (such as those found in olive oil).

Maharishi Ayur-Veda provides us with programs which help to protect our bodies against damaging free radical molecules. These rejuvenation programs utilize special herbal formulas and physical therapies (see chapter 12) to help protect the body against damaging free radical molecules. They go deeper than HRT. Despite its benefits, HRT does not correct the underlying imbalances in digestion and metabolism that are unmasked at menopause and that may eventually cause problems elsewhere in the body.

For some women undergoing menopause, hormonal changes create such upheaval and result in such severe symptoms that temporary HRT may be required while the psychophysiological imbalances are being addressed with Ayur-Vedic programs. For other women with less severe symptoms, regular Ayur-Vedic routines and Vata- and Pitta-balancing eating programs alone can help a woman enjoy a symptom-free menopause.

Ayur-Veda specifically addresses another concern about HRT. Since each woman's hormone levels are unique to her physiology and vary daily, the need to adjust the amounts of estrogen and progesterone coming in from outside is a continual dilemma. A synthetic hormone comes into your body in fixed amounts and at a fixed rate, whereas when your biological intelligence regulates the dosage, the amount and rate will vary in subtle and precise ways at different times of the day and under varying conditions. Therefore, many women undergoing HRT are receiving inappropriate amounts of hormones, to a greater or lesser degree.

The bottom line is this: Nature knows best. If you have not yet reached menopause, you can prepare yourself by following the Maharishi Ayur-Vedic treatment programs presented here. If you are going through menopause or are past it, follow the dosha-pacifying diets and cleansing routines, especially regular Panchakarma, to alleviate any specific menopausal symptoms and help you maintain vitality. If these symptoms persist, consult your physician about starting HRT. Be sure to gather a complete personal and family history covering heart disease, breast cancer, uterine cancer, and osteoporosis, since these conditions all have a bearing on your decision whether to begin HRT and how long to continue it. Recognize that this is not a decision to which you are bound: The therapy can begin and end at any time. However, if you are taking it for a certain severe problem, such as osteoporosis or heart disease, it can be continued indefinitely with good monitoring.

Almost all menopausal symptoms disappear spontaneously over time as your body adjusts to compensate for the hormonal and eliminatory changes. According to Ayur-Vedic principles, HRT treatment is an outside intervention that can cause your bodymind to be continually off-balance, with no opportunity to adjust from within. Whereas a short regime of HRT may be helpful, a long regime (unless serving to prevent serious illnesses for which you are at risk) prohibits this self-regulation from occurring. In light of the exciting initial research on Ayur-Vedic programs and the increase in antiaging hormonal levels, especially in women (which we discuss in the following section), we believe that a great deal more information on Ayur-Veda, hormone and estrogen production, and metabolism will soon be forthcoming. HRT, while certainly helpful now, may become an outdated intervention when we can learn to rebalance the body's loss of hormone production from our own natural inner pharmacy.

### The Ayur-Vedic Prescription for a Comfortable Menopause

The Ayur-Vedic routines ought to start prior to menopause, so that the doshas are balanced when a woman starts menopause. After the periods stop, Ayur-Veda suggests regular cleansing treatments to replace the purifying monthly cycle of menstruation. Internal cleansing treatments done at home (see chapter 9), daily oil massage, consistent exercise, a regular rest routine, and a proper eating program are essential elements to maintaining health and energy.

Here are some suggested interventions:

    1. Practice a stress-reduction technique such as TM daily, which enables your bodymind to produce its own anti-aging biochemicals.
    2. Engage in purposeful, enjoyable activity to enliven your mind and heart.
    3. Get enough rest; go to bed early and get up early.
    4. Eat plenty of fresh fruits, vegetables, grains, and legumes and follow the Ayur-Vedic dietary guidelines.
    5. Hot flashes represent a Pitta imbalance and are known to be aggravated by both stress and what we eat. Follow a Pitta-pacifying diet and the routine for Pitta-type PMS.
    6. Eliminate alcohol and caffeinated beverages.
    7. Vaginal dryness, emotional mood swings, and insomnia all represent Vata dosha imbalance. Follow a Vata-pacifying diet and the routine for Vata-type PMS to decrease these symptoms.
    8. Walk, swim, or bicycle and enjoy surya namaskar (see chapter 4) daily.
    9. Give yourself a daily oil massage (as described in chapter 12).
    10. Follow the monthly resting program (in chapter 9).
    11. Follow the internal cleansing instructions (in chapter 9). Not surprisingly, the program to reduce PMS symptoms (chapter 9) works equally well for reducing and relieving menopausal symptoms. To promote purification and the balancing of the doshas, follow the procedure monthly for three consecutive months if you are in good health. If you find that the symptoms have improved and you wish to continue, you may skip a few months, then repeat the program again for three months.

You've been given some ideas and programs to help your bodymind through the natural cycle of menopause, but we hope you'll appreciate that warm oil and hot water, while very helpful, do not take the place of the real contribution of Ayur-Vedic wisdom: the knowledge of the most substantive medical "field" yet discovered, the inner field of development.
In Ayur-Vedic terms, menopause is another opportunity to rede-

fine ourselves in concert with an ever new bodymind. It enables us to move into the more spiritual, expansive values of Vata and away from the more focused, controlling, driving qualities of Pitta. Vata often attunes us to our most intimate desires for creating and for expansion of the mind, to experience and express all kinds of poetry in every aspect of our lives, from the most personal to the most global and universal. At this stage, our nuclear families may need us less and less while our communities and our world need us more and more. We can expand our lives to embrace our world family, giving something creative and powerful back to life at every step. To accept these global challenges, we need to overcome any doubts or fears about maturing and aging.

## The Longevity of Women

What helps women live longer than men?

Until now, according to the National Center for Health Statistics, men succumbed to the effects of the fifteen leading causes of death in the United States more often than women. The life expectancy of women at birth still exceeds that of men by seven years. Even looking at the numbers among older citizens, when women no longer have the so-called protective hormonal advantage guarding them against heart attack, women still maintain a four-year longevity edge over men.

To even things out a bit, approximately 125 males are conceived for every 100 females. At birth, the numerical advantage of males is 105 for every 100 females born. Despite the fact that female newborns have a higher rate of "low birth weight," they survive better; newborn males have an 8 percent higher mortality rate. This higher rate continues throughout the entire life span. After seventy-five years of age, there are 100 females for every 65 males, and past eighty-five, there are 100 females for every 40 males.

Women did not used to live longer than men. Before the twentieth century, women died early, often during childbirth, or became so worn out from childbearing and raising children that a great many women died prematurely. In our era, however, women have had the chance to prove their endurance and now maintain a longer life span. Yet women do become ill and, in many cases, as recent statistics indicate, more ill than men. It is of interest that women live longer than men *despite* the fact that we experience far more chronic conditions.

Why *do* women live longer? Researchers believe the answer lies partly in the female X chromosome, partly in the differences between female and male sex hormones, and partly in women's immune systems. For example, the male hormone testosterone is correlated with higher blood pressure rates and higher amounts of stress hormones and the artery-clogging lipid LDL in cholesterol. Women apparently require less oxygen, use less energy, and metabolize more slowly.

Whether this longevity edge is a question of more favorable genetics because women are the carriers of the species, or of more favorable biology because women are the traditional care-givers and need to be longer-lived, is less important than what we do with what we are given. We don't present these findings to emphasize the differences between men and women but to ask what women can do to improve their health in light of specific female strengths.

One of our current health advantages is certainly behavioral; women address health concerns more directly than men. And we listen. A recent Harris Poll indicated that women are far more responsive than men to "good health-care" counsel. From the point of view of prevention, women seem to do what it might take to live longer.[8] From both a PNI and an Ayur-Vedic viewpoint, an active interest in being healthy is, in simple, practical terms, life-supporting.

A study conducted at Emory University identified fourteen primary causes of premature illness and premature death (defined as those occurring before age 65) and concluded that approximately two-thirds of early deaths are preventable.[9] We don't need medical breakthroughs alone to change the patterns of longevity in our nation; simply by using the knowledge we already have, we can become a far healthier nation. This is what many women today understand and, as a result, are taking on a greater degree of responsibility for their health, practicing the first line of defense, preventive medicine.

This is the kind of medicine in which Ayur-Veda specializes; all its programs and interventions are specifically geared toward a longer life for both women and men, based on a more comprehensive prevention which completely redefines aging.

## Becoming Ageless

*Age only matters when one is aging. Now that I
have arrived at a great age, I might as well be 20.*

Pablo Picasso (at 80)

Ayur-Veda proposes, and Western scientists are beginning to agree, that there is no theoretical limit to human longevity: In order to comprehend this possibility, we have to rethink what is called "the aging process" itself and ask the vital question: Do we really "age"?

According to modern medicine, we do so categorically. Chronological markers specify each phase of living and lead toward a collectively determined final end, otherwise known as death. The fear of this ending on the part of physicians themselves often promotes a kind of subtle and even a not so subtle form of malpractice. And patients learn to respond accordingly.

Belle S., eighty-five years old, has realized that if she tells her actual *chronological* age to the various doctors she sees, they may not treat her with the same committed care they would treat her with if she told them she was fifteen years younger. And she, along with the majority of older people, thinks of herself as at least fifteen years younger than her chronological age. In fact, it has been found that most advertisements directed at the "elderly" don't reach that audience because its so-called members don't identify themselves as elderly. Belle may be telling a deeper truth: She may indeed be many years younger *biologically*.

It's easy to see why she takes the years off. Many of her doctors envision her living only another hour or so solely because of the number eighty-five. In fact, a recent survey of U.S. physicians found that one-third of the surveyed group thought that once the average American woman has reached age seventy-five, she has less than five years to live. But, according to U.S. government statistics, she will actually live another twelve years on average, to age 87.[10]

Our real age—our biological age—is rarely accounted for in Western culture or medicine. If we were to calculate age properly, in biological terms, we might figure how much stress each individual had absorbed over a lifetime and how resilient his or her particular bodymind tends to be. We could not simply factor in environmental stress, because a physiologically balanced woman living in New York City might have absorbed far less stress than her out-of-balance counterpart on Maui.

The aging process is as individual as personality itself. Some of us age quickly, others slowly. Just attend a class reunion to see the startling physiological discrepancies between people born in the same year and coming from similar backgrounds. Standard thinking about aging tends to ignore these very significant individual differences. Most of us recognize that all eighty-year-olds are not the same age physiologically. Some have the physiology of (some) fifty-year-olds, or younger. Of course, you have to have a strong, intact sense of who you are to transcend cultural expectations of what you should look and feel like "at your age." When *Ms.* magazine founder and author Gloria Steinem turned forty, she responded to the observation "You're forty? You don't look forty!" with her now classic remark, "This is what forty looks like."

Beyond physical appearance, your *psychological* age may be far more important in considering the so-called aging process than your chronological age. In separating the biology of aging from the psychology of aging, researchers conclude that "many of the presumed psychological deficits of old age would occur to people of any age who are deprived of loved ones, close friends, meaningful activity, and intellectual stimulation."[11]

Actually, the research applies only to a minority. The vision of a *large* population of older people who are depressed and lonely is a myth. As a group, older people are as happy as and no more lonely than younger people. To questions such as "Do you have close friends?" or "Have you seen a friend in the last day or so?" people in their seventies and eighties answer similarly to those in their twenties or thirties. Nor are most older people ill. A study of 700 men and women aged fifty-five to eighty conducted at Stanford University School of Medicine found that the participants believed themselves to be far healthier than their parents were at the same age and attributed the improvement to life-style differences such as exercise and diet. And they are right.

In general, says Yale University endocrinologist Adrian Ostfeld, "About 75 percent of men and women over sixty-five remain healthy. Illness is concentrated in the other 25 percent and their diseases are generally related to life-style." Americans now live to an average of seventy-five years, whereas less than 150 years ago, the average American died at forty-five. People over eighty-five now constitute the largest growing segment of the U.S. population. In addition, there are approximately 36,000 centenarians in the United States; if the present trend continues, there will be 266,000 by 2020.

Research also shows that where the cultural expectation of a long life is prevalent, individuals resonate with that group expectation and live longer; their minds hold a picture of long life and their bodies respond accordingly. They are literally slowing the aging process to conform to cultural expectations. And that change in expectation is beginning to occur in our culture, as our present vision of possibilities shifts.

According to Dr. Edward Masoro, a physiologist at the University of Texas Health and Science Center, "If dietary restriction has the same effects in humans as it has in rodents, then human life span can be extended by at least 30% which would give us an extra thirty to thirty-five years, but once we understand the mechanisms that control aging, we may find it possible to extend the lifespan considerably more. Perhaps by 100%, which would give us an extra 100 to 120 years." Dr. Thomas Johnson at the University of Colorado agrees: "I think we may well be able to lengthen human life far beyond anything we ever dreamed possible. Based on what has been achieved in animal studies, it is conceivable that we may achieve human life spans of twice the current norm."[12]

Endocrinologists are finding that human growth hormone—a secretion of the pituitary gland that normally enables the body to heal wounds and break down fats, bolsters the immune system, and helps to build bone, muscles, and internal organs—is able to reverse body composition changes that occur in ten or twenty years of aging. A recent report published in the *New England Journal of Medicine* indicated that the effects of a genetically engineered growth hormone on older men with particularly low amounts of human growth hormone reversed a number of the effects of aging, resulting specifically in an increase in muscle mass, a loss of body fat, and increased energy. As the wife of one participant observed: "He's been looking fitter and trimmer and he's got more spree in his step." The annual cost of these hormones is around $14,000.[13] Pretty expensive "spree." What we really need is "free spree"—spree we can make ourselves, in our own bodies. And that is what research scientists are beginning to explore—how we can best use the substances we produce on our own.

Take DHEA-S, for example. DHEA-S is an adrenal hormone similar to human growth hormone, which floods the body while we are young and has powerful beneficial effects on the human system. Typically, the DHEA-S level in the body decreases very predictably with advancing age from a peak at age twenty-five until about 30 percent of its maximum level at age fifty to less than 20 percent over age seventy. However, new research is demonstrating that increased DHEA-S levels can reverse a number of age-related illnesses.[14]

On the basis of hormone and gene studies, researchers such as Dr. Michael Jazwinski at the Louisiana State University Medical Center believe that "it is possible that some people alive now may still be alive 400 years from now." Dr. William Regelson, professor of medicine at the Medical College of Virginia, concludes that "the possibilities of lengthening life appear practically unlimited."[15]

In essence, none of us, no researcher or medical expert, knows exactly why the bodymind couldn't continue indefinitely. What is required is a systematic way to slow, halt, and eventually reverse the aging process altogether. In one way or another, we need to access the underlying eternity, to become fully connected to the self-referential, unified field inside, where no energy is lost and no decay occurs. If your daily functioning could continue without entropy, established in a virtually stress-free physiology, then "the end" will be more a choice than a surprise. This is the immortal vision of Maharishi Ayur-Veda.

## Maharishi Ayur-Veda and the Reversal of Aging

*If for one instant we could come to understand
our universe and could perceive ourselves as
one with it. . . . we would see that there is
absolute immortality.*

Buckminster Fuller

In accordance with the Ayur-Vedic tenets, the human life span is not determined by conventional concepts of "young or old," but by the ability to remain fully conscious from beginning to end. We know that since birth, our body has been under continuous assault by chaotic influences from outside, has resisted them, and has maintained its integrity by constant reference to the natural sequence in our DNA. Aging occurs when the disorderly influences from the environment start to prevail. To reverse aging, we must fully reawaken nature's orderly biological intelligence throughout the bodymind. Every prescribed Ayur-Vedic treatment is thus designed to re-enliven this intelligence within to restore natural orderliness.

Scientific studies are already beginning to demonstrate that several of the approaches of Maharishi Ayur-Veda have the potential to halt and even reverse the aging process. In chapter 12 we will look at some studies on the effects of Ayur-Vedic rasayanas (herbal compounds) and bodily treatments such as Panchakarma on various diseases. Here we will now explore some effects from the daily practice of Transcendental Meditation (TM), the stress reduction program of Maharishi Ayur-Veda, on aging.

In chapter 5, we discussed a Harvard University study in which Transcendental Meditation was found to prolong life in people who learned to meditate while in their seventies or eighties. These findings suggest that the continued daily practice of the TM technique produces physiological results that slow or reverse the aging process.

Other research corroborates this possibility. For example, a study published in the *International Journal of Neuroscience* showed that five years of practicing TM was associated with an average reduction in biological age of 12.5 years, in tests of both men and women with a mean age of fifty-three years.[16] The subjects were divided into three groups: nonmeditators, short-term TM meditators (under five years), and long-term TM meditators (over five years). While the nonmeditating controls tested 2.6 years younger than their chronological age, the short-term meditators tested five years younger than their chronological age, and the long-term meditators, twelve years younger.

Another recent study, conducted by psychologist David Orme-Johnson, demonstrated that the practice of Transcendental Meditation significantly reduced medical utilization and costs, especially among adults over forty where illness rates are normally greater. Five years of insurance claims data for approximately 2,000 practitioners of the TM and TM-Sidhi program (see chapter 12) were compared with a normative data base of approximately 600,000 clients of the same health insurance carrier. Inpatient days for the TM group were 50.2 percent fewer than the norm for children (0–19 years); 50.1 percent fewer for young adults (19–39); and 69.4 percent fewer for older adults (40+). Outpatient visits were 46.8 percent fewer than the norm for children (0–19 years); 54.7 percent fewer for young adults (19–39); and 73.7 percent fewer for older adults (40+). Overall, hospital admissions were lower for the TM group than for other groups of comparable age, gender, profession, and insurance terms for all of seventeen major medical treatment categories.[17] The admissions rates for childbirth were similar to the norm, indicating that TM practitioners did not avoid medical care when needed.

In a recent eight-year longitudinal study of the medical expenditures of a group of 612 Canadian men and women before and after learning TM, it was found that three years prior to TM, this group had the same average total medical expenses as the norm for Quebec. After TM, there was an accumulative total decline of approximately 42 percent in expenditures over the following five years; those whose use of medical services was the highest decreased their total five-year expenditures by 68 percent.[18]

A number of studies have looked at specific physiological and biochemical changes resulting from participation in the TM program. One such change is the decrease in the repair efficiency of DNA that is thought to accompany aging. Dr. Hari Sharma and his colleagues at the Ohio State University College of Medicine studied the self-repair mechanisms of DNA in vitro by injuring lymphocytes through exposure to radiation. It was found that after five hours, the healing process in the DNA of lymphocytes taken from subjects practicing Transcendental Meditation was 100 percent complete, whereas for a control group of nonmeditating individuals it was only 80 percent complete.

Perhaps the most exciting recent study suggests that "people who meditate regularly have levels of an age-related hormone comparable to nonmeditators five to ten years younger." The study was conducted by Dr. Jay Glaser at the Maharishi Ayur-Veda Health Center in Massachusetts, in conjunction with researchers at the City University of New York. They compared the levels of DHEA-S in

423 TM meditators twenty to eighty-one years old with DHEA-S levels in 1,252 nonmeditators of the same age, ruling out the effects of diet, obesity, and exercise. A precursor of estrogen, serotonin, melatonin, and other hormones that tend to decrease with age, DHEA-S has been found to strengthen the immune system and help the body resist cancer. In Glaser's study, it was found to be present in much higher amounts than usual in older practitioners of TM. This research demonstrates not only that premature aging can be reversed but that it can be reversed outside the laboratory, by our own body manufacturing the proper chemicals and hormones. Glaser concluded that meditators participate in life "with more calmness, more tolerance, less physiological reaction to stress. If they go through the day in a more effortless way, they take on less stress, and what is aging, but accumulative stress?"[19]

One significant aspect of the Glaser study was that the results were consistently and strikingly higher among the women than among the men. The men over 45 had 23 percent more DHEA-S than their counterparts while the women over 45 had 47 percent more. In a similar study, physiologist Ken Walton looked at DHEA-S and other steroid hormones affected by chronic stress in TM meditators and nonmeditators. Levels of all hormones were significantly higher in the TM group and were far higher among the meditating women.[20] Both of these studies indicate that the daily practice of TM makes a significant difference in hormone production, especially for women. These studies also provide interesting avenues for future research on women's health because high DHEA-S levels have been associated with a lowered incidence of breast cancer and osteoporosis.

The results also corroborate other research on the differences in aging between men and women. But they take us a step farther. They suggest that if TM is as effective as it appears to be in dissolving and eliminating the long-term effects of stress and subsequent debilitation, the ability to retard and reverse the premature aging process (through production of the requisite hormones) will be more apparent in women than in men.

It is conceivable that by protecting ourselves from damaging environmental influences through stress-reduction programs like TM and by embracing Ayur-Veda and strengthening our naturally strong immune systems and bodymind functions, "the immortal woman," carved not out of marble, but out of the inner field of consciousness, is a real possibility.

### *Ayur-Vedic Bodymind Prescriptions for Reversing Premature Aging*

1. You've heard it before, but you are indeed as young as you think you are. Try not to experience life only in terms of a linear progression of age because that's just one reality; immortality is another.

2. Partake of a purpose or many purposes in life that really interest and excite you, bringing your mind, body, and emotions into harmony.

3. Enjoy some stimulating mental activity every day.

4. Enjoy inner silence on a daily basis.

5. Pay equal attention to what you eat, how you eat, and how you feel afterward as you digest.

6. Exercise but don't overcondition. Brisk walking, swimming, or a self-referral aerobic workout along with daily yoga exercise are the best (see next chapter).

7. If you remember to favor your positive emotions over your negative ones whenever possible, you'll be producing the best bodymind chemicals available for long life.

8. Be responsible for your own behavior and let go of trying to change others.

9. Be ever alert to be of help to others.

And finally, give yourself pause. Way beyond menopause. Allow yourself the luxury of conceptualizing a very long life span. Ayur-Veda brings a whole new outlook to any concerns we may have regarding midlife. The truth is, if our aging processes are even slowed down, much less reversed, we won't reach middle age until we're eighty or twice that. And we will be saying, "But this is what a hundred and sixty looks like!"

In the next chapter you'll find a suggested Maharishi Ayur-Veda daily program along with other approaches to bring your doshas into balance even more deeply—to prepare your bodymind for a disease-free life in the direction of immortality.

# Chapter 12

⚘

# SIMPLICITY

## Maharishi Ayur-Veda as a Daily Life Program

*To a steady mind*
*established in the Self....*
*mastery over the laws of nature arises.*

*Complete transcending is the best*
*among the sources*
*of health and happiness.*

Charaka Samhita

Health is not merely the absence of disease. Nor is it the absence of the awareness of disease. Being truly healthy starts within consciousness and is expressed on many different levels of your mind and body. Because it is a complete medical system, Maharishi Ayur-Veda treats every level of life, not only our psychophysical functioning, as an aspect of consciousness expressing itself. It is a life science, embedded in a universal perspective. Its purpose is to help you sustain a comprehensive awareness of the totality of natural law in every thing you do, in every thought and feeling you have. How the universe operates in you is as essential as how you operate in the universe.

To accomplish such deep bodymind care, Maharishi Ayur-Veda offers treatment approaches which contain both subjective and objective procedures for the development of consciousness in psychology, physiology, behavior, and in relation to the environment. We have already described the behavioral approach, and the approaches through eating, sleeping, and exercise. In this chapter, we'll consider some other approaches to healing.

First let's explore the essential bodymind health program offered by Maharishi Ayur-Veda. Of all the things you can do to promote the development and flow of consciousness within your bodymind, nothing appears to be more effective than the Transcendental Meditation program. By recognizing and "treating" your connection to the deepest level of consciousness through a simple technique of transcending body, senses, mind, intellect, and heart, you can effortlessly restore the smriti value to your bodymind: the memory of wholeness, the memory of total health.

## What Is the Transcendental Meditation (TM) Technique?

The Transcendental Meditation technique was brought to the West nearly forty years ago by Maharishi Mahesh Yogi, who has long been considered a great master in the Vedic tradition. What Maharishi teaches are the dynamics of how to structure the growth of the full potential of consciousness within our physiologies, on the basis of three Vedic principles: (1) A silent field of pure, unbounded consciousness underlies all our thoughts, perceptions, and feelings; (2) the natural tendency of the mind is to seek the bliss and freedom of its own unbounded status; and (3) as soon as the mind begins to take that inward direction, it starts to experience greater happiness and is drawn effortlessly to its own source in transcendental pure consciousness.

Because the practice of TM is based on these natural principles, the technique does not require any concentration or control of the mind. Therefore, it is easy for anyone to learn. The TM technique is a simple, natural mental procedure practiced for fifteen to twenty minutes in the morning and evening. It is practiced sitting comfortably at home, but can be done even on an airplane or at your office. It does not involve manipulation or suggestion. It is a technique rather than a philosophy or religion, and therefore people of all religions, including members of the clergy, practice TM and enjoy the benefits in terms of their own beliefs and life-styles.

These benefits include clarity of mind and thinking, health and vitality, and the capacity to enjoy life to its fullest. Research has shown that the results of TM can be seen immediately and accumulate over time. More than five hundred scientific research studies and papers from two hundred institutions in twenty-seven countries have documented significant results for mind, body, behavior, and environment.

What happens when you practice TM? The technique allows the mind to settle down effortlessly to a state of awareness where it is most calm, collected, and yet fully expanded and fully awake. This state of pure consciousness is the most essential form of human awareness. Because this experience is natural —not an altered state of consciousness—it is comfortable and enjoyable. As the mind settles down, the body gains a unique and profound state of rest and relaxation, allowing us to throw off stress and fatigue that has built up over the years. Without this deep rest, we can only hope to minimize the effects of stress and try to organize our lives to cope with problems. The goal of TM is not just to manage stress, but to eliminate it.

Although meditation is often associated with becoming reclusive and withdrawn, with the practice of TM you actually end up participating more fully in the world around you, better able to stay relaxed, healthy, and happy even in the midst of the most intense, dynamic activity. This is because the state of restful alertness experienced during TM simultaneously produces more peacefulness and more wakefulness, greater relaxation and greater energy. This state of restful alertness, originating with the deepest experience of pure consciousness, is where real bodymind healing must begin, not with practices such as visualization and positive thinking, which take place on the surface, producing a less profound effect. To support our positive desires and healing thoughts, we need to enliven the deepest level of awareness, the "being" level of complete health, prior to dealing with the specifics of illness.

No Ayur-Vedic program is therefore more essential to our health than a daily TM routine. There is no better way to maintain a healthy, integrated, ama-free bodymind and to avert disease. It can offer us deep rest, a heightened state of mental alertness, and the natural experience of bliss—a significant combination for invincible health.

As practitioners in the health field, we believe, based on the medical evidence alone, that anyone in the world who can find a TM instructor would do well to do so. The research demonstrates benefits in a wide range of areas: decreased in- and out-patient health-care usage; improvements in stress-related disorders such as insomnia, bronchial asthma, chronic headaches, chronic back pain, anxiety, and depression; reduction of major cardiovascular risk factors (high blood pressure, high cholesterol, cigarette smoking, and obesity); improved resistance to stress; and younger biological age.[1]

The bibliography lists books that can give you a more complete and thorough understanding of the practice and benefits of TM. If you want to learn the technique, it takes a total of about eight hours over four consecutive days and is taught by qualified TM teachers worldwide at the TM Centers and Health Centers listed in Appendix B.

## Maharishi Ayur-Veda Bodymind Approaches

Once you have been a TM meditator for at least two months, you may be able to learn another technique for the development of consciousness, known as the TM-Sidhi program. Transcendental Meditation can give the experience of transcendental consciousness, the state of restful alertness, enlivening the total potential of natural law. The TM-Sidhi program cultures the ability to think and act from this level. The result is that thoughts become far more powerful and more in harmony with natural law, which can enable you to have greater success in activity and in attaining your goals and aspirations. People often comment that this advanced program greatly accelerates the benefits of TM—improving health, increasing happiness, and enhancing the ability to gain more support from the environment in fulfilling one's desires.

One aspect of the TM-Sidhi program is called "yogic flying." During the first stage of yogic flying, the body lifts up and moves forward in short hops. Subjectively one may experience exhilaration, lightness, and bliss. EEG studies show that during this practice, at the moment the body lifts up, coherence is maximum in brain activity. According to Maharishi, "The mind-body coordination displayed by yogic flying shows that consciousness and its expression—the physiology—are in perfect balance." (The TM-Sidhi program, like the TM program, is available through the TM Centers listed in Appendix B.)

Several other approaches currently offered through Maharishi Ayur-Veda also produce a state of healing by enlivening consciousness from deep within. Primordial Sound Therapy is a technique designed to awaken in us the impulses of the Veda, the primordial sounds of nature that are capable of restoring balance in every aspect of our functioning, in our bodymind and in our interaction with the environment. The Psychophysiological Technique is a practice whose purpose is to bring our awareness back in touch with the bliss quietly awaiting us in every cell of our body. It is specifically taught for the purpose of reintegrating mind and body on the quantum level of healing. Both techniques are made available through the Maharishi Ayur-Vedic Health Centers and TM centers listed in Appendix B.

## Participating in the Maharishi Ayur-Vedic Home Programs

Just as weeding a garden a little every day keeps the flowers growing unrestricted, so a little internal weeding daily helps to keep us well and balanced. No doctor—Ayur-Vedic or otherwise—can do more for you than you can do for yourself, because only you can desire to awaken the healer and thereby the healing inside. And that desire is certainly there for many of us: A recent *People* magazine poll found that if we Americans had "an extra hour" a day, over one-third of us would use it to improve our minds and bodies.

Maharishi Ayur-Veda offers an extremely efficient yet highly pleasurable daily routine that we can do in about an hour per day to improve our minds and bodies. However, these are simply guidelines, not rigid rules, and should feel completely natural, as though you had thought of them yourself. It is not *what* we do, it is *how* we do it. All the "things to do" are best done with joy and ease. Pitta types especially need to counter the impulse to try to adopt a perfect Ayur-Vedic routine all at once, and to bear in mind that no routine is perfect, nor is there any competition to get "better," even with ourselves, remembering that *in Ayur-Vedic terms, we are already well; we are simply reminding our bodies of that situation.*

The key is effortlessness. The most important principle is that our health is essentially self-referral. The experience of awareness curving back on itself and regaining the resource of its own inner dynamics, organizing power, and intelligence is what heals us. Some of these programs can substitute for what you may already be doing. Consider that the essence of each program also implies that we do something *less:* that we *leave out* anything not health-promoting for us.

Take watching television as an example. Televisions in the United States are on about eight hours a day on average, whether we are watching or not. A third of us say we watch TV to relax, but does it really relax us? Even apart from the content, from the high-intensity stress and continual fear-producing violence, TV watching itself is extremely Vata- and Pitta-aggravating resulting from the flickering light and same-spot focusing. (It's not too great for Kaphas-on-the-couch, either.) Women in particular have been found to use TV mostly as an escape, especially as we get older. Although young teenage women watch the least (about eighteen hours a week), women over fifty-five watch an average of forty hours a week, more than any other group.[2] So when you are worrying about how to find additional time for a daily prevention program, also think about what you can leave out of your day to make it a healthy one.

### Maharishi Ayur-Veda Daily Program or *Dinacharya* (dih-nuh-chuh-reyah)

- Arise during Vata time, if possible (before 6:00 A.M.).
- Evacuate your bladder and bowels.
- After brushing and flossing your teeth, gently scrape tongue. You can use a small butter knife or a tongue scraper.
- Rinse your mouth with sesame oil, if desired (see instructions below).
- Drink some warm water, with lemon if desired.
- Abhyanga (see below).
- Bath or shower.

- Surya namaskar (see chapter 4) and other yoga exercise.
- Transcendental Meditation and TM-Sidhi program.
- Exercise according to constitutional type and other individual recommendations, as outlined in chapter 4.
- Light breakfast, before or after exercise; very light if before.
- Work, study, or other activities of the day.
- Lunch. Try to make this your main meal of the day, as your digestive fires are at their peak around noon. Eat according to your constitutional type and any other individual recommendations, as outlined in chapter 4.
- Take a brief rest after lunch.
- Work, study, and/or other activities.
- Transcendental Meditation and TM-Sidhi program.
- Exercise now if more convenient than in the morning.
- Supper. Try to keep it on the light side. Eat according to constitutional type and any other individual recommendations.
- Pleasant, relaxing activity such as an evening walk.
- Early to bed, during Kapha time before 9:30 or 10:00 P.M. if possible.

## SPECIFIC INSTRUCTIONS FOR DAILY PROGRAM

### DAILY MORNING MOUTH RINSE

The Ayur-Vedic texts recommend a daily sesame oil mouth rinse to prevent tooth decay and strengthen the gums.

1. Use a small amount of warm cured sesame oil (see next section).
2. After brushing and flossing, wash mouth out with comfortably hot water.
3. Take about a third of a mouthful of warm oil and swish vigorously for about a minute. Spit the oil out.
4. Rinse your mouth out with hot water.
5. Using a little more warm oil, swish it around again for about thirty seconds.
6. Rinse again with hot water.

### DAILY OIL MASSAGE (ABHYANGA)

The purpose of the daily oil massage is to assist in preventing the accumulation of physiological imbalances and to lubricate and promote flexibility of the muscles, tissues, and joints. The classical texts of Ayur-Veda also indicate that daily massage promotes softness and luster of the skin, as well as general youthfulness. Follow these simple instructions.

*1) Curing the Oil.* Unless a specific oil has been recommended for you, sesame oil should be used for the daily massage. If you find sesame oil unsuitable in some way, you may also try coconut or olive oil. To purify the oil, "cure" it by heating it to about 212° Fahrenheit, the boiling point of water. Adding a drop of water to the oil will tell you, when it boils away, that the proper temperature has been reached.

Please be aware that sesame and other oils are flammable; for this reason, they should be cured as follows:

- Always heat oil on low heat, never on high heat.
- Oil should never be heated unattended.
- Once oil reaches the proper temperature, it should be removed from the heat and stored in a safe place to cool gradually.
- When it is entirely cool, pour it into a quart or liter bottle.
- We suggest curing one quart or liter of oil at a time. This will suffice for about fifteen massages.
- Before each massage, reheat a small portion of the oil for a few seconds, in a pan on the stove or in a small plastic bottle under the hot-water tap.

*2) Preparation.* You might want to do your oil massage somewhere where the oil won't make a mess, like the bathroom. The oil should be heated and nearby. You should be completely free of all clothing and wearing no jewelry. Seat yourself on an old towel, which you will be designating for this purpose. (Be careful when drying an oily towel, even if washed, in an automatic dryer. Keep the temperature low or, better yet, dry it on a line or over the tub.)

*3) Head, Face, and Neck Massage.* Start by massaging your head. Place a small amount of oil on your palms and begin to massage the scalp vigorously. The entire massage should be done with the open part of the hands rather than with the fingertips. In the interest of time, you can just do your face and not your head, if you don't have time to wash your hair. But if you do have time, spend proportionately more time on the head area than on other parts of your body.

Next, apply oil gently with the open part of the hands to your face and outer part of your ears. You don't need to massage these areas vigorously. Massage the front and back of the neck and the upper part of the spine. Continue to use your open hands in a rubbing type of motion.

*4) Body Massage.* You may want now to apply a small amount of oil to your entire body and then proceed with the massage to each area. Massage your arms. The proper motion is back and forth in the direction of the length of the bones, and circularly over your joints. Massage both arms, including hands and fingers. Next do the chest, breasts, and abdomen. Use a straight up-and-down motion over your chest or sternum area; use a gentle circular motion over the breasts and also over your abdomen, following the bowel pattern from the right lowerpart of the abdomen, moving clockwise toward the left lower part. Massage your back and spine as best you can. Then massage your legs. Again use a back-and-forth motion in the direction of the length of the bones and a circular motion over the joints.

*5) Massaging the Feet.* Lastly, massage your feet. They are considered especially important, and, as with the head, proportionately more time should be spent here than on other parts of the body. Use the open part of your hands and massage vigorously back and forth over the soles of the feet.

When you are done, leave the oil on as long as you can, but wipe off excess oil before you bathe or shower, so as not to clog your tub drain.

Ideally, allow about ten or fifteen minutes each morning for the massage. If this time is not available on a particular day or even on a regular basis, it's better to do a very brief massage (two minutes or so) than to skip it altogether. According to all reports, once you have added this massage program to your daily life, the benefits will be so satisfying that you will quite naturally want to continue.

## Maharishi Sthapatya-Veda: Architecture in Accord with Natural Law

Our individual health is not really an isolated event. Maharishi Ayur-Veda considers the environment to be one single unified field that includes the innermost aspects of who we are—our consciousness, feelings, perceptions, thoughts, and bodies—and extends to the full range of all our surroundings. It thus seeks to awaken and harmonize the natural connection between the body, mind, and emotions and what we call the outer environment. Whether what we take in from the environment—food, air, sounds, color, perceptions, beauty, friendship, love—will be ama- or ojas-producing depends on what we are exposed to and how we interpret and absorb it.

*Sthapatya-Veda* (stuh-paht-yuh-vay-duh), like Ayur-Veda, is one of the disciplines of Maharishi's Vedic science. It is the science and art of Vedic architecture, a sophisticated and rich system in itself, and we mention it only briefly to offer you a taste of the wisdom it provides for creating a truly healthy environment, an environment that creates an influence of rest and balance. In this way, it helps fulfill the goals of Maharishi Ayur-Veda.

It is a very practical science that offers universal rules of design. One of its principles is that each room in a Sthapatya-Veda home maintains its own laws of nature; each room separately and in harmony with the others incorporates the influences of nature, creating an environment conducive to greater creativity, success, well-being, and health on all levels.

Another important principle of Sthapatya-Veda is that the quality of energy produced by the sun is different at different times of the day. Each quality of energy is most supportive of a particular kind of activity. So if the rooms in a home are oriented to the positions of the sun throughout the day, the energy produced by the sun will promote the success of the activities we perform in each room. For example, the dining room can be positioned so that appetite and digestion function most effectively at mealtimes; the bedroom can be located in the best place for a natural restful influence, and so forth.

Research shows that indoor pollution from artificial building materials and chemically treated products can be twenty times higher than outdoor pollution levels, even in such cities as New York and Los Angeles. This indoor pollution can cause a whole variety of discomforts and diseases, collectively known as the "sick building syndrome." Maharishi Sthapatya-Veda, favoring natural building materials, utilizes the principles of energy-efficient construction to provide protection from temperature changes without undue reliance on artificial heating or cooling. Circulation of fresh air in a home and ample green space in a city are considered essential to an ideal environment. Even more important than the use of natural building materials is the Vedic geometry and symmetry, which determines the right direction, the right proportions, and the best placement of buildings, rooms, gardens, lakes, etc. The constitutional types of the inhabitants are also carefully considered, so that the whole environment will help keep the doshas in balance. If we can live in a pollution-free and stress-free environment, in houses and cities built in accord with natural law, our health and happiness are nourished effortlessly throughout our daily lives.

Essentially, Sthapatya-Veda, like Ayur-Veda, is knowledge that takes the functioning of the parts and structures an integrated functioning of the whole. The whole and the parts—the individual and the universe—come into perfect alliance with each other.

## Maharishi Gandharva-Veda: The Music of Nature

Maharishi Gandharva-Veda is the classical music of the ancient Vedic civilization. It uses sound, melody, and rhythm to neutralize stress in the atmosphere and create a harmonizing and balancing influence. Gandharva-Veda was cognized thousands of years ago by sages who created instrumental and vocal sounds that matched perfectly with nature's own vibratory cycles. These ancient Vedic musicians understood the natural sound frequencies so precisely that they were able to create musical compositions to mirror the changing natural rhythms that prevail during the different times of the day and during the different seasons of the year. At the dawn of a new day, we'll notice that there is a special quality of freshness in the atmosphere; at noon there is a different quality, and in the evening yet another. By playing the appropriate music for each cycle of time, the physiology of the individual listener and the whole environment can gain further attunement with the laws of nature.

People report that when they play Gandharva-Veda music in their homes, the atmosphere feels more peaceful and relationships more harmonious and that Gandharva-Veda music quickly settles the mind if one is agitated or worried. Here is another useful tool we can incorporate into our daily routine to enhance our health and happiness. (For information on Maharishi Sthapatya-Veda and Maharishi Ghandarva-Veda music, please see the Appendix.)

## The Ayur-Vedic Physician and Pulse Diagnosis

We want you to be able to use this book for both knowledge and experience, and we have included as many Maharishi Ayur-Vedic home care programs as are currently available for you to do on your own.

However, you could have specific health questions or want an individualized prevention program that necessitates a consultation with an Ayur-Vedic physician. In one visit, you'll usually receive a pulse diagnosis and a personal eating, rest, and exercise program. The experience is quite different from a conventional medical assessment. It has been said that a great choreographer "can look at the way your body moves and find the medium, in dance, within which to move it." Similarly, the Ayur-Vedic physician can read your bodymind and find the healing medium within which to enliven and further balance it, identifying which bodymind approaches will work best for you, using a variety of diagnostic observations and tools. The most important one is pulse diagnosis.

Author Anatole Broyard wrote, "My ideal doctor . . . I can imagine . . . *entering* my condition . . . trying to see how he could make the premises more livable for me. He would see the genius of my illness. He would mingle his daemon with mine; we would wrestle with my fate together."[3] There are hundreds of medical tests that you could take to determine how sick or well you are at any given moment in your life. It might take months just to go through them, but by then your symptoms will probably have changed. Now imagine a physician who could perform a comprehensive diagnostic technique in a few moments and simultaneously compare your psychophysiology with that of thousands of others, a physician who could also prescribe specific daily routines for you and help reset your healing response precisely in tune with nature's program.

Such a physician is vaidya Dr. B. D. Triguna, who is the former president of the All-India Ayur-Vedic Congress and a renowned pulse diagnostician, considered among the most skilled and respected Ayur-Vedic physicians in the world.

> *While attending a conference in Washington, D.C., Dr. Triguna consulted with local physicians regarding the Maharishi Ayur-Vedic approach to care of their patients while examining patients. Without hearing any history or performing any physical examination, Dr. Triguna would gently grasp each patient's wrist for a few seconds and then describe the patient's health problems in minute detail—an impossible feat by any modern medical standards.*
>
> *One patient, himself a radiologist, entered the room and sat next to Dr. Triguna, who felt the radial pulse on his right arm. "Some blockage in the urinary system, on the right side," Dr. Triguna said, and then proceeded to draw a diagram of precisely where the blockage was occurring, approximately one-third of the way down the right ureter. The radiologist was stunned. Only through elaborate studies involving dyes and X rays would such a diagnosis be possible in modern medicine. He listened intently as Dr. Triguna explained its cause—"Too much heavy food, too much worry, irregular habits"—and nodded his head in agreement. He felt deeply known; he could easily make the changes Dr. Triguna suggested because they were familiar to him; he already knew what he was doing wrong in terms of eating and other daily behaviors.*

Dr. Triguna and other Ayur-Vedic physicians use pulse diagnosis routinely to feel imbalances in the physiology. But unlike a modern medical doctor or nurse taking a pulse reading, they are examining far more than heart rates. The pulse is taken at the junction point between consciousness and matter, where a thought becomes a neurotransmitter, a biochemical, or a hormone. At that deep level we can think of the pulse as an "im-pulse" of awareness. Because a pulse diagnosis may give results quite different from what the surface symptoms indicate, Ayur-Veda does not rely on expressed symptoms to determine cause.

An Ayur-Vedic doctor can identify several pulses, each related to the doshas. The Vata pulse, the "snake" pulse, is tested under the first finger and is associated with lightness; the Pitta pulse, the "frog" pulse, under the second finger, is jumpy; the Kapha pulse, the "swan" pulse, is heavier and more graceful. An experienced vaidya can discover within the pulse any disturbances in the doshas and any blocks preventing flow in the bodymind. He or she can also diagnose via the subdoshas within each dosha and evaluate the functioning of the seven dhatus. By analyzing the distribution and quality of all the impulses in the pulse, the Ayur-Vedic doctor is able to pinpoint precise imbalances.

During an Ayur-Vedic consultation, you are not kept in the dark about the diagnosis[4] and are never made to feel less a part of the treatment than the doctor. There is always respect for the underlying principle, that the healer inside *you* heals. In fact, you can be taught self–pulse assessment. (See Maharishi Ayur-Ved Health Centers listed in the Appendix.) Once you learn to read your own pulse, you can pay daily attention to changing health signals, a significant step in promoting self-sufficiency in personal health care.

You can feel the changes in the doshas in your pulse. At lunchtime you might notice a stronger Pitta pulse; at bedtime Kapha will be stronger. If you have a job interview, you may find the strength in the rapid Vata pulse. But more relevant than a specific diagnosis, self–pulse taking enables you to assess your immediate condition and simultaneously bring your awareness to any imbalance in your bodymind to start the healing process.

An Ayur-Vedic physician will make a diagnosis and, usually, recommendations for treatment. There is no wait between the two. Many Ayur-Vedic treatments have been described here, but there are a few that only an Ayur-Vedic physician can recommend, because patient situations and needs are so individual. He or she will also be alert to your willingness to carry out specific treatment programs, so you can discuss your treatment preferences openly.

One of the primary recommendations may be for specific herbs or rasayanas (mixtures of medicinal herbs).

## Ayur-Vedic Rasayanas and Herbs

*The persons using rasayana treatment in early ages lived for thousands of years unaffected by old age, debility, illness and death.*

Charaka Samhita

As Western doctors rely on their prescription pads to dispense cures through allopathic drugs, the Ayur-Vedic physician relies on his or her knowledge of plants and herbs to help balance the doshas. For an Ayur-Vedic physician, plants are the "holy healers." Ayur-Veda uses a large pharmacopeia of herbal (and mineral) preparations. Some of these are familiar to us: aloe vera for Pitta disorders, chamomile for Vata disturbance, ginger for Kapha imbalance. Many common spices such as saffron and turmeric do far more for us than simply flavor food. But most of the Ayur-Vedic herbs and rasayanas are less known in the West (although they are turning out to be of great interest to a number of researchers in the medical field).

Some of these are the plants, herbs, and minerals on which Western medicine has based its synthesized drugs. Because it is not possible to patent naturally-occurring plants or unprocessed plant extracts, the economics of the situation cause drug companies to spend their money on laboratory-created new extracts and not on making nonsynthesized natural products available. Examples abound of the medicinal use of naturally-occurring chemical compounds long before modern medicine discovered their use: Ayur-Vedic physicians were using herbs containing reserpine-like compounds to lower blood pressure, cardiac glycosides similar to digitalis to regulate heart arrhythmias, and fungal preparations similar to pencillin as antibiotics.[5]

These Ayur-Vedic natural substances have a number of advantages over allopathic drugs. Their approach is one of building and nourishing the system without debilitating side effects. One reason that side effects are so common with Western drugs is due to the "active ingredient" synthesis. Plants, like people, must maintain an overall homeostasis. The biochemical processes involved are similar, and in order to grow, the plant has to be balanced within itself. The apparently "inactive" ingredients are part of the plant's homeostatic mechanisms. Because the same laws of nature prevail in the plant world as in ours, these inactive substances in the plant actually help balance a human body's response to the active ingredient. Many modern drugs were developed by isolating a single active ingredient from an effective medicinal herb, but when we isolate the main substance from a medicinal herb, we interfere with the design that nature has perfected.

As ethnic medicine specialist Michael Weiner says, "Nature seems to be meant to be taken whole." When separated from its natural biochemical environment, the isolated active ingredient can produce serious side effects because the single ingredient disrupts the body's normal balance. As a result, many of the most common medications we take, such as cold relievers, often "merely trade one set of symptoms for another."[6] An article in *The Economist* reminds us that of the 5 billion people in the world, 4 billion depend to a certain degree on what are known as traditional remedies. Today, "the other billion are on the way to following them."[7] It seems that the ancient science of Ayur-Veda, because of the depth of knowledge it provides in so many other aspects of medicine, may offer us very safe and powerful herbal remedies that we ought not to ignore.

How do the rasayanas work? We know that most pharmaceuticals act through receptors in our cell walls, like keys fitting into locks. We know also that our receptors may respond better to natural plants than to active synthetic ingredients because the plant substances "fit" better, because the natural laws inherent in the plants correspond to and precisely correct the imbalances in our physiology. We can think of the Maharishi Ayur-Veda rasayanas as similar to physiological tuning forks resonating with particular parts of our body, helping each part to heal by resetting the orderly intelligence of natural law in that area and, at the same time, increasing overall balance in our bodymind.

On the surface, the rasayanas are not mysterious; they are nothing other than herbal compounds and are not considered "medicine" in modern Western pharmacology terms. Yet they are precisely formulated. A single rasayana may contain fifty ingredients, each of which must be meticulously handled this way and no other. Fortunately, Dr. Balaraj Maharshi, the preeminent Ayur-Vedic herbalist, working with Maharishi Ayur-Veda, has been able to reformulate many of the lost rasayanas described in the ancient texts. Of these, the most highly regarded is known as Maharishi Amrit Kalash (MAK). It is now available worldwide as an herbal supplement, and researchers are beginning to discover what are apparently some very important MAK effects. Preliminary results suggest that it may significantly strengthen the immune system, as measured by T-cell activity. Some cells, called macrophages, destroy unwelcome invaders, such as viruses; T-cells direct the macrophages to their targets, thus providing a sort of biological strategic intelligence. In one laboratory study, T-cell activity increased by 100 to 160 percent, depending on the amount of MAK used.[8]

There are also some beginning laboratory studies on breast cancer and MAK. In a pilot study to test the effects of MAK on animals, Dr. Hari Sharma, professor of pathology at Ohio State University Medical School, found MAK to be effective in preventing the formation of tumors in 80 percent of the cases and caused tumors to regress in 60 percent of the cases, with complete dissolution in half of those. MAK was found to cause no side effects or toxicity. From the results of another study, which demonstrated that MAK prevented inappropriate platelet aggregation, Dr. Sharma concluded that MAK may inhibit abnormal blood clots of the kind associated with strokes and heart attacks.[9]

Other laboratory research, conducted at the Massachusetts Institute of Technology by Dr. Tony Nader, demonstrated that certain Maharishi Ayur-Veda rasayanas block the ill effects of carcinogens and a highly deficient diet.[10] A recent study conducted at the University of Toronto Medical School confirmed these early results by demonstrating that MAK has a beneficial effect both at the initiation phase, when malignant cells first appear, and an even more pronounced effect at the promotion phase, when cancer cells begin to replicate out of control.[11]

Only recently have researchers even begun to study the effects

**306**

of the rasayanas and other Maharishi Ayur-Vedic interventions on disease. A number of universities and scientific organizations, including the National Institutes of Health, are currently participating in a variety of medical research studies on Maharishi Ayur-Veda.[12] Within the next few years, results of this ongoing research will be available to us.

### Maharishi Ayur-Veda Health Center Programs

A most wonderful way to be introduced to Ayur-Veda, whether you are feeling sick or well, is by visiting a Maharishi Ayur-Ved Health Center. Once there, you can experience the Panchakarma Treatment Program and other programs, enveloped in the careful, loving attention of trained Maharishi Ayur-Veda physicians and technicians.

According to Ayur-Veda there are two main types of medical therapy, pacification and purification. Pacification therapy exposes the physiology to therapies that address specific imbalances. Purification removes substances from the body, impurities that may have been causing illness.

*Panchakarma* (puhn-chuh-kahr-muh) is the essential Ayur-Vedic purification therapy. It is a necessary treatment because disease does not develop overnight, but comes about as the result of imbalances and impurities that amass in the bodymind over many years. Panchakarma removes these impurities and helps to restore balance.[13]

In one preliminary study, two Panchakarma treatments in one year produced a 4.8-year reduction in biological age, as measured by the Morgan Adult Growth Examination.[14] Another preliminary three-month study was conducted in the Netherlands on 126 patients utilizing several Maharishi Ayur-Veda treatment programs— the TM program, the Panchakarma program, and individualized herbal rasayanas—for ten chronic diseases, including rheumatoid arthritis, bronchial asthma, eczema, chronic constipation, headaches, chronic sinusitis, hypertension, psoriasis, diabetes mellitus, and chronic bronchitis. The subjects were independently rated by a physician employed by a Dutch health insurance company. The average duration of illness before treatment was twenty years. Significant improvements were seen in 79 percent of the patients after three months, and no harmful side effects were noted.

An eight-year epidemiological study of 650 men and women who were practicing TM, doing daily asanas, undergoing regular Panchakarma treatments, and following the Ayur-Vedic dietary routines indicated that they had 85 percent fewer hospital inpatient days than the national norm, and 59 percent fewer outpatient medical visits. The greatest differences were for older subjects. It is noteworthy that another group within the study, doing just the daily TM program, had a similar number of outpatient visits (58 percent below the norm) but 50 percent more inpatient days (42 percent below the norm) than those subjects doing TM and the additional Ayur-Vedic routines.[15]

Panchakarma treatment is based on constitutional type and is a carefully monitored program that requires the professional attention of an Ayur-Vedic physician and several technicians. (Indeed, the amount of mind-body medical attention one receives during this treatment is unheard of by Western standards.)

The average Panchakarma treatment takes about a week—which often passes all too quickly. As one woman described her first Panchakarma experience, "I felt as though a light had been switched on inside a dark, cramped closet—my body. It felt as though my body were remembering its own wisdom. A sensation of pleasure, warmth, and relief spread throughout my body, and I felt what I finally understood as 'bliss.' And that blissful feeling was coming from within myself."

Here are some of the most basic treatment modalities you may experience during Panchakarma:

***Snehana*** (snay-huh-nuh) or *oleation.* You start by taking some ghee (clarified butter) for a few consecutive mornings to prepare your physiology for purification.

***Virechana*** (vih-ray-chuh-nuh), or *laxative.* You take a laxative such as castor oil to give a good cleaning to the physiology, following specific instructions so you won't notice any unpleasant taste.

***Abhyanga*** (ah-bhyun-guh, loosely pronounced, "I'll be younger!"), or oil massage. Two technicians (women, if you are a woman) give you a specialized massage, each focusing on one side of your body, working symmetrically. An herbalized oil complementary to the requirements of your doshas at the time is used. The purpose is to help you get rid of ama within any part of your body to help balance the doshas. The loving, silent attention of the technicians is as significant a part of the treatment as the oil massage itself.

***Shirodhara*** (shih-roe-dhah-rah). You will most likely experience this specialized treatment during which a heated herbalized oil is gently poured onto your forehead by an Ayur-Vedic technician over a period of time, creating a sensation of such pleasurable, profound, and deep relaxation that many people lose all track of time. Shirodhara works to balance Prana and Apana Vata, the subdoshas of Vata that govern the activity of your mind and brain, calming your entire body through the central nervous system. It has been shown to increase coherence in brain functioning.

***Pizichilli*** (piht-zah-chih-lee). In this most luxurious treatment, the Ayur-Vedic technicians pour warm herbalized oil over your body, creating a most settling, balancing experience for Vata dosha.

***Svedana*** (svay-duh-nuh), or steam treatment. Lying swathed in sheets (except for your head) on a raised wood bed covered by a clear dome, you are bathed in hot herbalized steam to open the circulation channels and rid your body of ama through the skin. A technician applies cool compresses to your face and head to keep them cool.

***Udvartana*** (oohd-vahr-tuh-nuh). A full body massage given by two technicians that balances Kapha and is especially good for weight reduction.

***Vishesh*** (vih-shaysh). A deep, vigorous massage, suited to Kapha types, and particularly good for athletes.

***Pindasweda*** (pihn-duh-sway-duh). Rice boiled in milk and special herbs, wrapped in cloth, is massaged over the body by the technicians. This treatment balances all the doshas, but because it is cooling, it is most effective in balancing Pitta.

***Basti*** (buh-stee), or oil enema. Small, gentle, herbalized lubrication and elimination oil enemas, for removal of accumulated impurities.

***Nasya*** (nuh-syuh), or nasal cleansing. A facial rejuvenation and nasal congestion treatment, including massage, moist heat, herbalized vapor, and inhaled herbalized drops.

Many of the Maharishi Ayur-Ved Health Centers offer one-week and longer residential treatment programs that are truly designed to "re-create" you from the DNA up. The centers also provide delicious dosha-balancing meals, courses on Ayur-Veda, and other aspects of Maharishi's Vedic Science. You follow a prescribed daily routine to allow you to sink into blissful silence. You can also learn TM while there. However, if you don't have the opportunity for a residential stay, you can also have a similar experience on an outpatient basis at any of the centers.

We've attempted to introduce you to a number of aspects of a very large body of knowledge. But you no doubt have a few questions, and you can call or write us for some answers. You can also take a look at the questions and answers in Appendix A to see if one of your questions is at least partially answered there.

Our not-so-secret hope is that, as you go about your daily life, you will find yourself connecting to this inner resource of healing through all or any of the approaches to health offered through Maharishi Ayur-Veda. We hope you will immediately start experiencing the joyful "Aha" of recognizing what it feels like to be truly in good health, and that when you do, you'll start to feel even better. Wave after wave of awareness of the renewal of your healthiness will awaken deep joy in your heart and mind. And you will start to represent fully the health and healing that we as women can and must offer our world.

# Chapter 13

❀

# CONNECTION

## Maharishi Ayur-Veda, Women, and the World

*When we investigate the invisible mechanics of
nature, we find that everything in the
universe is directly connected with everything
else. Everything is constantly being
influenced by everything else. No wave of the
ocean is independent of any other.*[1]

Maharishi Mahesh Yogi

Vasudhaiv Kutumbakam.
*The world is my family.*

Maha Upanishad

According to the United Nations World Health Organization, health is "a state of complete physical, mental and social well-being and not merely the absence of disease or infirmity." We would go further and say that it's not really possible to separate our individual health from that of the society around us or of the environment or of the planet. Like many women in today's world, we feel this interdependence as a dual societal responsibility:

1. To be advocates for humanity—and to support those thoughts and actions which contribute individually and collectively to healing ourselves and others.

2. To be advocates for nature, to take steps to protect and heal the environment.

Maharishi Ayur-Veda offers women a deeply personal foundation for bringing health to the world, a platform for reciprocal healing. It supports the desire and ability to care for family, for friends, for the community, and for the world, by extending the inner ability to self-nurture to others. As one Indian woman saint counseled a disciple, "Learn to make the whole world your own; no one is a stranger, my child, the whole world is your own."

This unbounded vision of health to include the whole world is perhaps the ultimate secret of structuring the most dynamic health-care system of all: My good health is enhanced and maintained by yours (or diminished if either one of us is ill or unhappy). This sense of global healing is the most profound aspect of the real meaning of personal health.

"We must be fearlessly willing to manifest in our lives and healing arts what women have always known—the unity of being," writes author Jeanne Achterberg. But for this to happen, and for us to take on each of these great responsibilities, we need to put our own house in order.

To be effective agents of transformation, either quiet or active, we need to be in good health. To become more powerful healers, we first have to be healed. In order to make "the whole world our own" without causing strain, fragmentation, or illness, we must first be fully connected to the home of healing, to the fundamental laws of nature, which can guide and strengthen us. In order to produce a harmonizing influence, it is necessary for our bodymind to be established in the unified field of consciousness, so that we exude our own powerful atmosphere of harmony, happiness, and peace.

Sociologists and anthropologists have observed that the status of women is an index of the healthy development of society. When society is balanced, women are never second-class citizens who need to band together to seek respect and protection. When its women are healthy, then the society can truly be called healthy.

By providing us with the essential tools for self-sufficiency, Ayur-Veda enables us to learn to heal the way our minds, bodies, and hearts wisely want to heal, to become fully healthy women. It offers all of us the practical and specific knowledge to accept and even cherish the responsibility for our own health and the health of our friends, families, communities, and the world.

## Is There a Doctor in Your House?
## The Tradition of Woman as Healer

*Women are medicine.*

CheQweesh Auh-ho-oh
(Native American, Chumash tribe)

Women have always been healers, consistently serving as family and community care-givers. Where doctors have been a last and not a first resort, the "healing arts" have been considered the natural province of women, who have tended the sick, assisted at the births, prescribed the well-tested medicinal remedies. We have also been the mind and heart doctors, soothing the frayed nerves, mending the broken hearts, harmonizing the conflicts to avert the onset of further illness.

This healing tradition is still very much alive. What we are observing today is a growing trend toward women's *recognizing* their role as healers. If women are to continue to be the primary caretakers of children, parents, and friends, as well as of those lacking their own familial or social supports, societal acknowledgment and respect for that healing role is needed.

The tradition of women as healers is carried forward from the ancient cultures: from the goddess Isis tradition in ancient Egypt, from the Eleusinian mysteries of ancient Greece; from women healers persecuted for their knowledge in the Middle Ages and in seventeenth- and eighteenth-century North America, from the American Indian traditions such as White Buffalo Woman and Corn Woman, and from the development of midwifery and nursing as women's professions in the nineteenth century. Within these traditions, women have passed on the secrets of various practices through long chains of often undocumented oral lessons. The dispensers of this knowledge have been named everything from "old wives" to fortune-tellers, to omniscient grandmothers "from the old country" to shamans, to wise women.

**313**

The women's healing tradition continues today: Ecuadorean Indian women, "balm" practitioners in Jamaica, Puerto Rican *espiritistas,* Korean *mansins,* Hawaiian women healing in the Kahuna tradition, and other women the world over also maintain this "specialty," whether informally or formally.[2] In India, for example, women are often considered the family physicians. The tradition of woman as healer has also moved into the modern medical profession. After decades of being kept outside the physician kingdom, the percentage of American women doctors is rising rapidly and is estimated that it will reach nearly 50 percent by the year 2000. Already in Russia today, 90 percent of the doctors are women. Women in many nations see only women doctors for obstetrical and gynecological care, a trend which is also increasing in America.

It appears that women are indeed perceived as good medicine. There is evidence that in the United States, at least, women doctors are now generally preferred over male doctors by both men and women, in part because they are felt to be more concerned with their patients as individuals, not simply as embodiments of disease. Researcher Candace West found that perhaps because women physicians "suggest" whereas many male physicians tend to "command," patients of both genders follow health instructions from female physicians more readily than from their male counterparts.[3]

Similarly, American nursing professionals, the large majority of whom are women, are considered by patients to be the most vital source of care-giving in hospitals and other medical settings. Among medical professionals, nurses have perhaps best understood the multidimensional role of healer. The nursing profession was the first medical group to research the benefits of the holistic traditions and to incorporate holistic practices into their profession. Schools of nursing were also the first to teach the benefits of therapeutic massage and the healing value of love and attention as a part of medical training.

Moreover, the influence of woman-based health care is widening beyond the conventionally defined roles of doctors and nurses. The home-care movement, the number of hospices for severely ill patients, and the number of supportive AIDS clinics are all growing. All of these new institutions are primarily staffed by women. What has been increasingly recognized is that the basic requirement for a health practitioner—whether a doctor, a mother, or a dedicated friend—is the ability to bring healing attention to the bodymind awareness of the patient. What the health practitioner can do for the patient (or the healer-patient can do for herself) is to directly enliven the healing process through the power of focused care. By adding the attention of a nurturing, health-giving individual to the patient's self-healing process, the chances for a quick and complete recovery are greatly increased.

## Women in the Field of PNI

Woman as healer has also found an integrating and significant role in medical research today. It is of interest that, despite the dearth of women in medical research, the field of bodymind research, psychoneuroimmunology (PNI), has drawn a significant concentration of women, many at the top of the field.

For example, it was neuroscientist Karen Bulloch, now at the University of California at San Diego, who in the late 1970s first established the physiological connections between the brain and the immune system. Psychologist Janice Kiecolt-Glaser has been conducting important research at Ohio State College of Medicine on immune function and stress, especially on the long-term effects of stress on care-givers for Alzheimer's disease patients. Dr. Lydia Temoshok, while at the University of California at San Francisco, researched the link between immune system functioning and personality, particularly in AIDS patients; Dr. Carrie Millon and her colleagues at the University of Miami School of Medicine are studying the effects of psychological hardiness on physical hardiness in terms of bolstering the immune systems of individuals who have been exposed to the AIDS virus but have not shown symptoms. And finally, there is Dr. Candace Pert, former chief of brain biochemistry at the National Institute of Mental Health, the mother of the bodymind concept, whose research, now focused primarily on AIDS, continues to represent the cutting edge of the field.

Given what we know about women's harmonizing and abstracting characteristics, it is not surprising that women are drawn to and all highly creative within the field of PNI, which requires synthesis, the integration of body, mind, and heart, and a willingness to investigate the more abstract, nonlinear events. These PNI discoveries essentially reflect work which integrates formerly disparate fields through deeper connection. They are very much a part of the history of the discovery processes of women in particular, a process Virginia Woolf recognized in describing the work of a contemporary writer, Dorothy Richardson:

> *Her discoveries are concerned with states of being and not with states of doing. [She] is aware of "life itself," of the atmosphere of the table, rather than of the table; of the silence rather than of the sound.*[4]

## Women as World Healers: The Missing Peace of Healing

In light of the traditions that bring women into the domain of a healing role, with its attendant responsibilities and powers, it is understandable why women are actively involved as societal healers and as "healers of the world." Both consciously and instinctively—and these are not separate—women have understood that world peace is not really different from their own health or from the health of their families. According to Helen Caldicott, M.D., founder of the organization Physicians for Social Responsibility, it is women who innately understand the genesis of life. She reminds us that it is our responsibility now. This responsibility is recognized as part of a broader female quest for interconnection. Sociolinguist Deborah Tannen has written: "[I am] approaching the world as many women do; as an individual in a network of connections. Life, then, is a community, a struggle to preserve intimacy and avoid isolation."[5]

The desire for intimacy and connection lends itself to the development of a kind of emotional sensibility, a recognition of "where it hurts" and how to fix it. It is very likely that a natural ability to heal others has been cultured in the physiological responses of women. It is also apparent that many so-called "feminine" characteristics such as intuition, receptivity, surrender, harmony, and intimacy—whether enlivened in men or in women—balance the so-called masculine characteristics of rationality, focus, and specialization. Both are microcosms of nature's functioning and both need to be integrated in society, as well as in each of us. These female-principle qualities have not been fully valued or supported in our society, by men or by women. But that situation has been changing.

Harvard psychologist David McClelland's research on the psychology of war indicates that women or men who are most "warlike" have a high need for power and low empathy. We may suppose that a "peace personality" would have a low need for power and high empathy. If the deeper, more harmonizing laws of nature are ultimately to prevail, as well they must, kindness, love, nurturance, and cooperation are always going to outlast more superficial power tactics. As Lincoln observed, "Do I not destroy my enemies when I make them my friends?" Love and kindness disarm opposition by dissolving the boundaries between people and creating a true healing environment. As the research has been demonstrating, the real prevention of illness requires consistent ways to promote these healing values of the heart in both women and men.

A study at Stanford Research Institute (SRI) identified male and female styles of leadership. "Male" style, called "alpha," is characterized by a direct, linear, one-task-at-a-time, win-or-lose orientation. "Female" style, called "beta," is recognized as fluid, synthesizing, intuitive, contextual, and relational. The SRI researchers believe that a balance between these two styles is essential for good leadership. In a time of great change, however, female style may be more useful: The research indicated that beta thinking gets the job done more effectively, with its emphasis on group function, wholeness, interdynamics, and collective subtleties.[6]

According to the researchers, it is important to realize that these styles are not unique to each sex but have been polarized by role expectations, making beta-style behavior more prominent in women. For example, women who have entered the male power bastions, when observed in the competitive environment of corporate life, have been found to act as the harmonizers, the empowerers, and the nurturers. Some women lacking self-esteem may overdo this role. But it is women, especially those identified as "high in self-esteem," who are most often found to be the agents for improving health environments, whether advocating healthier air, better quality of life, or better working conditions at the office, in the community, or in the global environment.

Health and healing are not static, for the bodymind is ever changing, and changing within a group dynamic as well. Our good health is based on an interactive "flow" of health from the individual to the group and back again; from the individual to the group to the environment and back; from the individual to the universe and back. Maintaining the unrestricted flow of healthiness within this interdynamic harmony is the responsibility of every one of us.

Power, of course, is a necessary means to transformation. But real power comes most easily and most surely from getting nature on your side, on the inside, serving as the ultimate resource. Trying to operate from limits is the old, linear way of achieving influence; the "quantum" way requires going deeply, accessing wholeness, expanding, and forming new connections inside and out. This necessitates the ability to contact nature within and thus enliven the deepest power base in both individual and group consciousness.

## An Experiment in World Peace Through Collective Consciousness: The Maharishi Effect

Maharishi Ayur-Veda supports total health based on the development of consciousness, strengthening always from within. From this foundation of personal invincible health, any of us can make a worthy contribution to the creation of a stress-free, anger-free, disease-free, peaceful world. But it may be that we can do so collectively even more effectively.

We explored earlier how particles, in the quantum world, are seen as waves in the quantum field. Their existence has a localized aspect—the particle—as well as a universal aspect—the underlying field. In a parallel fashion, individuals can be likened to waves on an ocean. Each individual is the localized unique individuality of a wave and each is also the unbounded universal reality of the ocean. According to this model, individuals not only interact behaviorally but also *at a distance* via the underlying field or ocean, which is the common basis of everyone's existence. This same situation can be created in "collective" consciousness, another kind of internal milieu, whereby a small group could influence an entire population.

As early as 1960, Maharishi prescribed treating society *at its ba-*

*sis* in order to create a natural order and harmony in all the components of society and their interactions. He predicted that when one percent of the population practices the Transcendental Meditation technique individually, then an improved quality of life would be found in the entire society. This effect, known as the Maharishi Effect, has now been confirmed by a substantial body of scientific research. At least ten large-scale studies, carefully controlled for all demographic influences known to affect crime, have demonstrated that when one percent of a population practices TM, the crime rate in that city or country drops markedly, as do the suicide and accident rates. One study found a significant overall drop in crime rate in a sample of forty-eight American cities and reported results in the *Journal of Crime and Justice.*[7] In the mid-1970s, it was discovered that an even smaller number, the square root of one percent of a given population collectively practicing the TM-Sidhi program, is sufficient to produce a measurable and holistic influence of harmony and integration in the entire population. This would mean that a group of just slightly over 7,000 people would be enough to create an influence of peace for the whole world population.

To understand how such a small group could influence an entire population, we can look at analogous phenomena in physical systems. In quantum physics, there is a phenomenon known as "constructive interference." It suggests that in any given system, if a certain number of entities—the square root of the number of the elements in the system—are "coherent," the rest of the system will become coherent as well. We can look at this effect in terms of ordinary light versus laser light. The photons of ordinary light are random and disorderly, milling about with no particular pattern, whereas in laser light, the photons have all lined up synchronously, thereby emitting a beam of light so powerful it can cut through steel. It is the same light as your living room lamp, using the same energy, but *organized coherently.* Ordinary light is transformed into laser light through the coherent emission of a number of photons proportional to the square root of the total, causing the entire system to undergo a phase transition in which all the photons begin to interact coherently. This same kind of coherence effect can apply to other living systems.

The Maharishi Effect is a sociological application of this coherence effect, based on the coherence in the psychophysiological functioning of the TM and TM-Sidhi practitioners. The theory predicts that the coherent influence generated by the square root of one percent of the population experiencing the inner field of pure awareness will create coherence in world consciousness. (See Appendix B for research studies on this phenomenon.) To this end, a long-term global experiment is being conducted to secure the peace of the world permanently. Groups practicing the TM-Sidhi program are being studied to see if they are producing nonlocal global healing effects such as reduction in crime rate, violence, sickness, and wars, especially in areas where such negative experiences are most heavily concentrated. There have been over forty separate studies on this collective approach to reducing crime and hostilities which have indicated that when the square root of one percent of the population practice the TM-Sidhi program in a group, violence and crime decrease significantly throughout that population.[8]

The principle of the Maharishi Effect is prescribed in the Vedic texts as the mechanism for creating peace: "In the vicinity of coherence, hostile tendencies are eliminated." When this internal field of silence is accessed, we experience simultaneously our greatest resource for being healthy and our greatest resource for enlivening global health and global peace. The possibilities for a permanent world peace based on this coherence-creating phenomenon is very exciting news to modern researchers and theorists, as well as to government leaders, health professionals and peace researchers. With a focused, synchronous group consciousness large enough to fulfill the requirements for the Maharishi Effect on a global scale, world consciousness literally could be changed in a quantum moment.

## The Transformation of Medicine: Adding the Female Principle of Healing

*The new medicine doesn't turn its back on the old. It integrates that knowledge and then moves on, just like quantum physics integrates the laws of motion and of physics with the new*

*quantum mechanical law, bringing the whole
thing together in a new synthesis.*

Dr. Candace Pert

"To maintain a high level of fitness we must avoid physical decline, not repair it," writes author-physician Michael Crichton. All of us need guidelines on how to live daily life in a way that precludes decay and promotes a long and healthy life. But this knowledge must not be fragmentary or piecemeal. It must enable us to understand the connection between the universe and our health. You can't maintain the blessing of refined perception and accurate intuition when you are thoroughly worn out from a life in which you struggle to keep everything going at once. But when you recognize that you don't have to keep it together, that it *is* together *already,* life again becomes effortless, joyous, and healthy.

This nourishing wholeness is understood as the female principle, that which unites and heals mind, body, and heart, even when a part of the body is being treated for something as specific as a broken arm. It is this unified nurturance which has been missing from modern health care.

According to Dr. Vandana Shiva, a leading physicist and ecologist in India, the loss of the feminine principle in the high-tech world has resulted in the current ecological crisis: "It entails the disruption of nature's processes and cycles, and her interconnectedness."[9] Our health care too, as we've seen, has lost its connection to the female principle of nature. Modern medicine has been highly successful in combating "primary diseases" such as infectious ailments, but "secondary diseases"—those resulting from stress and degeneration, such as heart attacks and cancer—call for another approach, one we haven't been able to provide yet in mainstream medicine. The results are spiraling health-care costs, a loss of confidence in physicians, and doctors' frustration at their inability to do little more than treat symptoms. What biochemist Paul Ehrlich in 1910 called the "magic bullet" approach to medicine—a pill for every disease—although useful in some cases, is clearly outmoded as as entire medical system. Psychologist Deena Metzger has said that radiation and chemotherapy as medical treatments are the "natural responses from a society that thinks in terms of chemical warfare and nuclear power"; a belief system less oriented toward conquest might produce better cures.[10] Now, a global awareness of the need for female-principle medicine is growing.

We believe, along with a growing number of physicians, psychologists, and other health and mental health professionals, that Maharishi Ayur-Veda offers a sound and significant "next step" in health prevention and health care, exactly what we need to fulfill the new paradigm of medical care. And as women, we are physiologically ready and organized inside to access these deeper natural laws of harmony and love and to bring about this global healing which is already well in motion.

## A New Way of Healing Through Maharishi Ayur-Veda

By integrating all dimensions of healing, combining the subjective and the objective, Maharishi Ayur-Veda offers a comprehensive system of medicine for diagnosis, treatment, and prevention. It is the gift of "internal" medicine, based on the quantum model, which gives us access to a deeper set of natural laws from which healing can fully and effortlessly occur. For this reason, there is no theoretical model more egalitarian or more supportive of truly universal health care. But, more important, Maharishi Ayur-Veda provides us with a beautifully systematic way to understand and experience direct access to the healing field.

We feel women will appreciate and utilize a system of medicine that incorporates the ways in which women in particular think, behave, create, and ultimately heal. On the surface everything appears to be separate, but when we know the underlying reality, there are no differences, and everything is united. Maharishi Ayur-Veda offers the wholeness sought by women; it satisfies the longing for what writer Robin Morgan calls "the unified sensibility" and upholds "the insistence on the connections, the demand for synthesis, the refusal to be narrowed into desiring less than everything."[11] It is our responsibility as women and world citizens to contact and express this unity in our everyday lives, not to combat masculinity, but to complete it, so that every member of our world family can look around and say, "Yes, I am truly living in heaven."

Maharishi Ayur-Veda, with its emphasis on consciousness and self-referral health, is a complete medical system based on the wholeness of the male and female principles together. We see it as a deeply and fully intimate approach both to our personal health because it recognizes and relies on the inner field of healing, and as a means of global healing. "[It] is a simple way of living based on knowledge," says Dr. Brihaspati Dev Triguna. "Life should be pure, blissful, happy—not only our individual lives, but the life of the world. You have to have faith and good wishes for your nation—but not only for your nation, for the whole world."

We invite the women of the world to join us in bringing forth this beautiful resource, creating lifelong personal health and global healing in one simultaneous breath of interconnected purpose.

> *United be your purpose;*
> *Harmonious be your feelings,*
> *Collected be your mind,*
> *In the same way*
> *As all the various aspects of the universe exist*
> *In togetherness,*
> *Wholeness.*

Rig Veda

# APPENDIX A

## Answering Some Questions about Maharishi Ayur-Veda

*1. From the perspective of Ayur-Veda, what is the advice on going for regular medical tests such as the Pap smear?*

Since Ayur-Veda is first and foremost interested in prevention, it would support any tests, such as Pap smears or mammograms, that can give a patient accurate early diagnostic information. However, if you rely *only* on such "office" tests as a measure of your good health, and not on your intuition and feelings as well, you may be missing the most valuable diagnostic tool of all—your inner information system, since the tests only pick up the more well-established symptoms. So take the tests but also go by how you are feeling.

*2. Why is sesame oil used?*

Sesame oil is recommended by the ancient Ayur-Vedic physicians for many of the programs because it balances all three doshas. Recently, several researchers who were curious about the recommended use of sesame oil have discovered that sesame oil contains larger amounts than other oils of linoleate in triglyceride form. Linoleic acid is known for its antibacterial, antifungal, and anti-inflammatory properties, as well as its ability to halt the growth of cancer cells. (Drs. John Salerno and D. Edwards Smith are currently researching its usefulness in combating colon cancer, melanoma, and other forms of skin cancer, and gum disease, and have published preliminary results in *Anticancer Research*, volume 11, 1991.) For now, we know that it is a safe oil, good for all the treatment programs, and has prevention potential. Many mothers have also discovered that it soothes babies, especially those babies with Vata constitution.

*3. I find that even in my everyday life, I walk around with a great deal of fear. What does Ayur-Veda say to do about fear?*

Fear comes in two essential "flavors," one rational and the other irrational. Rational fear can be based entirely on intuition, and it's worth listening to. If you are in a potentially dangerous situation or environment, you can be supported and protected well by the heightened alertness brought about by even a subtle fear reaction. But irrational fear or free-floating anxiety can be life-damaging because it keeps the adrenaline pumping with no benefit to you. An imbalanced Vata dosha is usually the cause and can be addressed through the Vata-balancing programs. You may only need to change a few things in your daily life: For a start, consider eliminating Vata-aggravating substances such as caffeinated drinks, and getting more rest. Whereas modern medicine treats fear largely as a mental and emotional state, Ayur-Veda adds the dimension of physiology to psychological concerns (and the field of the mind to physical concerns), thereby offering a complete bodymind science.

*4. If my husband and children like one kind of food—usually not so healthy—and I'm trying to eat in an Ayur-Vedic way for my health, how do we resolve these family preferences? I want them to experience these benefits, too.*

Maintaining family harmony is sometimes a far better means of promoting good health than what we eat. We especially want to avoid any tensions at mealtimes. So it's fine for them to eat what they want, and you can have your own food program. They are probably eating out of habit, based on the "American Three-Taste Diet (sweet, salty, sour)." To move them toward a more taste-expanding eating regime, you can quietly introduce all six tastes at each meal. And encourage them to have a bigger lunch even when they are away from home, followed by a lighter dinner. If you can only orchestrate a few changes initially, discourage cold and/or carbonated drinks with meals; discourage TV during the meal; and encourage a quiet, settled mealtime, even if a short one.

*5. Does Ayur-Veda have a cellulite-reducing program?*

Fat is fat, but often an overproduction of fat within the superficial tissues along with a lack of circulation in certain areas can cause what some people call cellulite. It can also be understood as ama in that area. A special dry massage called *garshan* (gar-shahn), which stimulates flow and circulation, is suggested along with the other Ayur-Vedic programs, especially the ama-reducing eating program.

Garshan is best done with raw silk gloves or woolen mittens or gloves. You do the massage prior to abhyanga, or oil massage, for about five minutes. Use fairly vigorous strokes, except on your face and neck area. Use circular strokes on the joints and back-and-forth strokes on the long bones, twenty to forty times per area. Choose the areas where you may have some accumulated fat. Massage your abdomen and hip area horizontally and then diagonally. Use long vertical strokes on the thighs, circular strokes on the knees, back-and-forth vertical motions on the calf. Afterward, do your oil massage and take a warm bath or shower. Be sure you walk briskly every day and try to reduce or eliminate cheese, yogurt, and cold drinks from your diet.

*6. I eat a healthy diet, go to bed on time, and feel pretty good, but I can't seem to stop drinking my three cups of coffee daily, even though I do have insomnia quite often and know it would be better for me to give up the coffee.*

Actually, many Westerners drink coffee (and caffeinated tea) for one simple reason: To have the bitter and the astringent tastes of the six tastes needed for balance in their diet. A lack of purifying bitter herbs can make for an unhealthy condition, particular skin conditions. Our natural craving for this taste is a good one. Our bodymind is telling us something important. But overdoing coffee and tea can certainly create health problems as well. However, if we substitute bitter herbs such as aloe, senna, asaphoedida, and tumeric, or bitter foods such as romaine lettuce, endive, spinach, and lemon rind, we will notice that our coffee cravings start to disappear. Or we may find it is the "bean" value of coffee—its astringent taste—that our bodymind is craving, so if we substitute another kind of bean such as lentil or pinto, we can cut down on our coffee craving. If it's the heat and liquid value of coffee that you enjoy, hot water may turn out to be a good substitute.

*7. I'm a Vata-Kapha type, so why do I get irritated like a Pitta when I don't get my meals on time?*

We all have all three doshas active or we wouldn't be alive. So you do have some Pitta, and it sounds as though it may be working well.

*8. What does Ayur-Veda recommend with regard to milk?*

Milk is highly regarded in Ayur-Veda for its strengthening and nourishing properties, and for its ability to balance both Vata and Pitta doshas. If you boil the milk before drinking it, even if it has already been pasteurized, it will be much easier to digest and cause less congestion. Adding a couple of pinches of ginger or cardamom before boiling will enhance its flavor and aid in digestion. If you want to add raw sugar or honey, however, do so after the boiled milk has cooled down a bit. It's better to drink milk only in combination with other sweet tastes such as cereal, toast, or rice but not with salty foods or the other tastes. Wait for about half an hour to have milk after eating anything other than sweet foods.

9. *What do I do about craving foods that are not "Ayur-Vedically correct" for me? Should I follow my natural desire or the suggested diet?*

If the craving you feel is truly a natural one and not based on an addictive pattern that isn't satisfying your real hunger, then the advice is to go with your desire, as long as you aren't creating imbalances. Your bodymind is giving you specific information about how to bring it into balance through a particular nutrient or taste. The dietary recommendations for balancing each dosha are generally appropriate but not exclusive. Your well-being depends more on your self-referral knowledge at every moment. But you can test the accuracy of this self-knowing mechanism: If, after following your craving, you feel a sense of wholeness, satisfaction, lightness, and energy, your craving was "true" to your health needs. If, however, you don't feel very good after going with the craving, you may need to follow the dosha-balancing eating program more carefully until your bodymind information system is more reliable and trustworthy.

10. *What does Ayur-Veda say about microwave ovens?*

The amount of prana or breath or air in the food that we eat is a condition of how much real nourishment the food can provide for us. That's why Ayur-Veda recommends the freshest food possible. Microwaves tend to eliminate the prana in food, especially when the food is also prepackaged. So take a little more time to cook with your regular oven and stovetop. This will help eliminate the "extra" food you may feel you have to eat following your meal, because what your body was seeking in the food, its life-giving "breath," its orderly package of healing, was missing.

11. *Why does Ayur-Veda suggest for us to be happy when we are cooking? And what if that isn't always the case?*

The consciousness of the cook, say the Ayur-Vedic texts, flows into the food. So if we want our food to be maximally health-giving, we want the highest qualities of a loving nature to be transferred into the food. If we are feeling sick or irritable, these qualities of consciousness may transfer instead. Of course we can't pretend we are happy when we aren't. To release any stress we have before cooking, we could meditate first, or rest for a few minutes first, and/or say some nice things about the food—how beautiful the carrots look, how delicious the bread smells, etc. This sets up a nice feeling in the kitchen, and you'll feel better.

### 12. Should I refrigerate food?

Most Ayur-Vedic foods don't require much refrigeration and very little freezing. That's because, when following the Ayur-Vedic eating programs, we try to eat fresh and warm foods. Milk and cream are the only foods that need cooling and that's mostly to avoid spoilage. Our juices and other beverages should never be cold. Ghee, the clarified form of butter recommended by Ayur-Veda, does not need to be and should not be re-frigerated.

### 13. What is ghee and how do I make it?

Ghee is clarified butter, but although it's prepared from butter, its properties, according to Ayur-Veda, are very different from butter's. (However, although only the "good" cholesterol is found in ghee, it is still a good idea to check with your doctor before using ghee if you have a cholesterol problem.)

1. Place one or more pounds of unsalted butter in a deep stainless steel or Pyrex-type glass pan on medium or medium-low heat. (Watch to make sure that the butter doesn't scorch while melting.)

2. In the next thirty to forty minutes the water will boil away (butter is approximately 20 percent water) and milk solids will appear on the surface of the liquid and also at the bottom of the pan.

3. Be alert to remove liquid from heat when milk solids turn golden brown on the bottom of the pan. Otherwise, the ghee can burn. At this point, you may notice that the ghee may smell like popcorn and you may see tiny bubbles in the ghee rising from the bottom.

4. Strain the sediment from the ghee while it is hot, pouring it into a stainless steel or Pyrex-type pan. Strain by pouring through a cotton cloth placed over a stainless steel strainer. At this point it is very hot, so be cautious. Ghee should never be left unattended during this heating process.

5. Ghee can be stored at room temperature. Later, if the ghee becomes solid, just heat it slightly and it will return to liquid.

### 14. How do I choose proper Ayur-Vedic foods when I go to the market?

Food selection should start from a dosha-balancing perspective along with an awareness of the season. If you are following a particular dosha-balancing diet, just bring your list of foods and also a list of seasonal foods. The Ayur-Vedic seasonal foods correspond well to the foods that are likely to be freshest in the market, depending on the season. Favor foods that are native to the area in which you live and are in season there, because they have the local laws of nature most enlivened in them. As an overall principle, fresh food from anywhere is the best.

15. *Why does Ayur-Veda recommend hot water over other warm beverages, such as herbal teas?*

As Ayur-Vedic physician Dr. Raju has pointed out, "You don't wash your hands in tea or bathe in tea or wash the dishes with tea." Tea has a different effect on the body than pure water. Pure boiled water can improve digestion by eliminating ama and helping to balance the three doshas.

16. *How do I deal with disciplining the baby without incurring stress in her (or in myself)?*

According to Maharishi Ayur-Veda, you love the new baby with complete indulgence, trying to fulfill each of his or her desires until about age two, when it becomes the time to give the child some encouragement in the direction of setting boundaries. Regularity of life structured in love is what young children need most. Children need to learn what laws of nature are the ones to follow so they can be in tune with family and societal values. A child without boundary-setting guidance from the parents will start to become imbalanced and start eating poorly, sleeping irregularly, and losing a full sense of self. Clear discipline, carried out with sweetness, calmness, and love, is the key.

17. *What's the best way parents can incorporate Ayur-Veda into the lives of their children?*

They can do four things:

1. They can meditate regularly themselves and follow the other appropriate Ayur-Vedic programs, thereby offering their children healthier, less stressed interactions.

2. If the parents are meditating, the children can be instructed. There is a children's TM technique, which can be learned at age four and up, which is right for development at that age.

3. They can learn to read their children's pulses and then gear food, sleep, and other life-style considerations toward correcting any imbalances. If parents knew how to take their own pulses and the pulses of their children, they could pick up signs of imbalance before any disease manifests.

4. They can identify imbalances in their children and encourage specific food, rest, and exercise accordingly.

*20. What's the best way to travel and still maintain the Ayur-Vedic program?*

Travel itself—which is moving through space in whatever vehicle—increases Vata dosha. To get it back into balance, be sure you rest as much as possible during the trip; avoid cold food and drinks; eat smaller quantities to enable the body cycles to stabilize, especially if crossing a time zone; and continue your oil massage even if you are away from home. If you are on a plane, doing the TM program is a great way to feel rested following the trip, thereby avoiding jet lag. You can get off the plane and feel alert and ready to engage your physiology with "the physiology" of the new environment on the basis of deep rest.

*21. What are the essential Ayur-Vedic secrets of beauty?*

Quite simply, the deeper the contact with the inner structures of beauty, the more beautiful the outer surfaces. The production of ojas, the experience of bliss, and the desire to create a heaven on earth for everyone are the Lancôme, Revlon, and Estée Lauder products of the Ayur-Vedic world.

# APPENDIX B

## Maharishi Ayur-Ved Health Centers in North America

For the name of a physician trained in Maharishi Ayur-Veda in your area, call (800) 843-8332.

2101 W. Vineyard Ave., Suite 2111
Oxnard, California 93030
(805) 485-2883

470 San Antonio Rd.
Palo Alto, California 94306
(415) 857-0162

17308 Sunset Blvd.
Pacific Palisades, California
  90272
(310) 454-5531

Craig Perrinjaquet, M.D.
at the Breckenridge Medical
  Center
555 South Park Ave.
Breckenridge, CO 80424
(303) 453-9000

4910 Massachusetts Ave.
Suite 315
Washington, D.C. 20016
(202) 244-2700

3434 N. Washington Blvd.
Indianapolis, Indiana 46205
(317) 927-7252

The Raj
24th St. NW
Fairfield, Iowa 52556
(515) 472-9580
Out of State: (800) 248-9050

P.O. Box 282
Fairfield, Iowa 52556
(515) 472-5866

679 George Hill Rd.
P.O. Box 344
Lancaster, Massachusetts 01523
(508) 365-4549

33 Garden St.
Cambridge, Massachusetts
  02138
(617) 354-6764

Star Route 1, Box 196A
St. Genevieve, Missouri 63670
(314) 756-8011

19474 Center Ridge Rd.
Rocky River, Ohio 44116
(216) 333-6700

1929 43rd. Ave. E.
Seattle, Washington 98112
(206) 325-9280

347 Dolores St., Suite 221
San Francisco, California 94110
(415) 255-1928

Box 6500
Huntsville, Ontario P0A 1K0
Canada
(705) 635-2234

## Transcendental Meditation Centers in North America

2716 Derby St.
Berkeley, California 94705
(510) 548-1144

470 San Antonio Rd.
Palo Alto, California 94306
(415) 857-0108

17310 Sunset Blvd.
Pacific Palisades, California
  90272
(213) 459-3522

19 Prospect Hill Rd.
Stony Creek, Connecticut 06405
(203) 483-5180

250 Sandspur Rd.
Maitland, Florida 32751
(407) 539-2241

155 Stewart Dr. NE
Atlanta, Georgia 30328
(404) 250-9560

2407 Parker Place
Honolulu, Hawaii 96822
(808) 988-2266

3124 N. Southport St.
Chicago, Illinois 60657
(312) 477-0102

1601 North Fourth St.
Fairfield, Iowa 52556
(515) 472-4514

4818 Montgomery Lane
Bethesda, Maryland 20814
(301) 652-7002

33 Garden St.
Cambridge, Massachusetts
  02138
(617) 876-4581

1000 John R. Rd., Suite 201
Troy, Michigan 48083
(313) 583-7833

2700 University Ave. W., #80
St. Paul, Minnesota 55114
(612) 641-0925

6301 Main
Kansas City, Missouri 64113
(816) 523-5777

**333**

600 Camden Ave.
Moorestown, New Jersey 08057
(609) 231-0955

12 West 21st St., 9th Floor
New York, New York 10010
(212) 645-0202

23853 Hilliard Blvd.
Westlake, Ohio 44145
(216) 333-6700

234 South 22nd St.
Philadelphia, Pennsylvania
19103
(215) 732-8464

13789 Noel Rd., Suite 116
Dallas, Texas 75245
(214) 387-8686

801 Calhoun St.
Houston, Texas 77002
(713) 659-7002
For Maharishi Ayur-Veda:
(713) 659-7003

4317 Linden Ave. N
Seattle, Washington 98103
(206) 547-7527

1235 17th Ave. SW, Suite 308
Calgary, Alberta T2T 0C2
Canada
(403) 229-0406

6076 East Blvd.
Vancouver, British Columbia
B6M 3V5
Canada
(604) 263-2655

1498 Yonge St.
Toronto, Ontario M4W 3B8
Canada
(416) 964-1725

4205 St-Denis, Suite 320
Montreal, Quebec H2J 2K9
Canada
(514) 287-1501

For information about international Maharishi Ayur-Ved Health Centers, please contact:

Maharishi Foundation International
Hogeboekelweg 255
NL 7532 RE
Enschede, The Netherlands

Maharishi Ayur-Ved Universities are now being organized in the United States. The new universities and schools will provide professional training in Maharishi Ayur-Veda. Courses will be offered to train and qualify practitioners in all aspects of Maharishi Ayur-Veda, awarding degrees and diplomas in accord with state regulations, and will also provide health education courses open to the general public. For information, you may write to:

## APPENDIX B

College of Maharishi Ayur-Ved at
Maharishi International University
1000 N. 4th St., DB1155
Fairfield, Iowa 52557-1155
(515) 472-5866

For information on Maharishi Ayur-Ved Products International (MAPI):
P.O. Box 451
Lancaster, Massachusetts 01523
(800) 255-8332

For information on Maharishi Sthapatya-Veda, please write:
Maharishi Heaven on Earth Development Corporation
P.O. Box 2005
Fairfield, Iowa 52556
(310) 456-3670

Maharishi Ghandarva-Veda music is available through the Health Centers.

# NOTES

INTRODUCTION

[1] Maharishi Mahesh Yogi, *Life Supported by Natural Law* (Fairfield, Iowa: MIU Press, 1986), p. 114.

[2] Michael Crichton, "Greater Expectations," *Newsweek*, September 24, 1990, p. 58.

[3] Stephen Hall, "A Molecular Code Links Emotions, Minds, and Health," *Smithsonian*, June 1989, p. 64.

[4] Nancy Griffith-Marriott, "Body Mind: An Interview with Candace Pert," *Woman of Power*, Fall 1988, p. 25.


CHAPTER 1 WHOLENESS: REUNITING OUR PHYSICAL, MENTAL,
AND EMOTIONAL LIVES

[1] Maharishi Mahesh Yogi, *The Bhagavad-Gita: Translation and Commentary* (New York: Penguin Books, 1973), p. 147.

[2] Susan Blumenthal, Chief of the Behavioral Medicine Program, National Institute of Mental Health, quoted in Patricia Aburdene and John Naisbitt, *Megatrends for Women* (New York: Villard Books, 1992), pp. 134-35.

[3] Kenneth Walker, *Women Saints: East and West* (Hollywood, California: Vedanta Press, 1979), p. 227.

[4] Christine Gorman, "Sizing Up the Sexes," *Time*, January 20, 1992, p. 42.

[5] Charlene Spretnak, ed., from her introduction to *The Politics of Women's Spirituality* (New York: Doubleday, Anchor Books, 1982), p. xiii.

# NOTES

[1] *American Academy of Board Certified Physicians,* 1990.

[2] Lynn Payer, *Medicine and Culture* (New York: Penguin Books, 1989), pp. 17–20.

[3] Lawrence K. Altman and Elisabeth Rosenthal, "Changes in Medicine Bring Pain to Healing Profession, Demoralizing Doctors," *The New York Times,* February 18, 1990, p. 1.

[4] For women physicians, the trend is different. Although fewer than 20 percent of U.S. doctors are now women, it is predicted that by the year 2000, 50 percent of all doctors will be women. Thirty-eight percent of first-year medical students are now women. *New England Journal of Medicine,* November 30, 1989. According to Dr. Joyce Davidson at the Menninger Clinic in Topeka, Kansas, women doctors earn an average of 30 percent less than their male counterparts, but women are also more likely to go into the primary-care practices, which "have lower income expectations than highly paid specialties like surgeons." Altman and Rosenthal, p. 34.

[5] Robert Blendon and Humphrey Taylor, "A Health System That Needs Surgery," *The New York Times,* May 9, 1989, p. 3.

[6] Andrew Purvis, "A Perilous Gap," *Time,* special issue, 1990, p. 67.

[7] Nearly twice as many cesareans are performed at for-profit hospitals (30.5 percent) as at nonprofit hospitals.

[8] Kirkwood K. Shy, et al., "Effects of Electronic Fetal-Heart-Rate Monitoring, as Compared with Periodic Auscultation, on the Neurologic Development of Premature Infants," *New England Journal of Medicine,* March 1, 1990, pp. 588–93.

[9] One out of ten hysterectomies is performed as a treatment for uterine cancer.

[10] "Doubt Cast on Surgical Childbirth Procedure," *The New York Times,* July 2, 1992, p. 12.

[11] *Journal of the American Medical Association,* November 28, 1990, pp. 2648–53.

[12] Bill Lawren, "The Power to Stay Well," *Longevity,* June 1991, pp. 22–29.

[13] Barbara Ehrenreich, "Sick Chic," *Ms.,* February 1989, p. 28.

[14] "Women, Excess Weight and Longevity," *UC Berkeley Wellness Letter,* August 1990, p. 6. Yet women are more "protected" against their wish to end their own lives when they are terminally ill. In a study conducted by the American Society of Law and Medicine, the American court system supported the euthanasia preferences of men wishing to terminate their lives in six out of eight cases, while they allowed the same pa-

tient rights for women in only two of the fourteen cases before them. The study concluded that women were considered more emotional, immature, and in need of protection than men. "Death Bias," *Newsweek,* July 2, 1990, p. 6.

[15] "An Easy Monthly Breast Exam," *UC Berkeley Wellness Letter,* November 1986, p. 7.

[16] Gina Kolata, "NIH Neglects Women, Study Says," *The New York Times,* June 19, 1990; also, Sally Squires, "A Look at Research Involving Women," *The Washington Post,* December 12, 1989, p. 9.

[17] Nancy Touchette, "Estrogen Signals a Novel Route to Pain Relief," *Journal of NIH Research,* April 1993, Vol. 5, p. 53.

[18] Karen J. Armitage, et al., "Response of Physicians to Medical Complaints in Men and Women," *Journal of the American Medical Association,* May 18, 1979, pp. 2186–87.

[19] "The Female Factor," *UC Berkeley Wellness Letter,* March 1988, p. 1.

[20] Tamar Lewin, "Doctors Consider a Specialty Focusing on Women's Health," *The New York Times,* November 7, 1992, p. 1.

[21] *Journal of NIH Research,* February 1991, p. 28.

[22] *Medica,* March–April 1989, p. 4.

[23] Although as women we are more likely to be aware of our health than men are, we are also more likely to hand over healing responsibilities to doctors. This is a double-edged sword: If we have experienced effective treatment, we may come to rely unduly on the doctor and not engage in a responsible way in helping ourselves get better and make ourselves vulnerable to unnecessary drug or surgical interventions. If we are poorly treated, we may avoid getting the medical care we need.

[24] Jana M. Mossey, M.P.H., Ph.D., and Evelyn Shapiro, M.A., "Self-Rated Health: A Predictor of Mortality Among the Elderly," *American Journal of Public Health,* 72 (1982), pp. 800–807.

[25] Ehrenreich, *op. cit.*

[26] Quoted in Payer, *Medicine and Culture,* p. 12.

[27] Robert Ornstein and David Sobel, *The Healing Brain* (New York: Simon & Schuster, Touchstone Books, 1988), p. 160.

# NOTES

CHAPTER 3 KNOWLEDGE: IDENTIFYING YOUR AYUR-VEDIC CONSTITUTIONAL TYPE

[1] Robert Ornstein and David Sobel, *The Healing Brain* (New York: Simon & Schuster, Touchstone Books, 1988), pp. 30-32.

[2] John Hagelin, "Is Consciousness a Field? A Field Theorist's Perspective," *Modern Science and Vedic Science,* January 1987, vol. 1, no. 1, pp. 29-87.

[3] Jean Seligmann, "Tempermental Ills," *Newsweek,* August 13, 1979, p. 40.

[4] Tom Carney, "Hot Weather Triggers Aggressive Behavior, Psychologists Say," *Des Moines Register,* July 7, 1989, p. 2a.

[5] "Overheard," *Newsweek,* October 1, 1990, p. 17.


CHAPTER 4 BALANCE: IN THE BEST OF ALL POSSIBLE HEALTH

[1] One exception is MIT biochemist Dr. Judith Wurtman, whose research demonstrates individual differences in food needs: "Just like some people need nine hours of sleep a night, some people may need their carbohydrate every afternoon." Trish Hall, "Cravings: Does Your Body Know What It Needs?", *The New York Times Magazine,* September 27, 1987, p. 23.

[2] Douglas Stein, "Interview with Sarah Leibowitz," *Omni,* May 1992, p. 73.

[3] With thanks to Dr. John Douillard and Barbara Levinson McLaughlin.


CHAPTER 5 INTELLIGENCE: FACILITATING THE FLOW OF BIOLOGICAL
INTELLIGENCE TO RESTORE OUR HEALTH

[1] "When You Don't Know What to Say," *UC Berkeley Wellness Letter,* May 1990, p. 3.

[2] David Orme-Johnson et al., "Medical care utilization and the Transcendental Meditation program," *Journal of Psychosomatic Medicine* 49 (1988), pp. 493-500.

[3] M. J. Cooper and M. M. Aygen, "Effect of Transcendental Meditation on serum cholesterol and blood pressure," *Journal of the Israel Medical Association* (1987), pp. 1-2.

[4] Robert Ornstein and David Sobel, *The Healing Brain* (New York: Simon & Schuster, Touchstone Books, 1988), p. 258.

[5] "Little Problems/Big Stress," *UC Berkeley Wellness Letter,* November 1984, p. 1.

[6] Y. Niwa, "Effect of Maharishi 4 and Maharishi 5 on Inflammatory Mediators with Special Reference to Their Free Radical Scavenging Effects," *India Journal of Clinical Practice,* vol. 1, no. 8 (January 1991), pp. 23-27.

[7] J. Z. Fields et al., "Oxygen Free Radical Scavenging Effects of an Anti-Carcinogenic Natural Product, Maharishi Amrit Kalash (MAK)," *The Pharmacologist*, vol. 32 (1990), p. 155.

[8] *Newsweek*, February 12, 1990, p. 61.

[9] C. N. Alexander et al., "Transcendental Meditation, Mindfulness and Longevity: An Experimental Study with the Elderly," *Journal of Personality and Social Psychology*, vol. 57, no. 6 (1989), pp. 950–64.

CHAPTER 6 NOURISHMENT: CREATING THE TRANSFORMATIONS

FROM SICKNESS TO HEALTH

[1] Jane Brody, "Food Allergies: A Growing Controversy," *The New York Times Magazine*, April 29, 1990, pp. 18–19.

[2] *Archives of Environmental Health*, vol. 47, no. 2 (March–April 1992), pp. 143–46.

[3] Anastasia Toufexis, "Why Men Can Outdrink Women," *Time*, January 22, 1990, p. 61.

[4] Ronald Melzack, "The Tragedy of Needless Pain," *Scientific American*, February 1990, pp. 27–33.

[5] "Treating Substance Abuse Through Transcendental Meditation: A Review and Statistical Meta-Analysis," C. N. Alexander, P. Robinson, and M. Rainforth, *Alcoholism Treatment Quarterly* (in press).

[6] David O'Connell and C. N. Alexander, eds., *Recovery from Alcoholism and Drug Addiction Using Transcendental Meditation and Maharishi Ayur-Veda* (New York: Haworth Press, 1993).

CHAPTER 7 RESPONSIVENESS: FEELING AND HEALING IN

OUR EMOTIONAL BODYMIND

[1] Research conducted by sociologist David Phillips at the University of California at San Diego, reported in Sandra Blakeslee, "In Death, A Link to Birthdays," *The New York Times*, September 27, 1992.

[2] In another study, mortality among Chinese was found to dip by 35.1 percent the week before the Harvest Moons festival and peak at about the same amount the week after (34.6 percent). The same pattern does not appear in non-Chinese control groups for whom the holiday has no significance. David P. Phillips and Daniel G. Smith, "Postponement of Death Until Symbolically Meaningful Occasions," *Journal of the American Medical Association*, vol. 263, no. 14 (April 1990), pp. 1947–51.

[3] George Solomon and Rudolph Moos, "Psychologic Aspects of Response to Treatment in Rheumatoid Arthritis," *General Practioner,* vol. 32, no. 6 (December 1965), pp. 113-19.

[4] From a personal interview with neurophysiologist Ken Walton, Maharishi International University, Fairfield, Iowa, January 3, 1993.

[5] John W. Shaffer, et al., "Clustering of Personality Traits in Youth and Subsequent Development of Cancer among Physicians," *Journal of Behavioral Medicine,* vol. 10, no. 5 (1987), p. 441-47.

[6] *Natural Health,* January–February 1992.

[7] Robert Ornstein and David Sobel, *The Healing Brain* (New York: Simon & Schuster, Touchstone Books, 1988), p. 44.

[8] John Poppy, "Soothing the Savage Heart," *Esquire,* October 1989, p. 103.

[9] Maharishi Mahesh Yogi, *The Bhagavad-Gita: Translation and Commentary* (New York: Penguin Books, 1973), p. 236.

[10] Christopher Coe, *American Health,* March 1989, p. 48.

[11] "Family Attitude Results: Closeness to Parents," *Advances,* vol. 5, no. 2, pp. 50-52.

CHAPTER 8 LOVE: THE PHYSIOLOGY OF PERSONAL RELATIONSHIPS

[1] Maharishi Mahesh Yogi, *Love and God* (New York: Age of Enlightenment Press, 1978), pp. 16, 19.

[2] Carol Gilligan, *In a Different Voice* (Cambridge, Massachusetts: Harvard University Press, 1982).

[3] Danah Zohar, *The Quantum Self* (New York: William Morrow and Company, 1990), p. 137.

[4] Rudy Rucker, "The Powers of Coincidence," *Science 85,* February 1985, p. 54.

[5] Maharishi Mahesh Yogi, *The Bhagavad-Gita: Translation and Commentary* (New York: Penguin Books, 1973), p. 58.

[6] Robert Ornstein and David Sobel, *The Healing Brain* (New York: Simon & Schuster, Touchstone Books, 1988), pp. 103-04.

CHAPTER 9 PURIFICATION: THE MONTHLY CYCLE AS OUR HEALTH ADVANTAGE

[1] Howard J. Osofsky, M.D., "Efficacious Treatments of PMS: A Need for Further Research," *Journal of the American Medical Association,* vol. 264, no. 3 (July 1990), p. 387.

[2] D. R. Rubinow and P. J. Schmidt, "Mood Disorders and the Menstrual Cycle," *Reproductive Medicine,* vol. 32 (1987), pp. 389-94.

[3] From personal communication with the authors by Nick Argyl et al.,

Department of Physiology, Maharishi International University, Fairfield, Iowa, 1990.

[4] Hargrove and Abraham, *Journal of Reproductive Medicine,* vol. 27 (1982), pp. 721-24; also Siegel et al., *Journal of Reproductive Medicine,* vol. 32 (1987), pp. 395-99.

[5] Recent studies indicate that even a small amount of caffeine increases the severity of PMS symptoms. Annette Mackay Rossingnol, Sc.D., Heinke Bonnlader, R.N., M.S.N., "Caffeine-Containing Beverages, Total Fluid Consumption, and Premenstrual Syndrome," *American Journal of Public Health,* September 1990, pp. 1106-09; also Bruce Goldfarb, "Caffeine Increases Severity of PMS," *USA Today,* September 24, 1990, p. 1, section D.

[6] Judy Grahn, "From Sacred Blood to Curse and Beyond," in *The Politics of Women's Spirituality,* ed. Charlene Spretnak (New York: Doubleday, Anchor Books, 1982).

CHAPTER 10 NURTURANCE: PREGNANCY, CHILDBIRTH, AND OTHER CONCEPTIONS OF MOTHERHOOD

[1] Maharishi Mahesh Yogi, *Thirty Years Around the World* (Vlodrop, The Netherlands: Maharishi European Research University Press, 1986), p. 171.

[2] Adrienne Rich, *On Lies, Secrets and Silence* (New York: W. W. Norton, 1979), p. 77.

[3] Rig Veda, 10.13.125, verse 4.

[4] See, for example, Brian W. Jack, M.D., and Larry Culpepper, M.D., "Preconception Care, Risk Reduction and Health Promotion in Preparation for Pregnancy," *Journal of the American Medical Association,* vol. 264, no. 9 (September 1990), p. 1147.

[5] See the description of Dr. Alice Domar's Mind-Body Program for Infertility at New England Deaconess Hospital, as reported in Jennifer King, "The Mind-Body Connection," *New Age Journal,* August 1992, p. 95.

[6] Studies on pregnant American women indicate that they prefer saltier food like pickles, as well as milk and sweets, and dislike the taste of diet soda, coffee, beef, and alcohol. Trish Hall, "Cravings: Does Your Body Know What It Needs?," *The New York Times Magazine,* September 27, 1987, p. 64.

[7] Peggy Richardson, "Women's Important Relationships During Pregnancy and the Preterm Labor Event," *Western Journal of Nursing Research,* vol. 9, no. 2 (May 1987), p. 203.

[8] Robert Sosa, et al., "The Effect of a Supportive Companion on Perinatal Problems, Length of Labor, and Mother-Infant Interaction," *New England Journal of Medicine* 303 (1980), pp. 597-600.

⁹ A videotape that includes this program as well as other Ayur-Vedic guidance on the first few months of life entitled *Blissful Baby: The Maharishi Ayur-Vedic Mother/Baby Program* is available through the Maharishi Ayur-Vedic Health Centers (see Appendix B).

¹⁰ Tiffany M. Field, Ph.D., et al., "Tactile/Kinesthetic Stimulation Effects on Preterm Neonates," *Pediatrics*, vol. 77, no. 5 (May 1986), p. 654.

CHAPTER 11 FULLNESS: MENOPAUSE, LIFE SPAN, AND THE NEW AGING

¹ Lisa Davis, "The Myths of Menopause," *Hippocrates*, May–June 1989, p. 54.

² Jerilyn Prior, et al., "Spinal Bone Loss and Ovulatory Disturbances," *The New England Journal of Medicine*, vol. 323 (1990), pp. 1221-27.

³ Ann Voda et al., "Body Composition Changes in Menopausal Women," in *Women and Therapy*, vol. 2 (New York: The Haworth Press, 1991).

⁴ *New England Journal of Medicine*, vol. 325, no. 17 (October 1991), pp. 1189-95.

⁵ B. E. Henderson, M.D., et al., "Decreased Mortality in Users of Estrogen Replacement Therapy," *Archives of Internal Medicine*, vol. 151, no. 1 (January 1991).

⁶ Between 1979 and 1989, the death rate from myocardial infarction declined 30 percent. The nation's coronary heart disease death rate for white men was 155.8 per 100,000, and 5.6 percent lower for black men at 147.1 per 100,000. For black women the rate was 93 per 100,000 which is 24.5 percent higher than the rate for white women, 74.7 per 100,000. See "Cardiovascular Disease Remains Nation's Leading Cause of Death," *Journal of the American Medical Association* (January 1992).

⁷ Dean Ornish et al., "Can Lifestyle Changes Reverse Coronary Heart Disease?," *The Lancet*, vol. 336 (July 1990).

⁸ Albert Rosenfeld, "Why Women Live Longer Than Men—And How Men Can Start Catching Up," *Longevity*, July 1990, pp. 22-27.

⁹ "The Magic Bullet Is Prevention," *UC Berkeley Wellness Letter*, February 1986, p. 1.

¹⁰ "Fascinating Facts," *UC Berkeley Wellness Letter*, August 1989, p. 1.

¹¹ Carol Travis, "Old Age Is Not What It Used to Be," *The New York Times Magazine*, September 27, 1987, p. 24.

¹² Brad Darrach, "The War on Aging," *Life*, October 1992, p. 34.

¹³ Natalie Angier, "Growth Hormone and the Drive for a More Youthful State," *The New York Times*, July 6, 1990, p. A1.

¹⁴ For example, Dr. Arthur Schwartz at Temple University found that feeding high-dose DHEA-S to laboratory mice reduces their body fat by

one-third, prevents arteriosclerosis, alleviates diabetes, reduces the risk of cancer, inhibits the development of certain autoimmune diseases, and extends the normal life span of mice by 20 percent. See Darrach, "The War on Aging," p. 42.

[15] Darrach, "The War on Aging," p. 34.

[16] R. K. Wallace et al., "The Effects of the Transcendental Meditation and TM-Sidhi Program on the Aging Process," *International Journal of Neuroscience*, vol. 16 (1982), pp. 53–58.

[17] Specific findings included: 55.4 percent fewer for benign and malignant tumors; 87.3 percent fewer for heart disease; 30.4 percent fewer for diseases of the nervous system. See D. W. Orme-Johnson, "Medical Care Utilization and the Transcendental Meditation Program," *Psychosomatic Medicine*, vol. 49 (1988), pp. 493–500.

[18] Robert Herron, "The Impact of Transcendental Meditation Practice on Medical Expenditures," doctoral thesis, Maharishi International University.

[19] J. L. Glaser et al., "Elevated Serum Dehydroepiandrosterone Sulfate Levels in Practitioners of the Transcendental Meditation and TM Sidhi Programs," *Journal of Behavioral Medicine*, vol. 15, no. 4 (1992), pp. 327–41.

[20] Ken Walton et al., "Optimizing Adaptive Mechanisms: A Stress-Related Neuroendocrine Basis for Disease Prevention through Transcendental Meditation," *Psychoneuroendocrinology* (in press).

CHAPTER 12 SIMPLICITY: MAHARISHI AYUR-VEDA AS A DAILY LIFE PROGRAM

[1] In a study conducted in Israel, patients with high cholesterol levels who were instructed in the Transcendental Meditation technique showed a 20-percent reduction in cholesterol levels over an eleven-month period as compared to controls matched for sex, diet, weight, and starting cholesterol values. M. J. Cooper and M. M. Aygen, "Effect of Transcendental Meditation on Serum Cholesterol and Blood Pressure," *Harefuah* (journal of the Israel Medical Association), 1987, pp. 1–2.

[2] "TV: No Way to Relax," *UC Berkeley Wellness Letter,* April 1986, p. 1.

[3] Quoted by Pauline Kael in *The New Yorker,* February 11, 1991, p. 70.

[4] The one exception to this is if the patient is clearly terminally ill. Then the vaidya may on occasion choose to protect the delicate physiology from further stress.

[5] Alan K. Tillitson, *The Handbook of Ayurvedic Medicine* (Norfolk, Virginia: Bindi Press, 1986), p. 64.

[6] Maryann Napoli, "Cold Relievers," *The New York Times Magazine,* September 27, 1987, p. 8.

[7] "Medicinal Plants—Pills in a Haystack," *The Economist*, February 24, 1990, p. 87.

[8] V. Patel et al., "Enhancement of Lymphoproliferative Responses by Maharishi Amrit Kalash (MAK) in Rats," *FAESB Journal*, vol. 2 (March 1988), p. 20.

[9] H. M. Sharma, "Antineoplastic properties of Maharishi 4, against DMBA-induced mammary tumors in rats," *Journal of Pharmacology, Biochemistry, and Behavior*, vol. 35 (April 29, 1990), p. 19.

[10] In a study on rats already exposed to carcinogens conducted by Dr. Tony Nader, the rasayana group had 40 percent fewer tumors than the other animals. In another study, rats on a low-choline, high-fat, low-methionine diet—a diet known to accelerate aging and destroy the kidneys—who were fed the rasayana showed no kidney damage at all, in marked contrast to the other rats. A third study indicated that the rasayana helped recovery from brain damage (anto-rhinal cortical lesions, which affect memory and learning) more effectively than did ganglio-sides, the most powerful modern drugs known for reducing nerve deficits. Results of these studies are available through the Institute of Science, Technology and Public Policy, Fairfield, Iowa (see p. 357).

[11] Paper presented at the Annual Meeting of the American Society for Cancer Research, San Diego, 1992, abstract no. 75.

[12] Available from the Institute of Science, Technology and Public Policy, Fairfield, Iowa (see p. 357).

[13] The Maharishi Panchakarma program was studied at Albert Ludwig University in Freiburg, Germany, for its effects on blood lipids. Subjects were given a typical six- to fourteen-day treatment. Before-and-after comparisons showed a significant average decrease in total cholesterol of 10.5 percent, from 203.5 mg to 179.5 mg seven to ten days after treatment. There was an 8.7 percent decrease in LDL-cholesterol and a 17.5 percent decrease in the LDL-to-HDL ratio. The number of patients with high-risk profiles before treatment decreased by 43 percent for males and 35.8 percent for females. Using data from the Lipid Research Clinics Coronary Primary Prevention Trials study, the author calculated the reduction in risk for coronary mortality to be 17.4 percent based on a one- to two-week Panchakarma treatment program.

[14] Tim Stryker and R. K. Wallace, "Reduction in Biological Age Through an Ayur-Vedic Treatment Program" (paper presented at the *International Congress of Psychosomatic Medicine*, Chicago, September 1985).

[15] David Orme-Johnson, "Health Care Utilization and Maharishi Ayur-Veda" (paper presented at the annual meeting of the *American Psychological Association*, Toronto, 1993).

CHAPTER 13 CONNECTION: MAHARISHI AYUR-VEDA, WOMEN, AND THE WORLD

[1] Maharishi Mahesh Yogi, *The Bhagavad-Gita: Translation and Commentary* (New York: Penguin Books, 1973), p. 63.

[2] See Carol McLain, ed., *Woman as Healer: Cross-Cultural Perspectives* (New Brunswick, New Jersey: Rutgers University Press, 1989).

[3] Deborah Cushman, "Is There a Female Doctor in the House?" *Des Moines Register,* April 17, 1990, p. 1T.

[4] Michele Barrett, ed., *Virginia Woolf: Women and Writing* (New York: Harcourt Brace Jovanovich, Harvest Books, 1979), p. 191.

[5] *New York Times Book Review,* August 26, 1990, p. 27.

[6] Study reported in Betty Friedan, *The Second Stage* (New York: Summit Books, 1982), p. 40.

[7] M. C. Dillbeck et al., "The Transcendental Meditation Program and Crime Rate Change," *Journal of Crime and Justice,* vol. 4 (1981), pp. 25-45.

[8] See, for example, M. C. Dillbeck et al., "Consciousness as a Field," *Journal of Mind and Behavior,* vol. 8 (1987), pp. 67-104.

[9] Vandana Shiva, *Staying Alive* (Atlantic Highlands, New Jersey: Zed Books, 1989).

[10] Deena Metzger, *Ms.,* 1989, p. 63.

[11] Robin Morgan, "Metaphysical Feminism," in *The Politics of Women's Spirituality,* ed. Charlene Spretnak (New York: Doubleday, Anchor Books, 1982), p. 387.

# GLOSSARY

**abhyanga**        An oil massage

**agni**        Digestive fire, also one of the five basic elements of manifest creation associated with metabolism and transformation

**ahara**        Proper diet

**ahimsa**        Nonviolence or harmlessness

**ahita-ayu**        Actions that are disadvantageous to others and to society

**akasha**        One of the five basic elements of manifest creation associated with space

**ama**        That which blocks the flow of nature's intelligence in the bodymind

**Apana**        A subdosha of Vata associated with downward movement and the settling down of mental activity

**asana**        A bodymind posture, a yoga position

**asthi**        One of the body's seven basic constituents closely associated with bone

**bala**        Strength, immunity

**basti**        A gentle medicated oil enema

**Bhagavad-Gita**        A text of Vedic literature

**Charaka**        The most well-known of the ancient Ayur-Vedic physicians and author of the Charaka Samhita

| | |
|---|---|
| **dhatu** | One of the body's seven basic constituents, incorporating the Western concept of "tissue" |
| **dinacharya** | The Ayur-Vedic daily routine |
| **doshas** | The governing principles in nature |
| **duhkha-ayu** | Any type of life not good for the individual physiology |
| **Gandharva-Veda** | Music from the ancient Vedic tradition |
| **garshan** | A special massage that stimulates circulation |
| **ghee** | Clarified butter |
| **hita-ayu** | Any activity in life for the good and benefit of others, for the happiness of society |
| **Kapha** | The dosha expressing the natural laws associated with earth and water |
| **mahabhutas** | The five basic laws or elements of existence |
| **Maharishi Amrit Kalash (MAK)** | One of the Maharishi Ayur-Veda herbal preparations for longevity and rejuvenation |
| **majja** | One of the body's seven basic constituents closely associated with bone marrow's nervous tissue |
| **mamsa** | One of the body's seven basic constituents closely associated with muscle tissue |
| **manda agni** | Diminished digestive fire |
| **medha** | One of the body's seven basic constituents closely associated with fat tissue |
| **nasya** | A Panchakarma rejuvenation treatment for the head and nasal areas |
| **ojas** | The vital substance that bestows radiance and strength to the physiology |
| **Panchakarma** | A series of rejuvenating and cleansing therapies |
| **pindasweda** | A Panchakarma massage treatment |

# GLOSSARY

| | |
|---|---|
| **Pitta** | The dosha expressing the natural laws associated with fire and water |
| **pizichilli** | A Panchakarma oil treatment for the whole body |
| **pragya aparadh** | The mistake of the intellect, forgetting the underlying wholeness of life |
| **prakriti** | The essence of an individual's constitutional type |
| **prana** | Life force; a subdosha of Vata related to upward movement |
| **pranayama** | An Ayur-Vedic breathing exercise |
| **rakta** | One of the body's seven basic constituents, associated with blood |
| **rasa** | One of the body's seven basic constituents, associated with plasma; also one of the six tastes |
| **rasayana** | A mixture of herbs to rejuvenate the physiology and promote longevity |
| **Rig Veda** | An ancient Vedic text |
| **rishi** | The knower, the internal healer, a Vedic seer |
| **sama agni** | Balanced digestive fire |
| **sama dosha** | A bodymind type in which all three doshas are equally represented |
| **Samana** | Subdosha of Vata located in the stomach and duodenum; associated with digestion and assimilation |
| **samanya** | The principle of balance through similarity |
| **samhita** | The unified wholeness underlying all existence |
| **shirodhara** | A Panchakarmic treatment to soothe the central nervous system and promote increased brain coherence |
| **shukra** | The seventh dhatu, associated with ojas |
| **smriti** | Bodymind memory |
| **snehana** | A purifying oleation therapy |

| | |
|---|---|
| **srota** | Channel in the bodymind through which ojas flows |
| **Sthapatya-Veda** | The Vedic system of architecture |
| **sukta-ayu** | Any aspect of life which promotes bliss in the individual's physiology |
| **surya namaskar** | An Ayur-Vedic program |
| **swedana** | A Panchakarmic treatment to eliminate ama |
| **tikshna agni** | Overabundant gastric fire |
| **Udana** | Subdosha of Vata, associated with speech, general activity, strength, complexion, and the ability to make effort |
| **udvartana** | A Panchakarma massage |
| **vaidya** | An Ayur-Vedic physician |
| **Vak** | A Vedic woman seer |
| **Vata** | The dosha expressing the natural laws associated with space and air |
| **vayu** | One of the five basic elements of manifest creation, associated with air |
| **Veda** | Pure knowledge |
| **vikriti** | Imbalanced doshas |
| **virechana** | A Panchakarma therapy |
| **vishama agni** | Irregular digestive fire |
| **vishesh** | A vigorous Panchakarma massage |
| **vishesha** | The principle of balance through opposites |
| **Vyana** | Subdosha of Vata associated with movement, especially the circulatory system |

# SELECTED
# BIBLIOGRAPHIES

## General

Aburdene, Patricia, and John Naisbitt. *Megatrends for Women.* New York: Villard Books, 1992.

Achterberg, Jeanne. *Woman as Healer.* Boulder, Colorado: Shambhala Press, 1990.

Alexander, Charles N., ed. *Higher Stages of Human Development.* New York: Oxford University Press, 1990.

Allen, Paula Gunn. *The Sacred Hoop: Recovering the Feminine in American Indian Traditions.* Boston: Beacon Press, 1986.

Banchek, Linda. *Cooking for Life.* New York: Harmony Books (in press).

Barrett, Michele, ed. *Virginia Woolf: Women and Writing.* New York: Harcourt Brace Jovanovich, Harvest Books, 1979.

Brown, Melanie. *Attaining Personal Greatness: One Book for Life.* New York: William Morrow, 1987. Also on audiocassette: Nightingale-Conant Tape Series, 1993.

Campbell, Anthony. *TM and the Nature of Enlightenment.* New York: Harper & Row, Perennial Library, 1976.

Corea, Gena. *The Invisible Epidemic: The Story of Women and AIDS.* New York: HarperCollins, 1992.

Cutler, Winnifred. *Hysterectomy: Before and After.* New York: HarperCollins, 1990.

Dossey, Larry. *Recovering the Soul: A Scientific and Spiritual Search.* New York: Bantam Books, 1989.

———. *Beyond Illness.* Boulder, Colorado: Shambala Press, New Science Library, 1984.

Friedan, Betty. *The Second Stage.* New York: Simon & Schuster, Summit Books, 1982.

Gilligan, Carol. *In a Different Voice.* Cambridge, Massachusetts: Harvard University Press, 1982.

Greenwood, Sadja. *Menopause Naturally.* Volcano, California: Volcano Press, 1989.

Hagelin, John. "Is Consciousness the Unified Field? A Field Theorist's Perspective." *Modern Science and Vedic Science* 1 (1987).

Lawlor, Tony. *The Temple in the House: Finding the Sacred in Everyday Architecture.* New York: Tarcher/Putnam, 1994.

Mahaldar, Anjali. *The ILA MA Handbook.* Lancaster, Massachusetts: International Ladies Association of Maharishi Ayur-Veda, 1990.

Maharishi Mahesh Yogi. *Thirty Years Around the World.* Vlodrop, The Netherlands: Maharishi European Research University Press, 1986.

———. *Love and God.* New York: Age of Enlightenment Press, 1978.

———. *The Bhagavad-Gita: Translation and Commentary.* New York: Penguin Books, 1973.

———. *Science of Being and Art of Living.* New York: Signet Books, 1968.

McLain, Carol S. *Women as Healers: Cross-Cultural Perspectives.* New Brunswick, N.J.: Rutgers University Press, 1989.

O'Connell, David and Charles N. Alexander. *Recovery From Alcoholism and Drug Addiction Using Transcendental Meditation and Maharishi Ayur-Veda.* New York: Haworth Press, 1993.

Orme-Johnson, David, and John Farrow, eds. *Scientific Research on the Transcendental Meditation Program, Collected Papers.* Vol. 1. Rheinweiler, Germany: MERU Press, 1977. Vols. 2–6 (in press). Vlodrop. the Netherlands: MIU Press.

Ornstein, Robert, and David Sobel. *The Healing Brain.* New York: Simon & Schuster, Touchstone Books, 1988.

# SELECTED BIBLIOGRAPHIES

Payer, Lynn. *Medicine and Culture.* New York: Penguin Books, 1989.

Roth, Robert. *Transcendental Meditation: A New Introduction.* New York: Donald I. Fine, 1987.

Perrone, Bobette, H. H. Stockel and V. Krueger. *Medicine Women, Curanderas, and Women Doctors.* Norman, Oklahoma: University of Oklahoma Press, 1989.

Rich, Adrienne. *On Lies, Secrets and Silence.* New York: W. W. Norton, 1979.

Sharma, P. V., ed. and trans. *Caraka Samhita.* Delhi, India: Chaukhambha House of Orientalia and Antiquarian Books, 1983.

Shearer, Alistair, and Peter Russell, trans. *The Upanishads.* New York: Harper & Row, Harper Colophon Books, 1978.

Sheehy, Gail. *The Silent Passage.* New York: Random House, 1992.

Spretnak, Charlene, ed. *The Politics of Women's Spirituality.* New York: Doubleday, Anchor Books, 1982.

Steinem, Gloria. *The Revolution Within.* Boston: Little, Brown, 1992.

Svoboda, Robert E. *Prakruti.* Albuquerque, N.M.: Geocom Ltd, 1988.

Thomas, Lewis. *The Lives of a Cell.* New York: Bantam Books, 1975.

Walker, Kenneth. *Women Saints: East and West.* Hollywood, California: Vedanta Press, 1979.

Wallace, R. Keith. *The Maharishi Technology of the Unified Field: The Neurophysiology of Enlightenment.* Fairfield, Iowa: MIU Neuroscience Press, 1986.

Wilber, Ken, ed. *The Holographic Paradigm and Other Paradoxes.* Boulder, Colo.: Shambhala Press, 1982.

## Selected Research on Maharishi Ayur-Veda and the Transcendental Meditation Program

Alexander, C. N., E. J. Langer, J. L. Davies, H. M. Chandler and R. I. Newman. 1989. Transcendental Meditation, mindfulness and longevity: An experimental study with the elderly. *Journal of Personality and Social Psychology* 57: 950-64.

Alexander, C. N., P. Robinson, and M. Rainforth. 1993. Meta-analysis of nineteen studies on TM and substance abuse. *Alcoholism Treatment Quarterly* 11: (1-4).

Badawi, K., R. K. Wallace, D. W. Orme-Johnson, and A. M. Rouzere. 1984. Electrophysiologic characteristics of respiratory suspension periods occurring during the practice of the Transcendental Meditation program. *Psychosomatic Medicine* 46: 267-76.

Banquet, J. P., and M. Sailhan. 1974. EEG analysis of spontaneous and induced states of consciousness. *Revue d'electroencephalographie et de neurophysiologie clinique* 4: 445-53.

Bleick, C. R., and A. I. Abrams. 1987. The Transcendental Meditation program and criminal recidivism in California. *The Journal of Criminal Justice* 15: 211-30.

Brooks, J. S., and T. Scarano. 1985. Transcendental Meditation in the treatment of post-Vietnam adjustment. *Journal of Counseling and Development* 65: 212-15.

Chandler, H. M., D. W. Orme-Johnson, M. C. Dillbeck, and J. L. Glaser. June 1985. Improvements in memory, intelligence, psychomotor speed, and alertness in normal subjects from an Ayur-Vedic medicinal herbal-based rejuvenation therapy. Paper presented at the Twenty-eighth Annual Meeting of the Society of Economic Botany, University of Illinois, Chicago.

Cooper, M. J., and M. M. Aygen. 1987. Effect of Transcendental Meditation on serum cholesterol and blood pressure. *Harefuah* (journal of the Israel Medical Association) 95: 1-2.

Dillbeck, M. C., and D. W. Orme-Johnson. 1987. Physiological differences between Transcendental Meditation and rest. *American Psychologist* 42: 879-81.

Dillbeck, M. C., K. L. Cavanaugh, T. Glenn, D. W. Orme-Johnson, and V. Mittlefehldt. 1987. Consciousness as a field: The Transcendental Meditation and TM-Sidhi program and changes in social indicators. *The Journal of Mind and Behaviour* 8: 67-104.

Dwivedi, C., B. Satter, and H. M. Sharma. 1991. Anticarcinogenic activity of an Ayur-Vedic food supplement, Maharishi Amrit Kalash (MAK). *Pharmacology, Biochemistry and Behavior* 39: 649-52.

# SELECTED BIBLIOGRAPHIES

Eppley, K., A. Abrams, and J. Shear. 1989. Differential effects of relaxation techniques on trait anxiety: A meta-analysis. *Journal of Clinical Psychology* 45: 957–74.

Fields, J. Z., et al. 1990. Oxygen free radical scavenging effects of an anticarcinogenic natural product, Maharishi Amrit Kalash (MAK). *American Society for Pharmacology and Experimental Therapeutics* 32: 55.

Gelderloos, P., H. H. B. Ahlstrom, D. W. Orme-Johnson, H. I. Msemaje, P. H. Goddard, J. Glaser, and R. K. Wallace. April 1988. The influence of an Ayur-Vedic herbal preparation on visual discrimination of a field with interfering stimuli. Paper presented at the Iowa Academy of Science.

Gelderloos, P., K. Walton, and D. W. Orme-Johnson. 1990. Effectiveness of the Transcendental Meditation program in preventing and treating substance abuse: A review. *International Journal of the Addictions* 26: 293–325.

Glaser, J. L., J. L. Brind, M. J. Eisner, and R. K. Wallace. August 1992. Elevated serum dehydroepiandrosterone sulfate levels in older practitioners of an Ayur-Vedic stress reduction program. *Journal of Behavioral Medicine* 15: (4), pp. 327–41.

Hanissian, S. R., H. M. Sharma, and G. A. Tejwani. February 1988. Effect of Maharishi Amrit Kalash (MAK) on brain opioid receptors. *Federation of American Societies of Experimental Biology (FASEB) Journal* 2.

Hauser, T., R. K. Wallace, and K. G. Walton. April 1987. Platelet imipramine receptor binding of Maharishi Amrit Kalash. Paper presented at the meeting of the American Association of Ayur-Vedic Medicine, Fairfield, Iowa.

Herbert, J. R., and D. Lehmann. 1977. Theta bursts: An EEG pattern in normal subjects practicing the Transcendental Meditation technique. *Electroencephalography and Clinical Neurophysiology* 42: 397–405.

Kasture, H. S., S. Rothenberg, R. Averbach, K. Cavanaugh, D. K. Robinson, and R. K. Wallace. September 1985. Improvements in mental and physical health with the Maharishi Ayur-Veda Panchakarma program. Paper presented at the Eighth World Congress of the International College of Psychosomatic Medicine, Chicago.

Nader, T. June 1987. Maharishi Ayur-Veda Bhasma rasayana: Its safety and effectiveness in animal models of diet-induced tissue damage, in surgically induced brain lesions and in chemically induced cancer lesions. Paper presented at the Twenty-eighth Annual Meeting of the Society for Economic Botany, University of Illinois, Chicago.

Nader, T., D. Bueche, and P. Neuberne. Ayur-Vedic rasayana prevents kidney and liver damage caused by a low lipotrope high fat diet in rats. Paper presented at the Federation of American Societies of Experimental Biology, Washington, D.C. *Federation Proceedings* 46.

Niwa, Y. January 1991. Effect of Maharishi 4 and Maharishi 5 on inflammatory mediators, with special reference to their free radical scavenging effects. *Indiana Journal of Clinical Practice* 1: 8.

Orme-Johnson, D. W. 1988. Medical care utilization and the Transcendental Meditation program. *Psychosomatic Medicine* 49: 493–500.

————. 1973. Autonomic stability and Transcendental Meditation. *Psychosomatic Medicine* 35: 341–49.

Patel, V., J. Wang, R. N. Shen, Z. Brahmi, and H. Sharma. March 1990. Reduction of mouse Lewis lung carcinoma (LLC) by M-4 rasayana. Annual Meeting of the Federation of the American Societies for Experimental Biology, Washington, D.C.

Patel, V., X. N. Dileepan, D. J. Stechschulte, and H. Sharma. 1988. Enhancement of lymphoproliferative responses by Maharishi Amrit Kalash (MAK) in rats. *FASEB Journal* 2: 20.

Prasad, K. N., J. Edwards-Prasad, S. Kenrotti, C. Brodie, and A. Vernadakis. 1992. Extracts of Maharishi Amrit Kalash-5, an Ayurvedic herbal preparation induces differentiation in neuroblatoma cells in culture. *Neuropharmacology* 31: 599–607.

Schneider, R. H., R. K. Wallace, H. S. Kasture, R. Averbach, S. Rothenberg, and D. R. Robinson. 1990. Physiological and psychological correlates of Maharishi Ayur-Veda psychosomatic types. *Journal of Social Behavior and Personality* 5: 1–27.

Sharma, H. M., C. Dwivedi, B. C. Satter, H. A. Gudehitihlu, W. Malarkey, and G. A. Tejwani. 1990. Antineoplastic properties of Maharishi-4, against DMBA-induced mammary tumors in rats. *Journal of Pharmacy, Biochemistry and Behavior* 35: 767–73.

Sharma, H., et al. April 1990. Effect of MAK (M4 & M5) on DMBA-induced mammary tumors. Paper presented at the Annual Meeting of the Federation of the American Societies for Experimental Biology, Washington, D.C.

Sharma, H. M., et al. 1992. Inhibition of human LDL oxidation in vitro by Maharishi Ayur-Veda herbal mixtures. *Pharmacology, Biochemistry and Behavior* 43: 1775–82.

Sharma, H. M., Y. Feng, and R. V. Panganamala. 1989. Maharishi Amrit Kalash (MAK) preventing human platelet aggregation. *Journal of the International Atherosclerosis Society* 3: 227–30.

Stryker, T., and R. K. Wallace. September 1985. Reduction in biological age through an Ayur-Vedic treatment program. Paper presented to the International Congress of Psychosomatic Medicine, Chicago.

Wallace, R. K., M. C. Dillbeck, E. Jacobe, and B. Harrington. 1982. The effects of the Transcendental Meditation and TM-Sidhi program on the aging process. *International Journal of Neuroscience* 16: 53–58.

Wallace, R. K., J. Silver, P. Mills, M. C. Dillbeck, and D. E. Wagner. 1983. Systolic blood pressure and long-term practice of the Transcendental Meditation and TM-Sidhi program: Effects of TM on systolic blood pressure. *Psychosomatic Medicine* 45: 41–46.

For information on current research on Maharishi Ayur-Veda, please contact:

> The Institute of Science, Technology and Public Policy
> 1000 N. 4th St.
> Fairfield, Iowa 52557-1137
> (515) 472-1200
> Fax: (515) 472-1165

# INDEX

# ABOUT THE AUTHORS

NANCY LONSDORF, M.D., received her M.D. from the Johns Hopkins School of Medicine, and did postgraduate work in psychiatry at Stanford School of Medicine, where she also served as a research fellow in psychiatry and neurophysiology. She studied Maharishi Ayur-Veda in India. She is a practicing primary-care physician and medical director of the Maharishi Ayur-Ved Health Center in Washington, D.C.

VERONICA BUTLER, M.D., received her M.D. from Howard University College of Medicine, did postgraduate work in public health at the University of Michigan, and studied Maharishi Ayur-Veda in India. She is a board-certified family practitioner; director of Women's Programs for the College of Maharishi Ayur-Ved in Fairfield, Iowa; co–medical director of Maharishi Ayur-Ved at the Raj Health Center; and director of the Family Practice Center in Ottumwa, Iowa.

MELANIE BROWN, PH.D., the author of several books, received both her doctorate in educational psychology and her M.S.W. in psychiatric social work from the University of California at Berkeley. A former psychotherapist, she worked with Maharishi in the fields of education and psychology. She is president and founder of My Baby U., Inc., producing a multimedia curriculum on infant development, on which she is conducting research under a grant from the National Institute of Child Health and Development.

Printed in the United States
by Baker & Taylor Publisher Services